Evidence-based Patient Choice

Evidence-based Patient Choice

Inevitable or impossible?

Adrian Edwards
Glyn Elwyn

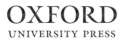

OXFORD
UNIVERSITY PRESS

OXFORD
UNIVERSITY PRESS

Great Clarendon Street, Oxford OX2 6DP

Oxford University Press is a department of the University of Oxford.
It furthers the University's objective of excellence in research, scholarship,
and education by publishing worldwide in

Oxford New York

Athens Auckland Bangkok Bogotá Buenos Aires Cape Town
Chennai Dar es Salaam Delhi Florence Hong Kong Istanbul Karachi
Kolkata Kuala Lumpur Madrid Melbourne Mexico City Mumbai Nairobi
Paris São Paulo Shanghai Singapore Taipei Tokyo Toronto Warsaw

with associated companies in Berlin Ibadan

Oxford is a registered trade mark of Oxford University Press
in the UK and in certain other countries

Published in the United States
by Oxford University Press Inc., New York

© Oxford University Press, 2001

The moral rights of the authors have been asserted

Database right Oxford University Press (maker)

First published 2001

British Library Cataloguing in Publication Data

Data available

Library of Congress Cataloging in Publication Data
ISBN 0-19-2631942

10 9 8 7 6 5 4 3 2 1

Typeset in Times Ten
by Florence Production Ltd, Stoodleigh, Devon
Printed in Great Britain
on acid-free paper by
Biddles Ltd., Guildford and King's Lynn

Contents

Contributors

Richard Ashcroft (England) is lecturer in medical ethics at Imperial College School of Medicine. He read mathematics and history and philosophy of science at Cambridge University, before going on to complete a PhD on the ethics of research in the natural sciences, also at Cambridge. He spent just over a year at Liverpool University, as lead researcher on an NHS Health Technology Assessment project on the ethics of clinical trials. The special focus of this project was the relevance of social, cultural, and economic factors to the ethics of design and recruitment in trials. For three years he was lecturer in ethics in medicine at Bristol University. He has published widely on the ethics of medical research, genetics, and health technology assessment. His current interests are in the theory and ethics of rational choice.
Email to richard.ashcroft@ic.ac.uk

Hilda Bastian (Australia) has been a health consumer advocate for seventeen years, since becoming involved with maternity consumer groups when her first son was born. For a few years she has been the chairperson of the Consumers' Health Forum of Australia, a national coalition of consumer and community groups with an interest in health. She is also an international convenor of the Consumer Network of the Cochrane Collaboration, and was until recently the co-ordinating editor of the Cochrane Consumers and Communication Review Group.
Email to hilda.bastian@flinders.edu.au

Paul Bellaby (England) is a sociologist, with central interests in the impact of labour markets and work patterns on health and behaviour in illness: *Sick from Work* (1999) is a publication of his in this area. He has also sought to develop and apply the cultural theory of risk. He is currently Reader in Sociology and Associate Director of the Institute for Public Health Research and Policy at the University of Salford, having taught sociology previously at the Universities of East Anglia and Keele.
Email to p.bellaby@salford.ac.uk

Judith Belle Brown (Canada) is an Associate Professor in the Centre for Studies in Family Medicine, Department of Family Medicine at the University of Western Ontario and the School of Social Work at King's College, London, Ontario, Canada. Following a PhD in social work from Smith College, she now conducts research in the areas of patient–doctor communication, physician well-being, physician practice behaviour (obstetrics, palliative care, clinical practice guidelines, cancer care), empowerment of the chronically ill elderly, the influence of culture on health, and women abuse. Dr Brown has published widely on the patient-centred clinical method, and co-ordinates courses on patient-centred communication at UWO at postgraduate and masters levels.

Cathy Charles (Canada) is an Associate Professor at the Department of Clinical Epidemiology and Biostatistics, McMaster University. Cathy received her first degrees in sociology at the University of Toronto and her PhD in socio-medical sciences from Columbia University. Her research interests include: public and patient participation in health care decision making, the use of research information to improve the organization and delivery of health care, the health professions and public policy, and resident classification systems for long-term care. She is currently undertaking a study on shared decision making with women with early stage breast cancer and their physicians. Cathy also has teaching interests in medical sociology, health policy analysis, and qualitative research methods.
Email to charlesc@mcmaster.ca

Angela Coulter (England) is Chief Executive of the Picker Institute Europe, which works with European health care providers to survey patients' experience and promote patient-centred care. A social scientist by training, Angela has a doctorate in health services research from the University of London and has published widely on a variety of topics including user involvement in health care, primary care development, clinical effectiveness, women's health, public health, and evaluating health system reforms. She holds visiting professorships in the medical schools at Oxford and University College, London. From 1993–9 she was an Executive Director of the King's Fund in London leading their work on health policy analysis, research, and service development. Prior to that she worked for twelve years at the University of Oxford where she established and directed the Health Services Research Unit. She is the founding editor of *Health Expectations*, an international journal of public participation in health care and health policy.
Email to angela.coulter@picker-europe.com

Martin Eccles (England) is Professor of Clinical Effectiveness at the Centre for Health Services Research, University of Newcastle upon Tyne. He leads

a programme of research into 'Effective Professional Practice' within which he runs the North of England Evidence-Based Guideline Development Programme. He also works one day a week as a general practitioner (family physician) in Northumberland. He is chair of the Guidelines Advisory Committee at the National Institute for Clinical Excellence, a member of the NHS R&D Health Technology Assessment Commissioning Panel, and a member of the NHS R&D 'Methods to promote the uptake of research findings' Research Commissioning Panel.
Email to martin.eccles@newcastle.ac.uk

Adrian Edwards (Wales) is a part-time general practitioner (family physician) in South Wales and also a senior lecturer at the University of Wales College of Medicine. His principal research interests are in systematic reviews and the communication and discussion of research evidence with patients. Amongst these there is a particular interest in the use and efficacy of decision aids, and he leads the first major UK trial of decision aids in general practice. He is one of the founding members of RADAR (Research About Decisions And Risk). Several authors of this volume perceived the value of drawing together the various perspectives and evidence about 'evidence-based patient choice' into one publication. Others side-stepped the task with the nimble-footedness that we like to see in a Welsh rugby player (but seldom do, even among the Australasian ones). After doggedly pursuing the task, he takes the credit (shared with Glyn Elwyn) and blame (not shared) in equal measure.
Email to edwardsag@cf.ac.uk

Glyn Elwyn (Wales) is a senior lecturer in general medical practice at the University of Wales College of Medicine, a director of research within the CAPRICORN Primary Care Research Network, and director of CeReS, a Research Support Unit in Wales. His academic interests focus on referral analysis and shared decision making between patients and doctors. He studied at INSEAD, European management school in 1999 as part of the European Strategic Leadership Programme and is involved in research collaborations in Europe, led by Professor Richard Grol at Nijmegen. He has published widely on shared decision making and is one of the founding members of RADAR (Research About Decisions And Risk).
Email to elwyng@cf.ac.uk

Vikki Entwistle (Scotland) is a senior research fellow at the Health Services Research Unit, University of Aberdeen, Scotland, where she directs a programme of work on consumer participation in health care. She has published widely on the development and assessment of consumer health information materials, patient and consumer involvement in health care, and

media coverage of health and medical issues. Vikki serves on the editorial teams of *Health Expectations*, an international journal of public participation in health care, and of the Cochrane Consumers and Communication Review Group.
Email to Vae@hsru.abdn.ac.uk

Gunther Eysenbach (Germany), MD, is a medical informatics and public health researcher at the Department of Clinical Social Medicine, University of Heidelberg. His main research interests are consumer health informatics and the challenges and opportunities of e-Health and the Internet for evidence-based medicine and public health. He has written widely in the field of consumer health informatics. Among others, he is author of a German textbook for computers in medicine, was editor of a German loose-leaf book on computers for physicians, founding editor of the international *Journal of Medical Internet Research*, and editor of an English-language book on *Medicine and Medical Education in Europe*. He serves on the executive board for the Society of Internet in Medicine, and is co-chair of the International Medical Informatics Association, and the Workgroup on Consumer Health Informatics.
Email to Gunther_Eysenbach@med.uni-heidelberg.de

William Godolphin (Canada) is Professor in the Department of Pathology and Laboratory Medicine at the University of British Columbia. His research, teaching, and service has ranged across breast cancer, toxicology, laboratory automation, and medical education. He is half of the Director (with Angela Towle) of the Informed Shared Decision Making project in the Office of the Co-ordinator of Health Sciences at UBC. He sees his interest in evidence-based patient choice as a rational reaction, in a moderately intelligent person who also scores low on the Right Wing Authoritarian scale, to a long career in academic pathology.
Email to wgod@unixg.ubc.ca

JA Muir Gray was born and educated in Glasgow but then strayed South to spend English money on health care. He has worked in all aspects of public health, and thence to R&D. His earlier responsibilities included being Secretary of ASH (Action on Smoking and Health), co-ordinator of the National Breast and Cervical Cancer Screening Programmes, establishing the Centre for Evidence-Based Medicine (Oxford), and being Regional Director of Research and Development for the Anglia and Oxford Region of the NHS Executive. Currently he is Director of the Institute of Health Sciences, University of Oxford, Director of the National Screening Committee (UK), associate editor of the *Journal of Evidence-Based Health Care*, and Director of the National electronic Library for Health.

Trisha Greenhalgh (England) is a part-time general practitioner (family physician) in North London and senior lecturer in primary health care at University College, London. She is involved in a number of teaching and research projects relating to effective communication and evidence-based practice in primary health care. She is co-editor of the book *Narrative-based medicine – dialogue and discourse in clinical practice*.
Email to p.greenhalgh@ucl.ac.uk

Richard Grol (Netherlands) holds chairs at the Universities of Nijmegen (in 'Quality in Health Care') and Maastricht (in family practice). He is Director of the Centre for Quality of Care Research (WOK) and president of the European Working Party on Quality in Family Practice (EquiP). He has a considerable record of research in this area and more recently his research interests have developed to include public participation in health care. He is chairman of the European Task Force on Patient Evaluations of General Practice (EUROPEP). He has published widely in these fields, and is a member of the editorial boards of the journals *Quality in Health Care, British Medical Journal*, and *Health Expectations*. He is also a lead editor of the forthcoming Oxford Textbook of *Primary Medical Care*.
Email to r.grol@hsv.kun.nl

Margaret Holmes-Rovner (USA) leads the Division of Health Services Research, Michigan State University. Her research for the past twenty years has focused on patient and physician decision making. She served as President of the Society for Medical Decision Making and now chairs the Health Care Technology and Decision Sciences Study Section of the Agency for Health Care Research and Quality. She is presently the North American associate editor for *Health Expectations*. Dr Holmes-Rovner has developed decision aids and decision aid evaluation measures, and participated in a systematic review of decision aids. She recently began two studies related to evidence-based patient choice. The first examines patient understanding of information in decision aids, and the second seeks to develop web-based and paper-based decision aids for women aged 40–9 considering breast cancer screening.
Email to Margaret.HolmesRovner@ht.msu.edu

Tony Hope (England) is Professor of Medical Ethics at the University of Oxford and an Honorary Consultant Psychiatrist. Since 1990 he has led the Oxford Practice Skills Project. This involves education in ethics, communication skills, and the law for clinical medical students. He took up the newly created post of university lecturer in practice skills in 1996. This work has led to a considerable amount of postgraduate educational commitment and to collaboration with several Eastern European countries for similar

educational initiatives. In 1997 he co-founded the Oxford Centre of Ethics and Communication Skills in Health Care Practice (Ethox).
Email to Tony.hope@ethox.ox.ac.uk

Alex Jadad (Canada) obtained his medical degree in Columbia in 1986, specializing in anaesthesiology. He was a leading medical expert on cocaine in Colombia and an internationally sought after speaker. In 1990 he moved to the UK and joined the University of Oxford, where he developed and evaluated analgesic interventions for the treatment of acute, chronic, and cancer pain, and witnessed and contributed to the birth of the Cochrane Collaboration. In 1995, he moved to Canada and joined the Department of Clinical Epidemiology and Biostatistics at McMaster University. In 2000 he moved to become Director of the Program in Health Innovation and holds the Rose Family Chair in Supportive Care (Department of Health Administration and Anaesthesiology) at the University of Toronto. Among several areas of continuing interest he is an editor of the Cochrane Consumers and Communication Group, is involved in many initiatives to promote patient–professional participation in health care, and is a leading light in the new and emerging discipline of health informatics.
Email to ajadad@uhnres.utoronto.ca

Hilary Llewellyn-Thomas is a Canadian who recently assumed a professorship in the Department of Community and Family Medicine, Dartmouth Medical School, USA. She is a past President of the Society for Medical Decision Making. Her research career in Canada focused on: patients' attitudes toward their health state; their preferences for treatment alternatives and for involvement in treatment decisions; their attitudes toward waiting for, under-going, and recovering from treatment; and their understanding of the risks and benefits of different treatment options. At Dartmouth's Center for the Evaluative Clinical Sciences, Dr Llewellyn-Thomas leads a research programme concentrating on the evaluation and dissemination of interventions designed to support shared decision making.
Email to Hilary.A.Llewellyn-Thomas@dartmouth.edu

Annette O'Connor (Canada) obtained her nursing education at Ottawa and Toronto Universities. She is a professor at the University of Ottawa School of Nursing in the Faculties of Health Sciences, and in the Department of Epidemiology and Community Health in the Faculty of Medicine, and leads the Clinical Epidemiology Unit at the Ottawa Hospital Loeb Health Research Institute. Dr O'Connor's research programme focuses on under-standing and improving the decision making of people facing health care choices, and improving the support provided by health professionals who counsel them. This work has culminated in numerous publications, a concep-

tual framework of decision support, 20 decision aids for patients or practitioners, a widely used evaluation measure of 'decisional conflict', and several
educational courses on shared decision making. Dr O'Connor has also
contributed internationally to several scientific societies, notably the
Cochrane Collaboration, and projects in China and Chile to promote
evidence-based decision making.
Email to aoconnor@lri.ca

Máire O'Donnell (Scotland) is a research fellow at the Health Services
Research Unit, University of Aberdeen. Her particular research interests are
in the development of evidence-based patient information materials and
involving people in health care decision making.
Email to m.odonnell@abdn.ac.uk

Michael Parker (England) is a lecturer in medical ethics at the University of
Oxford. He is also Honorary Clinical Ethicist at the Oxford Radcliffe
Hospitals Trust. He has written on a wide range of topics in bio-medical
ethics including, *Ethics and Community in the Health Care Professions*
(Routledge, 1998) and *The Cambridge Medical Ethics Workbook* (with
Donna Dickenson, Cambridge University Press, 2000). He currently holds a
Wellcome Trust grant for a project leading to the development of an elec-
tronic web-based bio-ethics resource on the ethical and social implications
of biotechnology (the UK Bio-ethics and Society Network).
Email to michael.parker@ethics-and-communication-in-health.oxford.ac.uk

William Rosenberg (England) is a senior lecturer in medicine and Consultant
Physician at Southampton University Hospitals Trust. He is a specialist in
hepatology with a particular interest in viral liver disease but also works as
a general physician in the University Hospital which provides care for the
population of Southampton. He trained in clinical epidemiology and when
previously at Oxford was a leading member and author at the Centre for
Evidence-Based Medicine. He retains an ongoing interest in the use of
evidence-based medicine in clinical practice and education at all levels.
E-mail to wmr@soton.ac.uk

David Rovner (USA) is Professor Emeritus of Medicine and Endocrinology
at Michigan State University. His original research interests were in
endocrine hypertension and Primary Aldosteronism. More recently he has
focused on clinical decision analysis and cost-effectiveness analysis in health
care. Under these themes he has addressed a number of specific areas
including referral practices regarding obesity, hormone replacement therapy,
patient decision making, medical decision making, medical informatics, and
evaluation of the patient decision support videos from the Foundation for

Informed Decision Making. With Arthur Elstein he developed and taught
one of the USA's first courses in clinical decision analysis that became part
of the core curriculum in medical schools. He continues to teach in this
course to the present. David Rovner has just finished five years as associate
editor of the journal *Medical Decision Making*.
Email to rovner@msu.edu

Theo Schofield (England) is a general practitioner (family physician) in
Shipston on Stour, Warwickshire. He is also a lecturer in general practice,
and Director of Communication at the Centre for Ethics and Communication
in Health Care Practice, University of Oxford. He has a long-standing interest
and involvement in the teaching of communication skills for medical students
and general practitioners, and was one of the authors of *The Consultation:
an approach to learning and teaching*, (OUP, 1984). He is currently involved
in research on evidence-based patient choice, as well as other aspects of
improving quality of care in general practice.
Email to theo.schofield@dphpc.ox.ac.uk

Anthony Scott (Scotland) is a Senior Research Fellow in the Health
Economics Research Unit, University of Aberdeen. Tony is co-ordinator of
the HERU's 'Behaviour and Incentives in the Supply of Health Care'
research programme. His research interests are in the economics of primary
care, particularly factors influencing medical decision making and the interaction between patients' and doctors' preferences in the doctor–patient
relationship. He is also involved in work examining patients' preferences for
primary care services using discrete choice experiments and a range of other
projects.
Email to a.scott@abdn.ac.uk

Moira Stewart (Canada) leads the Centre for Studies in Family Medicine
and the Thames Valley Family Practice Research Unit at the University of
Western Ontario. She is an epidemiologist who, for the past twenty years,
has conducted research on the quality of primary care and on communication
between patients and doctors. She has published widely on these issues
(including *Patient-Centered Medicine: Transforming the Clinical Method*
(1995)) and has also been particularly active in fostering an international
network of teachers and scientists of communication in medicine.
Email to moira@julian.uwo.ca

Angela Towle (Canada) had an early life as a zoologist but has worked for
the past fifteen years in medical education, particularly at undergraduate
level. She also worked for several years at the King's Fund, London where
she became an enthusiast for evidence-based patient choice. Upon moving

to Canada, she joined forces with Bill Godolphin to establish the Informed Shared Decision Making project at the University of British Columbia. Together they direct a number of research and development projects which aim to teach medical students, physicians, and patients how to engage in making informed and shared decisions about treatment options.
Email to atowle@unixg.ubc.ca

Foreword

Richard Grol

There is an increasing awareness that patients can and should play an important role in deciding on their care, in defining optimal care, and in improving health care delivery. New popular concepts, such as patient-centred care, patient empowerment, patients as partners, shared decision making, and informed choice illustrate this emancipation of the patient. Its relevance is underlined in different theoretical perspectives. From an ethical perspective, more autonomy of patients is regarded as a basic value and important goal in health care. From a psychological perspective, more involvement of patients is seen as leading to better adherence to advice and treatment and, thus, to better health outcomes. From an epidemiological viewpoint, patients are seen as rational beings who can, after being informed about the benefits and risks of treatment alternatives, decide on optimal management of their condition. Whichever perspective one wants to adopt, involving patients in decisions about health care and improvement of care is important for a number of reasons. Many patients are well informed, much more than in previous years; they often have experiences relevant for optimal management but unknown to their health care professionals; their needs and preferences can differ considerably to those of the professionals; and, essentially, the effectiveness of care provision often depends on the co-operation of the patient.

Many different methods are used to empower and involve patients, such as communication training for professionals, needs assessment tools, interactive education on video or CD-ROM, information sites on the Internet, the use of risk tables, and decision aids. Usually, the best evidence on clinical effectiveness is used in these tools. However, the area is new, and theory and anecdotal experiences still dominate the debate and continuing developments. Research evidence on the value and effectiveness of such approaches is scarce. Nevertheless, we are dealing with an extremely interesting and challenging area, which may change the landscape of health care in the next decade. We see, for instance, inconsistent and sometimes conflicting results in studies on Shared Decision Making (SDM): some patients want to be involved, others not; involving patients is effective in some studies and not in others. Clearly many questions need to be answered in the years to come. Crucially, we need to identify which approaches of involving patients should be used for which patients, with what problems, and at what moment in time.

It is difficult to predict the future, but we may also expect considerable changes in the relationship between patients or consumers and their care providers in the years to come, all arising from the emancipation of the patient in health care. For a long time there was concern about paternalistic attitudes among health care professionals, and that this fostered dependent attitudes among patients. Now, there is an additional concern about unrealistic patient autonomy and consumerism, and that this may foster *laissez-faire* attitudes and loss of morale among professionals. Professionals need to learn to strike a balance between these two extremes so that they neither lose their clients nor fail to cope with the new consumerist patients. The public needs to achieve a balance in which consumerist expectations (fuelled by the ever-increasing potential of health care delivery) can be expressed, and yet they can still have a health care system which provides appropriate support (usually via professionals) when addressing their health problems.

Education of the public on what is 'appropriate' care is therefore very urgent. We need a bridge between evidence-based medicine and guidelines on the one hand, and empowering and involving patients on the other. New methods and approaches to the interaction between health care professionals and patients or consumers need to be developed and evaluated. We also need a new conceptualization of patient-centred care, perhaps as 'dialogue-centred care', in which there are shared responsibilities for the care process between patients and professionals, and mutual rights and obligations. Such a dialogue between patient and professional can differ per patient and problem. When hard evidence for a specific problem is available, the approach to the problem will be different from cases where such evidence is lacking and the professional does not have strong views about the best treatment. It also makes a difference whether individual patients adopt dependent, leading, or participating roles in the decision making. For all these different situations we need specific decision making and patient involvement models of proven effectiveness.

So, an enormous challenge lies before us. In this new and challenging field this book about 'evidence-based patient choice' (EBPC) is manna from heaven. It summarizes the current state of knowledge about these new patient involvement approaches. Insights from different disciplines (medicine, epidemiology, economics, ethics, sociology, and psychology) are included. It is probably by far the most comprehensive account of scientific and ethical thinking about patient choice at this moment. And, it manages to show us the way to a potential future: health care provision where patients and professionals operate as real partners with shared goals, playing an equal music in deciding on the best management of the health problems.

Abbreviations

AIDS	auto-immune deficiency syndrome
AZT	azidothymidine
BMJ	British Medical Journal
BSE	bovine spongiform encephalopathy
CME	continuing medical education
EBM	evidence-based medicine
EBPC	evidence-based patient choice
EU	European Union
FIFE	feelings, ideas, functioning, expectations
GM	genetically modified
HBM	health belief model
HMO	health maintenance organization
HRT	hormone replacement therapy
ISDM	informed shared decision making
NELH	National electronic Library for Health (UK)
NHS	National Health Service
NICE	National Institute for Clinical Excellence
NNH	number needed to harm
NNT	number needed to treat
OMNI	Organizing Medical Networked Information
OPTION	observing patient involvement in treatment choices
PAMs	professions allied to medicine
PG	postgraduate
PSA	prostate specific antigen
QALY	quality adjusted life year
R&D	research and development
RCT	randomized controlled trial
RDF	resource description framework
SDM	shared decision making
SDP	Shared Decision making Programs®
SG	standard gamble
SID	supplier-induced demand
TTO	time trade-off
UG	undergraduate

UK	United Kingdom
USA	United States of America
WTP	willingness to pay
WWW	World Wide Web
XML	eXtensible Markup Language

Section 1
Evidence-based health care

1 Evidence-based patient choice?

Glyn Elwyn and Adrian Edwards

Defining the frame

This book's focus is on the decisions taken in consultations between health care patients and professionals. We mention this here because we are all too aware of the frame we have placed around the discussions. These eighteen chapters consider one of the most complex issues of all – human decision making – and, in addition, do so within the politically sensitive contexts of health care systems as they test the ability of their collective financing arrangements to meet the demands placed on them.

Decision making by individuals has been widely discussed in economic texts where the dominant theory is that of *rational choice* engaging in a free market environment. But this literature is riddled with assumptions that are being challenged by alternative models proposed by theorists from cognitive and political science (Green and Shapiro 1994). Heap touches on some of the assumptions when he states that 'the typical autonomous agent seems like a sovereign customer with a coherent shopping list and a fat wallet in a well-stocked market' (Hargreaves Heap *et al.* 1992). These assumptions are decidedly shaky when we consider images of patients, fearful for their well-being, in awe of medical expertise, faced with difficult concepts, yet suspicious of motives as they become aware of the struggle to provide access to basic treatments, never mind novel advances. Add to this disparity the previously mentioned critique of the rational choice model as an explanatory framework for human decision making (Etzioni 1993), and we begin to appreciate the contested analysis of the interactive processes within consultations.

Although this book concentrates on individual choices within clinical consultations we nevertheless recognize that this process cannot, and should not, be considered in a vacuum but should be placed in the wider discourse of health care delivery to populations. Most of the examples in this book are from medical settings in the developed world, where professionals and patients are engaged in the process of redefining roles (Elwyn *et al.* 1999). Although the detail of these examples will seem hypothetical to four of the

six billion people on the globe who live in grinding poverty, the basic principles at the heart of the relationship between the professional and patient
are just as relevant (Charles *et al.* 1997), even if the choices available are
more restricted. In many ways, this is the dilemma that faces any discussion
about choice. The globalization of trade and the digitalization of data, riding
the wave of free market philosophy is shaping societies across the world.
Electronic access to the World Wide Web will increase the borderless nature
of trade and, given the fall in the cost of electronic connectivity, the future
netizens of Africa, South America, and China (to name a few regions) will
soon be able to search for information about health care interventions with
ease. Disparities will be sharpened by the arrival of windows onto worlds
where choices are abundant and therefore relevant topics of concern. We do
not yet know how the enhancement of individual autonomy and reflexivity
will be tackled in economies where the pressing concerns revolve around
basic necessities.

Nevertheless, even in developed consumer economies, the issue of
providing individual choice is bound to cause tension between individuals
and society (Eddy 1991). The arguments in political science and economics
about *public choice* and the extent to which 'free riding' occurs on collectively organized benefits are issues that deserve much more attention than
we have been able to give them in this volume (Buchanan and Tullock 1962).
It is instructive to consider how *public choice* scholars think about this area.
Choice, they state, is the act of selecting from alternatives. 'Public' refers to
people. But people do not choose. Choices are made by individuals, and
these may be private or public. Private choices are made in the course of
daily living, and are usually narrowly circumscribed. Public choices are made
when an individual selects among alternatives for others as well as for
himself. Traditional economic theory has been narrowly interpreted to
include only the private choices of individuals in the market process and
traditional political science has rarely analysed individual choice behaviour
and how it is to be regulated to ensure a wider good. As Hardin notes, 'the
narrow rationality of self-interest that can benefit us all in market exchange
can also prevent us from succeeding in collective endeavors [sic]' (Russell
1982).

Some choices in health care are cost neutral (where options take up equal
resources). In others, conservative decisions are made which take up minimal
interventions, such as the aptly named watchful waiting approach, and patient
preferences often reduce costs (Barry *et al.* 1995). But this is not always the
case, and it is in fact an increasingly unlikely outcome as new drugs and
surgical interventions become available. Who will be the arbiter of whether
expensive new technology or heroic yet futile interventions are made available to individuals within collectively funded health care systems? Placing a
publicly declared barrier on what will and will not be included in any given

system will inevitably open the debate about an individual's freedom to purchase preferred treatments privately. What effect will this have on health care systems, which inevitably have interdependencies that are not so easily compartmentalized into public and private boxes?

Evidence-based patient choice

The phrase 'evidence-based patient choice' (EBPC) belies its origin in the heyday of 'evidence-based medicine' (EBM) – the middle 1990s – when the ironic suggestion that health care decisions should be based on 'evidence' was at the same time a novel *and* contested process in medicine. In truth, as Muir Gray (Chapter 2) points out, EBM was a carefully chosen term, designed to jolt complacency about medical decision making, and to present biostatistics in a way that was fundamental to all aspects of patient care and relevant to health care professionals (including policy makers and managers) throughout their careers. 'Clinical epidemiology' never captured (and never will) the imagination of so many people. The arguments which surrounded EBM – the admissibility, constitution, and hierarchy of evidence in health care, disparagement of the 'medical' and by association 'reductionist' paradigm, the subversive dismissal of expertise and seeming evangelization of Sackett – need not be rehearsed in more depth here, although the debates were great fun (Grahame-Smith 1996). Marvel at the force of this attack: 'The EBM protagonists are dazzled scientists who set out to dazzle, rejoicing like acrobatic children vaulting through the statistical stratosphere, casting down meta-analyses and systematic reviews to clinicians below' (Miles *et al.* 1997). This reaction was probably more common than is generally acknowledged, and captures the sour bemusement of the 'good old boys sat around the table' (GOBSATs) when confronted by 'SPins, SNouts and NNTs'.

In tandem with this emphasis on 'evidence' (or often a realization of its absence) as a guide to decision making, there was a parallel dimension advocating the role of patients and appreciating their increasing 'power' within health care settings. The most often quoted definition of EBM states that:

> [it is] the conscientious, explicit and judicious use of current best evidence in making decisions about the care of individual patients. The practice of evidence-based medicine means integrating individual clinical expertise with the best available external clinical evidence from systematic research. By individual clinical expertise we mean the proficiency and judgement that individual clinicians acquire through clinical experience and clinical practice.
> *(Sackett et al. 1996)*

and reveals that the approach did not appreciate that patients had important parts to play in clinical decision making. EBM, as presented in the original texts at least, was based on medical paternalism: professionals make decisions and patients follow orders.

It appears slightly odd that the original protagonists of 'evidence-based medicine' seemed to have arrived with this blind spot in their field of vision. Perhaps it is because they arrived from a 'biomedical' camp, arguing as they do, a pedigree that extends back to Magendie and Bichat in the mid-nineteenth century (founders of pathophysiology). It is clear that the EBM texts (Sackett *et al.* 1997) do not acknowledge the literature that has positioned patients at the centre of the clinical process, work that has played a fundamental part in the development of modern clinical practice (Laine and Davidoff 1996).

Over the past three centuries, historians have attributed the success of medicine to advances in the understanding and control of biological processes, brought about by expanding knowledge in the relevant sciences. It may be argued that this 'biomedical model' of how ill health is conquered is overestimated (Yardley 1997). Despite the undeniable power of modern medicine to cure and to prevent illness, the reduced morbidity and mortality rates in Western populations are actually due in large part to socio-economic and lifestyle factors such as improved diet, housing, hygiene, and safety. The biomedical model has dominated medicine as it forms part of the basis of the 'realist view' of the world. This view holds that by accurate observation and rational deduction humans can attain an objective knowledge of the nature of reality that will enable us to predict and control nature.

From a realist perspective, biological phenomena (objective facts) tend to be seen as more reliable (and also more controllable) than the psychosocial context. The result has been a dominant biomedical model based on 'biological reductionism' where bodily events are best explained exclusively in physical processes. As Yardley (1997, p.4) notes:

> ... whereas physicians and healers in previous non-Western cultures might see the social, subjective or spiritual significance of illness as an intrinsic and significant part of the phenomenon (a view often shared by the afflicted person and his or her associates), modern Western diagnostic practices are designed to exclude, or at least isolate, these aspects of illness in order to focus more clearly on the biological processes, which are regarded as of primary importance.

But the dominance of this approach has never been total. In the 1920s Freud and others contributed to an awareness of the psyche (albeit a mistaken one). Towards the end of the twentieth century, as the costs and limitations of scientific medicine have become increasingly apparent, an appreciation of the need to consider psychosocial influences on health has grown. In the 1970s the application of behavioural principles to health problems gave rise to new disciplines such as 'health psychology'. It was Engel (1960) who proposed the 'biopsychosocial model' drawing on an approach used in 'systems theory' (Weiss 1969; von Bertalanffy 1968). The model was welcomed by social scientists (and by those in generalist clinical work) as it affirmed the importance of psychosocial factors and allowed an expansion in biopsychosocial research. By employing a range of methodologies (quantitative and qualitative) it has been possible to achieve widespread recognition in medical circles that psychosocial factors significantly influence health status.

It was within this context that McWhinney (1972), described a paradigm shift for clinicians who worked in primary care. He recognized that at the heart of the biopsychosocial model was the issue of understanding the patient perspective on illness. Analytic descriptions of the professional–patient relationship (Balint 1957) and the consultation process were published (Stott and Davies 1979; Pendleton *et al.* 1984). Gradually a 'patient-centred' consulting style (Brown *et al.* 1986; Levenstein *et al.* 1986; Stewart *et al.* 1995) was described and promoted (Tuckett *et al.* 1985) (for further details see Chapter 7). At the heart of patient-centredness is the recognition that there needs to be an assessment of the disease (the biological process) and the illness (its effect on the individual and how they function in society). The professional actively seeks to enter into the patient's world to understand his or her unique experience of illness. Of central significance to this volume, their views about how their health should be investigated and managed need to be fully explored.

EBM's blind spot was inevitably noted and in 1996, as part of the King's Fund *Promoting Patient Choice* series, a booklet was published in which Hope used the term 'evidence-based patient choice' (Hope 1996). He defined it as follows: 'the use of evidence-based information as a way of enhancing people's choices when those people are patients'. It is not the most elegant of titles, yet it does two things. It reveals the rather awkward engagement of these two concepts and at the same time, anchors the term to a time when patient choice was accepted, unquestioningly it seems, as a 'good thing'. As we turn the page on a new millennium, choice is not nearly as benign a concept as it at first appears. For this reason, we have stuck with the title of evidence-based patient choice, but have added a question mark.

The context for evidence-based patient choice

It is helpful, we think, to be aware of the context during the late 1990s in which the issue of 'patient choice' emerged so clearly. We can now confidently state that the gap between resources and identified health care needs is widely recognized, if not coherently tackled. Within this acceptance is a groundswell opinion that wishes to see medicine move 'forward as a sound applied biological and social science', drawing together the themes of evidence and patient-centredness that we outlined earlier (Ellwood 1988). Added to these almost opposing dynamics are three other interlocking trends: a rhetoric that has promoted a change in how providers of services are perceived. They are no longer merely producers but now need to be aware of consumer demands and needs, with the necessary added involvement in planning and policy making. Secondly, there is an increased accountability of public services which are starting to envelop the professionals and managers who work in them. Thirdly, there exists an increasing emphasis on patient rights and autonomy.

If we then view this complex, and often combative, interaction of forces in the recent political framework, it is possible to discern an overall pattern. The certainties that defined socialist and conservative politics have given way to a middle ground that seems to be redefining the relationship between the individual and the state. Concentrating for the moment on the UK, the country has emerged in the late 1990s from a relatively long period of Conservative government, a recognizable neo-liberal administration where state industries were privatized, individuals were encouraged to become householders and stockholders, to be responsible for their own well-being, arrange personal pensions, choose schools – in short, to develop as much self-reliance as possible. The National Health Service (NHS) remained relatively stable, if undernourished, and could be viewed almost as a defining enclave of the welfare state. Nevertheless, even the NHS was subjected to market forces and split into purchasers and providers. Hospitals became free standing Trusts with boards modelled on commercial structures. Purchasers were downsized Health Authorities or general practitioners (family doctors) provided with budgets (fundholders).

Even after the introduction of a centre-left administration in the UK in the mid 1990s, the structural framework of the purchaser–provider split continued. Hospitals (and recently community services) are organized on commercial models (Trusts). This preservation of the market ethos in the health care system serves well to emphasize the distinction between the 'old' and 'modernized' social democracies that are now installed in many countries, and the extent to which the centre ground of politics and policy is fiercely contested.

This has led to the suggestion that there is now a 'third way' (Giddens 1998) – a middle path where the state encourages a culture of enterprise yet intervenes judiciously to provide safety measures for the vulnerable or dependent and policies to prevent social exclusion. The state has withdrawn its influence in many spheres (such as in heavy industry and the provision of utilities such as telecommunications, broadcasting, water, and electricity) and market forces are encouraged as a means of generating wealth. There is encouragement of individual determination and financial independence, especially in terms of obtaining higher education and pension provision. The 'third way' advocates remain committed to state provision of social welfare services, child education, and health care, provided they respond appropriately. As Giddens (2000) states: 'in the reform of state and government, as well as in economic policy, third way politics looks to respond to the great social transformations of the end of the twentieth century: globalization, the rise of the new knowledge-based economy, changes in everyday life and the emergence of an active, reflexive citizenry'. Health care has to adapt to the needs of this 'reflexive citizenry' which is exactly why 'choice' is playing such a central part in the evolution of new services. It exemplifies the complexity of balancing individual rights to self-determined choices against pooled resources that are, in principle at least, available equally to all.

The introduction of genuine choice into health care settings, especially into those such as the NHS which is a loosely organized (and geographically diverse) bureaucratic organization with recognized rules governing access and referral, is beset with problems. Choice at policy levels would entail a debate about how health services were organized and 'prioritized' (the favoured term): decisions would have to be made between services – more child health provision versus cardiac surgery for example – or within services – for example, reducing waiting times for hip rather than for knee replacements. The task of how best to engage the wider public in these issues remains unresolved.

Introducing patient choice in areas of public health policy requires a willingness to modify the traditional paternalistic, partly persuasive approach taken by screening and immunization campaigns (e.g. financial incentives are offered to UK professionals to obtain maximum childhood immunization coverage and to ensure that at least 80% of eligible women have had a cervical smear performed). Genuine patient choice at the provider level would entail encouraging informed decisions on these issues, freedom to move between clinicians, health care organizations, even to opt for services in other European countries (where waiting times in some regions are significantly lower). At the level of individual consultations, choice means being offered a menu of options, and sufficient information to allow informed decisions. What impact could this have on the organization of clinical services? What should professionals – or more appositely perhaps, managers – do when patients choose to have treatments that are too expensive or not available locally? Choice, whilst on the surface appearing to be a desirable pathway to fairness, equity, and individual freedom, can suddenly become perversely impossible to manage, and divisive. A good example is the risk inherent in providing individuals with the possibility of access to genetic testing. This could well lead to a group that, unwittingly perhaps, are at significant disadvantage in the insurance market.

Erosion of expertise

Alongside these political and ethical debates, is the tendency for the gap between expert and lay knowledge to narrow, especially in those countries where stable educational structures have enabled more than one generation to become literate and, of late, electronically coupled to the Internet.

This levelling process inevitably accelerates the de-professionalization of medicine. Johnson has described three phases to professional organizations, namely, patronage, collegiate, and mediated (Johnson 1972). It was patronage that largely supported physicians in the seventeenth century, when the wealthy sought their advice. By the eighteenth century, physicians had engineered a 'collegiate profession'. This trend was fuelled by the rise of hospitals, colleges, and medical schools – a process that had been successful in generating a 'club' attitude to the way medicine was practised and governed. The third phase is becoming increasingly tangible and involves third party mediation and accountability. Doctors are now managed, appraised, directed by guidelines, and the basis of their expertise – access to a unique bank of knowledge – is undermined as the World Wide Web becomes an ubiquitous source of information. Add to these accelerating trends the move to investigate professional activities (as in Bristol for example where audits of paediatric cardiac surgery outcomes revealed clinical performance below comparable standards) and it becomes obvious that professionals face the prospect of medicine being redefined as a tightly monitored and regulated discipline. It is no coincidence that in parallel with the declining power and authority of professionals is realization that the patient role is gaining ground.

This concerted move to discuss increased patient involvement occurred in the late 1980s. Variations in medical practice were being highlighted (Wennberg *et al.* 1988) and the potential conflict between individuals and society in collectively funded health systems were being debated (Eddy 1991). In the UK, in the same policy breath as the internal market initiative, the NHS policy makers were promoting the wisdom of patient involvement. *The Patient's Charter* (Department of Health 1991) was published in 1991, followed by *Local Voices* (Department of Health 1992) and the publication of hospital league charts. Almost unnoticed in *The Patient's Charter* was the statement that 'you (the patient) have a right to have any proposed treatment, including any risks involved in that treatment and any alternatives, clearly explained to you before you decide whether to agree to it'. In 1996, *Patient Partnership: building a collaborative strategy* (NHS Executive 1996) emphasized the intention to 'promote user involvement in their own care, as active partners with professionals.' These processes are not unique to medicine. The corporate world has long recognized the added value of 'co-opting customer competences' (Prahalad and Ramaswamy, 2000) so that individuals actively engage in the customization of products in the just in time delivery systems that now characterize many modern retail systems. Specifying the exact configuration of your personal computer using Dell's online facilities is a good example of this trend and a glimpse perhaps of the interactive future that could lie ahead for health systems.

Patients, clients, users, consumers and citizens

This book collects together the work of those who are interested in the potential partnership between people and professionals in health care services. We use the word *people* here to point out one of the defining semantic issues of the evolving relationships – what is the generic term that should be used to describe individuals in health care contexts? As health care advances in predictive testing occur, and with the prospect of extensive genetic prediction ahead, the term *patient* with its associated images of passive individuals who seek and follow professional advice is seen by many as dated and inappropriate. But as editors, to avoid distracting readers, we had to ask what term is the most acceptable? The word *client* has connotations of trade or references to relationships that have long-term therapeutic contracts. The term *users* and *consumers* have been suggested. Perhaps these new terms are acceptable in some health care contexts. Users of health care services are *using* facilities when they immunize their children or attend organized screening services. Consumers are perhaps defined by those who seek health care in active, even proactive ways, as in situations when new services and lifestyle modifying drugs are expected, if not demanded. Health care is no longer defined by people receiving services when they are ill – the stereotypical *patient*. It seems we have to accept that a number of terms will become commonplace. We eventually adopted the term 'patient' in this book for the sake of consistency and defined this to include any individual who interacts with a health care professional or service. Only one chapter was given leeway. Eysenbach and Jadad in their forward-looking chapter (Chapter 17) were determined to view people as consumers and professionals as providers. Maybe that is the future and who are we to argue?

Overview of the book

Section 1   Evidence-based health care

The book has been compartmentalized into sections, using chronology and related themes as the two guiding principles. The next two chapters set the scene. Muir Gray outlines the development of evidence-based medicine (Chapter 2) and reflects on the often hostile reactions of many professionals to the concept, particularly in those who practice medicine by a mixture of experience, opinion, and out-of-date assumptions. He draws attention to the fact that systematic reviews and the emphasis on 'evidence' could not have occurred without the revolutionary access to electronic information. Reviewing and summarizing this empirical data has resulted in a wealth of generalizable statements about clinical practice, drawn from groups and populations of patients. Ironically, this itself poses a problem. This body of evidence, eminently applicable to populations, is not automatically applicable to individuals. The challenge of individualizing care, based on the best possible data, is what lies ahead for clinicians in the twenty-first century. Entwistle and O'Donnell (Chapter 3) pick up this challenge and explore the roles of patients in this more open, reflexive relationship where there are transparent acknowledgements of the borders that distinguish certainty from uncertainty. As reviews of the roles patients wish to play in decision making reveal, their preferences vary. But it is unsafe to make assumptions, especially at the individual level, and we do not know whether preferences are stable over time or consistent for different problems (Schneider 1998). If, as it seems likely, they do vary, then the onus it seems has to be on an interactive determination of role preference, at each consultation.

Section 2   Theoretical perspectives on evidence-based patient choice

The next section contains discussions from the disciplines of ethics, economics, and sociology. Veracity, autonomy, and beneficence are amongst the ethical issues raised by Ashcroft and his colleagues (Chapter 4) as arguments in favour of facilitating patient choice. But as they reveal, *choice* is not an innocent. Allowing, encouraging, or even insisting that patients engage in the task of choosing preferred tests and, eventually, treatments, opens up debates about costs, possible conflict with professionals and the potential futility of pursuing ends beyond means, and the resulting tension between individual benefits and wider societal priorities.

The ethical position itself is not clear-cut because the principle of autonomy is not necessarily beneficial (de Haes and Molenaar 1997) and may conflict with the equally valid principle of beneficence. When professionals withdraw from providing guidance about decision making it is known that many patients experience anxiety and feel abandoned (Quill and Cassel 1995). This approach would characterize the enforcement of *mandatory* patient autonomy, in distinction to the more usual deployment of *optional* patient autonomy used by most professionals, where they adapt to preferred levels of involvement. Models of decision making can be mapped on to these ethical stances – paternalism denies autonomy, the informed choice model (see Chapter 8) corresponds to mandatory autonomy. The middle ground, known as shared decision making (SDM), is best characterized by optional autonomy. Shared decision making requires the professional to use his or her expertise and experience to guide the patient and make decisions if required. Consequently, SDM would appear to be consistent with the new ethical principle of relationality proposed by Bottorff *et al.* (1996). This principle promotes the provision of accurate honest information in the context of the individual situation, examining the ethics of care in terms of such factors as response, interpretation, accountability, and social solidarity, often counterbalanced against other values such as truth and confidentiality.

We enter here the realm of economics and Scott (Chapter 5) makes the point that much of economic theory is concerned with measuring consumer preference, influences on decision making, and the 'analysis of informational asymmetries between economic actors'. The discussion is enriched by the fact that the typical assumptions of economics, those of rational individuals with access to comparable data, are torpedoed by patient distress, lack of understanding, mis-comprehensions, and missing data (whether withheld or unavailable). The power and informational imbalances exist to such an extent that the models have to be adapted and the concept of the professional as the 'perfect agent' is debated. Bellaby (Chapter 6) grapples with the issue of risk and the difficulty posed when this concept means different things to different groups of people. A scientist's understanding and perception of risk for certain events, particularly in his or her specialist area, will be different to the public's understanding.

Perceptions of risks are exaggerated when the hazard is exceptional, and the probability of exposure is low, but depreciated · when the hazard is familiar, but the probability high. Recent concern about bovine spongiform encephalopathy (BSE) and the effect on the meat market are just one example of the capacity to generalize risk aversion. Bellaby cites the current use of the term 'risk society' and that the role of science is fast becoming that of predicting and preventing unnecessary risk, even though some determinants are seemingly beyond the realms of control. There is a certain irony in the fact that *evidence-based patient choice* calls for the gap between public and scientific perceptions of risk to be narrowed yet, at the same time, this appraisal of evidence usually increases the levels of uncertainty when attempts are made to predict the probability of outcomes at a specific individual level from population-based data.

Section 3 Conceptual development for clinical practice

We have already described the two big ideas that have combined to form EBPC. The first stems from the empirical tradition initiated by Locke, which has recently acquired the label 'evidence-based medicine'. The second flow is as old as the hills and is based on respect for the spirit, the whole person, and the rights to individual self-determination. These ideas were encapsulated in Kirkegaard's work (1988), where he argues that the most important human activity is decision making, because it is through the choices we make that we create our lives and become ourselves. This focus on the individual, and the way people experience the world in unique ways led to the philosophy of phenomenology that rejected the Cartesian dualism of mind and body as separate entities. Although these ideas were being debated in the 1930s it was not until 1960 that Engel described a 'biopsychosocial' framework for clinical practice (Engel 1960). It was as part of this realization of the need to integrate different facets that the concept of putting the patient at the centre of the medical process was described (Levenstein 1984), and the next section of this book sketches some of the more recent developments of this approach. Stewart's influential group have summarized their work over the last three decades, both in teaching and research in this area (Chapter 7). They describe a search for 'common ground' where patients and professionals agree on problems and discuss how they should be managed. The Ontario group had not however considered patient involvement in decision making to the depth that is now emerging in the literature and a firmer conceptual frame is now available for examining the interactive decision making processes between professionals and patients.

Elwyn and Charles (Chapter 8) summarize recent publications about shared decision making, in contrast to other approaches such as paternalism and informed choice. Recent developments in this field, such as the determination of competences and ways of measuring these professional skills, are highlighted. As Edwards and Bastian (Chapter 9) point out, one of the key skills of involving patients in decisions is to be able to share information about risk in ways that they readily grasp the relevant issues. One of the difficulties here is the fact that risk information is susceptible to errors of interpretation and the inherent dangers of manipulation, typically by unrecognized framing effects. This chapter summarizes the existing literature and describes how to ensure that information can be presented in as accurate and balanced a way as possible. An interesting approach, more formal and rational, to decision making is decision analysis (Elwyn *et al.*, Chapter 10). This method combines the assessment of event probability and the value (translated into numerical terms) that individuals put on future outcomes in order to arrive at what is argued to be a rational choice. But as the authors suggest, there are many slips between cup and lip, especially in the busy complexity of service settings where the time required to engage in stepwise deliberations is at a very high premium.

Section 4   Evidence-based patient choice in practice

Using the NHS in the UK as their contexts, Schofield (Chapter 11) and Rosenberg (Chapter 12) compare and contrast how evidence-based health care and patient choice could be incorporated into typical service environments. Primary care is typified by high volume undifferentiated problems in short time frames but where many typical strands are seen, such as acute infections, chronic diseases, exacerbations and, increasingly, preventive and predictive interventions. Secondary care works with more selected populations and works at a greater level of depth in terms of investigations and procedures. Both settings provide unique challenges to professionals who wish to develop EBPC. Greenhalgh provides an example from practice and, drawing on her eclectic basket of interests, tells a story about a patient who was concerned about a milky discharge from her breasts (Chapter 13). The chapter describes the search for evidence (arduous journey), its appraisal (a balance of probabilities), and the assessment of its applicability to an individual patient (shared judgements). This *narrative* account of medicine in action is both an intellectual thriller and a guided tour of what it would be like for both professionals and patients if medicine were guided by the principles of EBPC.

Taken as examples of the best that can be achieved in the practice of EBPC, these three chapters illustrate the practical hurdles to get over. Patient preferences clearly need to be considered but the general trends seem obvious enough. Patients want more information in health care settings and as they become more aware of the complexity and uncertainties which underlie most decisions about tests or treatments their desire for active participation increases. Faced with this demand and aware of their increasing accountability to set standards of care (both of their communication skills and technical outcomes), health care professionals are struggling to meet expectations. There is no easy answer to these issues but it is noticeable that one potential way of meeting at least a part of this increasing demand for tailored information is the development of decision aids. O'Connor and Edwards cover this field (Chapter 14) and cite both the most recent evidence of effectiveness and allude to the next phase of research.

Section 5   The next and possible future developments

The last section of the book speculates about the future. Towle and Godolphin consider the changes in knowledge, skills, and attitudes that are required for EBPC to establish itself as a way professionals routinely approach their practice (Chapter 15). Their emphasis is on the need to place education and training programmes deep within the ethical framework of respecting patient autonomy so that undergraduate and postgraduate curricula, and the resulting role models produced, are not out of tune with espoused policies. Holmes-Rovner *et al.* (Chapter 16) widen this debate and ask why it is that EBPC is not entering the mainstream of professional practice? Are health care professionals unwilling to relinquish their power? Are there some covert obstacles, hidden perhaps in a caring collusion between professionals and patients who recognize the genuine difficulty of facing uncertain futures, particularly when illness or anxiety weaken the decision making processes?

Eysenbach and Jadad draw us further into these arguments and announce the arrival of a new science of *consumer heath informatics* (Chapter 17). This is a world where an individual's personal health record is instantly available on the Web, updated when individuals make contact with their health provider. It acts as a customized portal to the expanding world of health information, validated by quality assurance guarantees. They conclude wistfully that 'the vast potential of the Internet to promote health information and to foster consumer–professional communication is far from realized' and note how the influence of information networks, now accelerating as wireless access increases, accelerates the shift of power within clinical consultations (Jadad 1999).

Coulter in the final chapter agrees (Chapter 18), and drives home the message that profound changes will occur in the relationship between health care professionals and their patients in the next decade. She cites the basic ground rules of effective communication – exchanges of accurate information, explorations of fears and concerns, opportunities for expressing empathy, participation in treatment options, and a negotiation of different views. However she then brings us firmly down to earth by the reminder that the average duration of primary care consultations is 8 minutes and that outpatient appointments in secondary care are seldom much better. The question is stark and obvious: how can all these components be accommodated without fundamental changes in the organization of care? Evidence-based patient choice is a clumsy phrase perhaps. But whatever the merits of the label, it conveys the underlying principles, and they are more than fashionable new ideas: they describe a frame shift that will transform the landscape of medicine (Kuhn 1962).

References

Balint M (1957). *The doctor, the patient and his illness*. London, Tavistock.

Barry MJ, Fowler FJ, Mulley AG, Henderson JV and Wennberg JE (1995). Patient reactions to a program designed to facilitate patient participation in treatment decisions for benign prostatic hyperplasia. *Medical Care* **33**(8): 771–82.

Bottorff JL, Ratner PA, Johnson JL, *et al.* (1996). Uncertainties and challenges: communicating risk in the context of familial cancer. British Columbia, School of Nursing, University of British Columbia.

Brown J, Stewart M, McCracken EC, *et al.* (1986). The patient-centred clinical method. 2. Definition and application. *Family Practice* **3**: 75–9.

Buchanan JM and Tullock G (1962). *The calculus of consent: logical foundations of a constitutional democracy*. Ann Arbor, University of Michigan Press.

Charles C, Gafni A and Whelan T (1997). Shared decision making in the medical encounter: what does it mean? (Or it takes at least two to tango). *Soc Sci Med* **44**: 681–92.

de Haes HC and Molenaar S (1997). Patient participation and decision control: are patient autonomy and well-being associated? *Medical Decision Making* **17**: 353–4.

Department of Health (1991). *The Patient's Charter*. London, HMSO.

Department of Health (1992). *Local Voices*. London, HMSO.

Eddy DM (1991). The individual v society. Is there a conflict? *JAMA* **265**: 1446–50.

Ellwood PM (1988). A technology of patient experience. *New England Journal of Medicine* **318**: 1549–56.

Elwyn G, Edwards A and Kinnersley P (1999). Shared decision making: the neglected second half of the consultation. *BJGP* **49**: 477–82.

Engel GL (1960). A unified concept of health and disease. *Perspect Biol Med* **3**: 459–85.

Etzioni A (1993). Normative-affective choices. *Human Relations* **46**: 1053–69.

Giddens A (1998). *The third way*. London, Polity Press.

Giddens A (2000). *The third way and its critics*. Cambridge, Polity Press.

Grahame-Smith D (1996). Evidence-based medicine: Socratic dissent. *BMJ* **310**: 1126–7.

Green DP and Shapiro I (1994). *Pathologies of rational choice theory*. New Haven, Yale University Press.

Hargreaves Heap S, Hollis M, Lyons B, Sugden R and Weale A (1992). *The theory of choice*. Oxford, Blackwell.

Hope T (1996). *Evidence-based patient choice*. London, King's Fund Publishing.

Jadad AR (1999). Promoting partnerships: challenges for the Internet age. *BMJ* **319**: 761–4.

Johnson TJ (1972). *Professions and power*. London, Macmillan.

Kierkegaard's writings III. Edited and translated by Hong HV and Hong EH. 1st Edition 1988. Princeton University Press.

Kuhn T (1962). The structure of scientific revolutions. Chicago, University of Chicago Press.

Laine C and Davidoff F (1996). Patient-centered medicine: a professional evolution. *JAMA* **275**: 152–6.

Levenstein JH (1984). The patient-centred general practice consultation. *South African Family Practice* **5**: 276–82.

Levenstein JH, McCracken EC and McWhinney IR (1986). The patient-centred clinical method. 1. A model for the doctor–patient interaction in family medicine. *Family Practice* **3**: 24–30.

Locke J (1999). *An Essay concerning human understanding.* London, Penguin Classics (Reprint Edition). Editor Roger Woodhouse.

McWhinney IR (1972). Beyond diagnosis: an approach to the integration of clinical medicine and behavioural science. *New England Journal of Medicine* **287**: 384–7.

Miles A, Bentley P, Polychronis A and Gray J (1997). Evidence-based medicine: why all the fuss? This is why. *Journal of Evaluation in Clinical Practice* **3**: 83–68.

NHS Executive (1996). *Patient partnership: building a collaborative strategy.* Leeds, NHS Executive.

Pendleton D, Schofield T, Tate P and Havelock P (1984). The consultation: an approach to learning and teaching. Oxford, Oxford University Press.

Prahalad CK and Ramaswamy V (2000). Co-opting customer competence. *Harvard Business Review* January–February: 79–87.

Quill TE and Cassel CK (1995). Non-abandonment: a central obligation for physicians. *Annals of Internal Medicine* **122**: 368–74.

Russell H (1982). *Collective action.* Baltimore, Johns Hopkins University Press.

Sackett D, Scott Richardson W, Rosenberg W and Haynes RB (1997). *Evidence-based medicine. How to practice and teach EBM.* New York, Churchill Livingstone.

Sackett DL, Rosenberg WMC, Muir Gray JA, Haynes RB and Richardson WS (1996). Evidence-based medicine: what it is and what it isn't. *BMJ* **312**: 71–2.

Schneider CE (1998). The practice of autonomy: patients, doctors, and medical decisions. New York, Oxford University Press.

Stewart M, Brown JB, Weston WW, McWinney IR, McWilliam CL and Freeman TR (1995). *Patient-centred medicine: transforming the clinical method.* Thousand Oaks, CA, Sage Publications.

Stott NCH and Davies RH (1979). The exceptional potential of the consultation in primary care. *Journal RCGP* **29**: 201–5.

Tuckett D, Boulton M, Olson I and Williams A (1985). *Meetings between experts: an approach to sharing ideas in medical consultations.* London, Tavistock.

von Bertalanffy L (1968). *General system theory.* New York, Braziller.

Weiss P (1969). The living system: determinism stratified. In: *Beyond Reductionism* (ed. A Koestler and JR Smythies). New York, Macmillan Publishing Co.

Wennberg JE, Mulley AG, Hanley D, Timothy RP, Fowler FJ and Roos NP (1988). An assessment of prostatectomy for benign urinary tract obstruction. Geographic variations and the evaluation of medical care outcomes. *JAMA* **259**: 3027–30.

Yardley L, (ed.) (1997). *Material discourses of health and illness.* p. 4. London, Routledge.

2 Evidence-based medicine for professionals

JA Muir Gray

Introduction

Ludwig Wittgenstein was a very able medical laboratory technician, working in Newcastle General Hospital during the Second World War, and in addition was one of the twentieth century's most influential philosophers. His contribution in his latter, better-known, job was to linguistic philosophy and although his text is often dense and difficult, his basic messages were, and are, simple and clear. Words, he said, are simply tools, and most causes of disagreement arise from the fact that those who were arguing were using the same term with different meanings. For Wittgenstein, what can be said is the same as what can be thought, as the famous aphorism from his key work the *Tractatus* says, 'the limits of my language are the limits of my world' (Wittgenstein 1922). He also pointed out that words, as they become more widespread in their use, pick up many different meanings and may eventually cause more confusion than clarity. All these observations relate to the term 'evidence-based medicine' since it was first introduced five years ago.

The most widely cited definition of EBM is that it is:

> ... the conscientious, explicit and judicious use of current best evidence in making decisions about the care of individual patients. The practice of evidence-based medicine means integrating individual clinical expertise with the best available external clinical evidence from systematic research. By individual clinical expertise we mean the proficiency and judgement that individual clinicians acquire through clinical experience and clinical practice.
>
> *(Sackett et al. 1996)*

There are, however, many other definitions of EBM, and, in addition to the explicit definitions, there are also obvious implications in the term that have led some to see the concept as one imbued with negative and pejorative connotations (Grahame-Smith 1996; Polychronis *et al.* 1996; Stradling and Davies 1997). Evidence-based medicine has been portrayed as 'cookbook medicine', as medicine by the rules, as a style of clinical practice which devalues the individual clinician. Nothing could be further from the truth, at least in the minds of those who penned the definition cited above. If others have a different interpretation, then the responsibility must rest with the individuals who coined and promoted the term 'evidence-based medicine' because it is a rule of communication that where there is a problem in communication the primary responsibility rests with the sender and not the recipient of the message.

Evidence-based medicine and evidence-based health care

Evidence-based medicine or clinical practice describes the use of best current evidence to provide the most appropriate health care for individual patients. In the UK, where responsibility for the health of populations is clearly allocated to health authorities and to management, the concept of *evidence-based health care* was invented. This may be defined as the use of best current knowledge as a basis for decisions about groups of patients or populations (Muir Gray 1996). An example of the use of evidence in policy making was the decision by the Department of Health that prostatic cancer screening should not be introduced, based on two systematic reviews of the evidence about prostatic cancer screening.

The origins of evidence-based decision making

One of the claims frequently made by people critical of the concept of EBM was that they had always been practising EBM, and many of those who had been in practice in the later decades of the twentieth century were confident that they had seen the birth and development of modern scientific medicine – rational, empirical, and, as they believed, evidence-based. There were, however, a number of factors that shook this faith and led to a reappraisal of the part that evidence played in decision making.

Studies of variation in service delivery and clinical practice

A number of studies of clinical practice and service delivery have shown that the variation in the rate at which a service is provided or an intervention is used is frequently far greater than can be explained by a variation in the incidence or prevalence of disease. Variations have been shown:

- between countries;
- between services in the one country;
- between services in the one geographical locality;
- between clinicians in the one team.

Furthermore, clinicians were usually unaware of the range of variation or where they stood in the ranking. These studies of variation cast doubt upon the claims, and beliefs, of clinicians and service managers that they were all practising rational and empirical medicine.

Identification of gaps

The development of audit in the late 1980s led to studies of service delivery which compared clinical practice and service delivery with best current practice. Audit revealed that there were frequent gaps between what was known and what was done. Two types of gap were identified:

- failure to start interventions or services that did more good than harm at reasonable cost, e.g. stroke units after stroke, or aspirin after myocardial infarction;
- failure to stop interventions that had been shown to be of low value, e.g. annual cervical smear tests.

These audit studies made it clear that people were not acting systematically or promptly on research findings.

Economic pressures

All societies face three important trends that influence need and demand – population ageing, new technology, and rising expectation. In every society these trends result in need and demand increasing at a rate faster than the resources that are available (Eddy 1993). As a consequence, decision makers, whether clinicians or managers, are under greater pressure for decisions to become more open and explicit. In justifying decision making, managers and clinicians have used evidence to a greater degree (Eddy 1994).

There appear to be two necessary pre-conditions for evidence-based decision making to flourish within a policy framework – a fixed budget and a commitment to cover the whole population. When budgets are expanding, it is often possible for decision makers to slide away from tough decisions; similarly where there is no need to cover the whole population, decision makers faced with tough choices can respond by excluding coverage to heavy users of services. Where, however, there is a commitment to the whole population with a fixed amount of resources, there is pressure. Where there is pressure on decision makers, evidence becomes increasingly important in decision making.

The UK National Health Service Research and Development programme

In the UK, the development of evidence-based health care was stimulated and facilitated by the NHS R&D Programme. This had as one of its explicit objectives the promotion of an evaluative culture. The ability to focus resources on the development of evidence-based decision making has been crucial for the growth of this approach in the UK.

Key individuals

In social change, key individuals have a part to play and the contribution of Professor David Sackett, one of the founders of the evidence-based movement in North America, merits special mention, for the work he did at the Centre for Evidence-Based Medicine – the annual workshops to provide support and inspiration to teachers, the publication of the book *Evidence-Based Medicine* (Sackett *et al.* 1997), and the complementary journal of secondary publication, *Evidence-Based Medicine* and its sibling journals, notably *Evidence-Based Mental Health*, *Evidence-Based Nursing*, and *Evidence-Based Health Care* – has been very significant.

The knowledge revolution

These pressures and trends created a context in which evidence-based decision making could flourish. In parallel another set of changes was taking place which changed fundamentally and forever the confidence that was formerly placed in the data used by clinicians.

Peer review – feet of clay

In the first decades of the second half of the twentieth century, the scientific establishment appeared to be confident, unstoppable, and self-regulating. It perhaps reached its zenith in the 1960s but a number of factors influenced the self-confidence of the scientists and physicians.

There was growing concern about the adverse effects of science, as epitomized in Rachel Carson's classic *The Silent Spring* (1962). This book was first published in 1962 and criticized the widespread ecological degradation that was occurring with the use of insecticides, weed killers, and other common products as well as the use of sprays in agriculture. The book opened more than a few eyes about the dangers of the modern world and stands today as a landmark work. In medicine and health care there were increasing examples of the unintended harmful side-effects of medicine and health care, of which thalidomide was perhaps the most dramatic and best publicized. These events shook the confidence of the scientific community. However, confidence in the process of peer review, regulation of scientific quality by the criticism of articles submitted for publication, remained strong for somewhat longer until empirical studies of scientific articles in journals demonstrated just how misplaced this faith actually was.

Flaws in books

Most busy clinicians tended to turn to textbooks for expert knowledge but textbooks gradually became larger and, by moving from single author textbooks to multi-author tomes, appeared to cope with the trend of increasing specialization. However, a landmark study by Antman and his colleagues (Antman *et al.* 1992) showed just how slowly textbooks responded to new knowledge. This study showed that treatments that did more good than harm took many years to enter the standard texts, whereas treatments that had been demonstrated as being at best ineffective continued to be recommended by prestigious authors long after their use had been discredited scientifically.

Flaws in editorials

Those clinicians who had appreciated that books could quickly become out of date, and were often slow to respond to new developments, had traditionally relied on editorials and review articles to keep up to date, but two classic papers, one by Cindy Mulrow from the San Antonio Veterans Medical Center, now the San Antonio Cochrane Center (Mulrow 1987), and Andy Oxman and Gordon Guyatt from McMaster whence so much of the energy for evidence-based medicine flowed (Oxman and Guyatt 1988), demonstrated that these review articles and editorials were themselves unscientific, biased, and unreliable. This was for reasons such as:

◆   the authors gave no indication about the methods used to find the evidence cited in the editorial;

◆   citation was selective with authors tending to cite only those articles that supported their views.

Thus, the busy clinician would have no alternative but to depend on supposedly up-to-date expert articles, but there was little comfort to be found when these articles were subjected to epidemiological scrutiny. Brought up to revere the peer review process, it was assumed that the reader could rely on the quality of original articles within a journal. However, objective scrutiny of journal articles repeatedly demonstrated significant flaws, of which the greatest was probably the bias towards positive results. Table 2.1 lists five contributions to positive bias.

   The net effect of these flaws is usually to make a new treatment appear more effective (or harmful) than it actually is. That is, it exaggerates the effect of treatment, and this influences both clinicians and patients.

The evolution of the systematic review

Recognizing that editorials and reviews were often biased, usually to the positive, a number of workers started to develop a new method of

Table 2.1 Published research: five positive biases

Bias	Cause
Submission bias	Research workers are more strongly motivated to complete, and submit for publication, positive results
Publication bias	Editors are more likely to publish positive studies
Methodological bias	Methodological errors such as flawed randomization produce positive biases
Abstracting bias	Abstracts emphasize positive results
Framing bias	Relative risk data produce a positive bias

synthesizing evidence – the systematic review. The key characteristics of a systematic review, and of one sub-type, the Cochrane Review, are set out in Table 2.2.

As with EBM, the term 'systematic review' is open to a number of meanings. Some people regard it as being synonymous with meta-analysis. However, meta-analysis, the combination of data from different studies, is often done but is not a necessary feature of a systematic review. Secondly, it is sometimes assumed that systematic reviews can only be done on randomized controlled trials (RCT) but this is not true, and any type of research, including qualitative research, can be the subject of a systematic review.

Table 2.2 Key characteristics of a systematic review

All systematic reviews:
- state their objectives
- ascertain as much of the available evidence as possible
- use explicit quality criteria for inclusion or exclusion of the studies found
- use explicitly stated methods for combining data
- produce reports which describe the processes of ascertainment, inclusion and exclusion, and combining data

In addition, Cochrane Reviews:
- are prepared by multidisciplinary groups, including consumers
- conform to the procedures laid down in the Cochrane Collaboration Handbook
- are based on hand searching of the literature
- are published in the Cochrane Library
- are kept up to date when new evidence becomes available

Keeping systematic reviews up to date – the wonder of the Web

One of the problems encountered by those who sought information from books and journals was caused by the limitations that paper imposes on the searcher. So far as textbooks are concerned, paper imposes a major constraint because it is not possible to correct a mistake or update a part of a book without reprinting the whole book, a costly procedure which usually means that several years elapse between editions of a book. Journal articles, of course, can be more regularly and quickly updated, but most readers of a journal pay less attention to the letters page than to the summary and titles of articles. They may therefore miss corrections in the letters page. Furthermore, even if they see the correction, the edition of the journal in which the original article was published may not be to hand. Fortunately the knowledge revolution coincided with the Web revolution.

The Web revolution

Like the railways in 1850, the World Wide Web is making fortunes for some, transforming society, stimulating the economy, and leading to competition and parallel developments. It also employs, like the railways, thousands of low-paid workers, although the navvies of the Web have less physically arduous a task than the navigators who built the railways on vast amounts of bravery and beer but little money. The Internet stimulated the development of a number of software tools which allowed international organizations such as the Cochrane Collaboration to function efficiently. Software was developed to run the Web, particularly Web page publishing tools, which allowed everyone who can type to become a publisher. The browsers, which facilitate searching and communication, have transformed the way in which knowledge is produced, distributed, found, stored, and used. The Web revolution in turn, facilitated the EBM revolution. It has also transformed the availability of information for patients – and this will be examined in depth in Chapter 17 (Eysenbach and Jadad).

The EBM revolution

The spread of EBM took place with dramatic speed, both within the UK and worldwide. Its appeal was different to different individuals, and it is important to appreciate that it did not appeal to everyone.

The appeal to clinicians

For the ordinary clinician before the advent of EBM, the world was sharply divided into research and practice. However the proponents of EBM always emphasized the need for both research *and* practice to be based on a careful appraisal of best current knowledge. In a world in which there was increasing emphasis on guidelines, the leading figures in EBM were able to demonstrate how individuals did not always fit neatly into guidelines. They therefore emphasized that clinicians had to use their scientific training and their judgement to interpret them, and individualize care accordingly. Cost containment can be fairly easily obtained in health care governed by managers: one simply has to have a fixed budget and fire any manager who is unable to stick to budget. Within most systems of contained costs, however, the value obtained from resources invested is determined not by managers but by clinicians, whose decisions, in sum over the range of services, determine the actual expenditure on health care.

The work of David Eddy, illustrated in Fig. 2.1, demonstrated that the major *manageable* factor responsible for an increase in health care costs, or in the pressure on decision makers where costs were fixed, was a change in the volume and intensity of clinical practice (Eddy 1993).

For a population of one million there may be hundreds of managerial decisions but there are many millions of clinical decisions. If clinicians introduce multiple small changes into their practice the net effect is huge. The types of change that increase the volume and intensity of clinical practice are shown in Table 2.3.

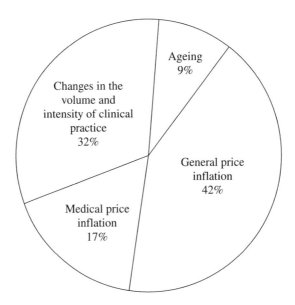

Fig. 2.1 Factors contributing to increased health care costs.

Table 2.3 How innovations in clinical practice increase costs

◆ Treating conditions that were previously untreatable.

◆ Treating people who would previously have been untreated because of changing professional perceptions of need and appropriateness and changing public expectations. These may result from:
   increasing safety of intervention;
   more acceptable, less invasive, more pleasant interventions;
   changing attitudes to chronological age as a reason for refusing treatment;
   changing expectations about health and disease.

◆ Providing more expensive types of treatment:
   more expensive drugs;
   more expensive imaging;
   more expensive tests;
   more expensive staff.

◆ More intensive clinical practice:
   longer duration of stay;
   more tests per patient;
   more professional interventions per patient;
   more treatments per patient.

Thus for managers and policy makers, EBM offered the opportunity to switch the mix of interventions offered to a population from that depicted in Fig. 2.2(a) to Fig. 2.2(b). Such a move would greatly increase the value obtained from the resources invested.

The value of EBM to patients

When one of the founders of the Centre for Evidence-Based Medicine was going to speak at a British Medical Association debate against the motion that EBM was deplorable, a not uncommon occurrence, he phoned Iain Chalmers, Director of the UK Cochrane Centre, for support and advice. Dr Chalmers' advice was simple: 'Just tell the audience that when patients form a movement against evidence-based medicine, then we will take your concerns seriously'. The response of patients to the concept of EBM was usually one of surprise. Patients had thought that doctors had always based their decisions on best current knowledge. It also came as a shock that even the knowledge, where it was available, was often deficient (or commonly not even utilized by doctors who had been left behind the knowledge frontier). They therefore welcomed EBM enthusiastically and it is remarkable how quickly that access to information has turned the table on professional expertise and power. It is no longer feasible to feign knowledge: patients are just as likely to have searched for the evidence before they consult a clinician.

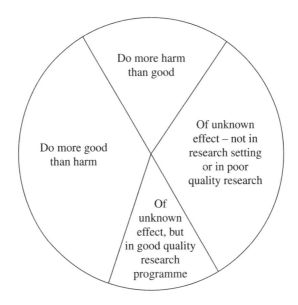

Fig. 2.2(a) The mix of interventions offered before the evidence-based paradigm.

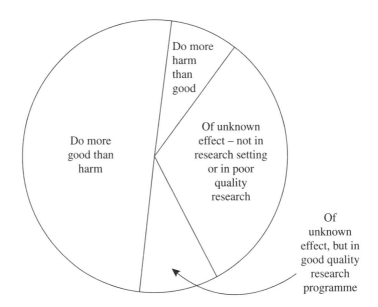

Fig. 2.2(b) The mix of interventions offered during the evidence-based medicine era.

Revolution and counter-revolution

The term 'evidence-based medicine' was selected with some care and in the knowledge that it would raise some hackles. The group involved had evidence that clinicians were not basing their decisions on best current knowledge and could see great political and public concern when this fact was more widely appreciated. Convinced of the importance of clinical freedom, those who founded the Centre for Evidence-Based Medicine wished to stimulate the clinical professions to recognize that they needed to adopt the five steps of evidence-based decision making much more frequently (Table 2.4). It seemed clear that clinicians should campaign vigorously for the skills and resources to practice EBM.

At the time the Centre was founded, there were many health care professionals who had no access at all to a library service, and for many health care professionals easy access to a library was impossible during the working day. In the evenings or at weekends, if they were able to visit, the most valuable resource – the librarian – was not present.

One option had been to call the Centre a 'Centre for Clinical Epidemiology', but working on the principle that there was little difference between stimulation and irritation they decided to adopt a term that would announce their intention clearly and unequivocally. The reaction was mixed and in general older physicians were less enthusiastic than younger physicians, in part because a decision making system based on 'expert' opinion is inevitably much more tied up with personality and power than decision making based on evidence. When the decision making in an organization moved to the right as shown in Fig. 2.3, personal opinion and personality became less significant in decision making. Such a shift was interpreted by some as a loss of power and control.

The question, 'What is the best current evidence?', which would usually be interpreted as a value-free question, was also interpreted by some senior members of staff as indicative of a loss of respect by younger professionals for their older colleagues. Some of the terms that were used to described the EBM movement are listed in Table 2.5.

Table 2.4 The five steps of evidence-based decision making

- Asking the right questions.
- Finding the relevant evidence.
- Appraising the evidence to select the best.
- Decision making based on the evidence.
- Storing the evidence for future use.

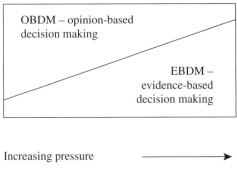

Fig. 2.3 The shifting basis for decision making.

Table 2.5 Terms used to describe the evidence-based medicine movement

◆ cookbook medicine
◆ arrogant
◆ faddish

Journals were split; the *New England Journal of Medicine* and *The Lancet* were less enthusiastic than the *British Medical Journal*, the *Journal of the American Medical Association* and *The Annals of Internal Medicine*, but even *The Lancet* changed its opinion and stated in an editorial that: 'The concept of evidence-based medicine has emerged as one of the fundamental elements in Western-style clinical medicine' (1998).

Individualization – the great challenge for evidence-based medicine

Knowledge, whether expressed as facts or guidelines, is usually information that has been derived from the study of groups of patients or populations. The statement that 'screening for high blood pressure is an effective means of preventing stroke' is certainly true when applied to populations. However, the question of interest to the individual clinician or patient is: 'what will be the effect, both good and bad, on this individual?'

In *The Third Way* Anthony Giddens has identified individualization as a central trend in modern society, a trend in part due to the dissolution of the 'welfare consensus' that dominated in the industrial countries up to the late 1970s and the final discrediting of Marxism, coupled with the profound social, economic and technological changes that helped bring these about. This emphasis on the 'individual' complements (perhaps results from) the apparently opposite trend of globalization (Giddens 1998). We are all members of a global society but this does not diminish the individual. In fact there now appears to be much stronger emphasis on the rights of the individual.

Thus, for example in screening, it is not possible to undertake a form of utilitarian social accounting in which the benefits that will accrue to a thousand people are compared with what would be felt by a hundred. That is, it is not accepted that net profit of 900 people benefiting, provides an incontrovertible reason for starting a screening programme. The individual in the twenty-first century expects, and has a right to be offered, information about the probability of risk and benefit as it affects them as an individual. The fact that this leads to real policy making dilemmas is a reflection of the unresolved nature of the debate. For example, a cervical cytology screening service only achieves a reduction in female mortality from cervical cancer when at least 80% of the eligible population is screened: lesser degrees of coverage are not effective. Yet, if individuals are given accurate information about pros and cons (rather than encouraged to attend under the current incentive schemes) it is very likely that the percentage willing to be screened will drop substantially, thus reducing the 'effectiveness' of the programme.

The number needed to treat

Different approaches are being taken by epidemiologists to try to express data in ways that may be more relevant to, and perhaps more comprehensible to, individual patients. One of these approaches is the number needed to treat (the NNT). This has been complemented by the NNH – the number needed to harm – allowing the calculation of the probability of being helped or being harmed. This and other issues about the presentation of data will be explored in Chapter 9 (Edwards and Bastian).

Clinical practice as a social action

The work of the clinician is, however, not simply a matter of statistical manipulation of data. The clinician deals with the individual patient in a human interaction, particularly those clinicians who are in face-to-face contact with patients, as opposed to pathologists or radiologists who still have to make decisions about individuals but not on the basis of a face-to-face encounter.

Fig. 2.4 illustrates one way of thinking about the individual decision. This shows that the evidence, however presented, has to take into account the condition of the individual patient and that patient's values.

In the words of Mr Gates, the arrival of the digital age does not diminish the need for human beings. But it does force us to ask the question, 'what is the function of the human being in the digital age?', whether that individual

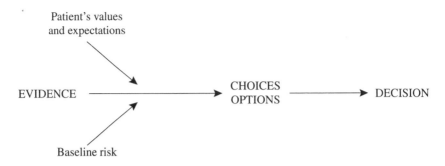

Fig. 2.4 The contributions to an individual decision.

is a travel agent or a banker or a doctor. What is clear is that individuals cannot keep up to date except in the most highly restricted and specialized areas of knowledge. The job of the human being is to become skilled at locating relevant valid data for their needs. In the sphere of medicine the required skill is to be able to relate the knowledge generated by the study of groups of patients or populations to that lonely and anxious individual who has come to seek help.

References

Antman EM, Lau J, Kupelnick B, Mosteller F and Chalmers TC (1992). 'A comparison of results of meta-analysis of randomized control trials and recommendations of clinical experts.' *JAMA* **268**: 240–8.

Carson R (1962). *The silent spring*. London, Penguin.

Eddy DM (1993). Three battles to watch in the 1990s. *JAMA* **270**(4): 520–5.

Eddy DM (1994). Principles for making difficult decisions in difficult times. *JAMA* **271**(22): 1792–8.

Giddens A (1998). *The third way*. London, Polity Press.

Grahame-Smith D (1996). Evidence-based medicine: Socratic dissent. *BMJ* **310**: 1126–7.

Lancet (Editorial) (1998). Patients' records on the Internet: a boost for evidence-based medicine. *Lancet* **351**: 751–2.

Muir Gray JA (1996). *Evidence-based health care*. New York, Churchill Livingstone.

Mulrow C (1987). The medical review article: state of the science. *Ann. Intern. Med* **106**: 485–8.

Oxman AD and Guyatt GH (1988). Guidelines for reading literature reviews. *Can Med Assoc J* **138**: 697–703.

Polychronis A, Miles A and Bentley P (1996). The protagonists of 'evidence-based medicine': arrogant, seductive and controversial. *Journal of Evaluation in Clinical Practice* **2**: 9–11.

Sackett D, Scott Richardson W, Rosenberg W and Haynes RB (1997). *Evidence-based medicine. How to practice and teach EBM*. New York, Churchill Livingstone.

Sackett DL, Rosenberg WMC, Muir Gray JA, Haynes RB and Richardson WS (1996). Evidence-based medicine: what it is and what it isn't. *BMJ* **312**: 71–2.

Stradling JR and Davies RJO (1997). The unacceptable face of evidence-based medicine. *Journal of Evaluation in Clinical Practice* **3**: 99–103.

Wittgenstein L (1922). *Tractacus Logico-Philosophicus*. London, Routledge.

3 Evidence-based health care: what roles for patients?

Vikki Entwistle and Máire O'Donnell

Introduction

In this chapter, we explore the roles that patients and consumers might play in evidence-based health care. Evidence-based health care may be criticized by some for appearing paternalistic but it has potential to incorporate greater patient and consumer involvement.

We begin by considering the roles of patients that have been described in the literature to date. We will explore the types of contribution that individual patients can make at each of the key steps of a 'classic' evidence-based approach to health care. We then consider how research evidence about the effects of health care may affect the choices that are offered to people and the choices that they make, and how people may find other types of information, in addition to 'conventional' evidence of effectiveness, helpful.

In the later parts of the chapter, we consider some of the implications of evidence-based health care for the provision of information to patients. We conclude with a brief look at how consumers can help to ensure the future potential of evidence-based health care by enhancing the relevance and quality of research that is done and information that is produced for patients.

We would like to stress that the forms that evidence-based health care might take and the roles that patients might play within it vary considerably across different health care situations. We wrote this chapter primarily with conscious, competent patients and 'key' health care decisions in mind – decisions such as whether or not to have a hysterectomy, and possibly what type of hysterectomy to have. We do not address the many decisions that are routinely made in the process of implementing these decisions, for example which suture materials and wound dressings are to be used.

Roles for patients in evidence-based health care: some views from the literature

The theory and practice of evidence-based health care have been described in various ways. The idea that health care practice should be guided by rigorous research evidence about the causes and courses of health problems and the effects of health care interventions is central to most accounts. However, the processes by which research evidence might guide health care practice have been envisaged in diverse ways.

One of the features that varies across accounts of evidence-based health care is what role(s) if any are envisaged for patients. Some descriptions of evidence-based health care have illustrated patients playing particular roles in specific scenarios. They have not always discussed whether the patient roles illustrated would be applicable in other situations. Other writings have made more general recommendations about how health care providers and patients should interact. The roles that have been portrayed or advocated for patients include:

♦ passively receiving an evidence-based justification for interventions given;

♦ asking questions that prompt health care professionals to search for research evidence;

♦ expressing preferences for particular interventions and their likely outcomes; and

♦ actively selecting a course of action after being given evidence-based information about the various options.

Early descriptions of evidence-based health care focused on what was seen to be new about the approach: the types of information that should influence clinical decisions about which tests, treatments, and forms of care individual patients would or would not receive. In a classic introductory article, the Evidence-Based Medicine Working Group claimed that EBM was emerging as 'a new paradigm for medical practice'. This paradigm involved using the medical literature, and particularly evidence from clinical research, more effectively (Evidence-Based Medicine Working Group 1992).

The scenario used in this article to illustrate an evidence-based approach involved a 43-year-old man who had experienced a first grand mal seizure. The man was admitted to hospital, where physical examinations showed no abnormalities and he was prescribed an anti-epileptic drug. He was concerned about his risk of seizure recurrence. The evidence-based approach to care that was described involved a junior doctor searching Medline for relevant articles about seizure recurrence. She then critically appraised the single directly relevant article found, and determined that the results of the study reported were applicable to her patient.

The junior doctor gave the man the information that she had found (that the risk of recurrence at one year is between 43% and 51%, but that after a seizure free period of 18 months his risk of recurrence would likely be less than 20%). The advantage claimed for the evidence-based approach in this case was that the man left the hospital with a clear idea of his likely prognosis (which had been concerning him). The authors argued that if he had been given information based on the opinions of the senior doctors, with his risk of seizure recurrence being described as 'high', he would probably have left the hospital 'in a state of vague trepidation about his risk of a subsequent seizure' (Evidence-Based Medicine Working Group 1992).

A scenario in another article involved a 77-year-old woman with well-controlled high blood pressure and mild heart failure. Her doctors were debating whether or not to offer her long-term warfarin therapy. In this scenario, the medical team formulated two clear questions:

1. 'How great is the annual risk of embolic stroke in a 77-year old woman with non-rheumatic atrial fibrillation, hypertension, and moderate left ventricular enlargement if she is not given anticoagulants?'

2. 'What is the risk reduction for stroke from warfarin therapy in such a patient, and what is the risk of harming her with this therapy?'

They then searched the literature for relevant clinical articles and appraised the available evidence for its validity and usefulness.

The team 'discussed the evidence with the patient and she decided to start taking warfarin'. The discussions were not described, and it is not clear how much of a recommendation the woman was given before making her decision. This article did not discuss patients' roles in decision making in any detail. It did note, though, that an evidence-based approach to health care could lead to 'better communication with patients about the rationale behind management decisions'. This perhaps suggests that the authors did not necessarily envisage that patients would actively deliberate different treatment options and make the final selection of therapy themselves (Rosenberg and Donald 1995).

More recent writings by the advocates of evidence-based health care have emphasized that health professionals' individual clinical expertise should be integrated with the best available evidence from clinical research that was the focus of earlier articles. Individual clinical expertise is taken to include 'the more thoughtful and compassionate use of individual patients' predicaments, rights and preferences in making decisions about their care' (Sackett *et al.* 1997).

These more recent writings stress the need to take patients' views into account when interpreting and applying research evidence. They encourage health care professionals to assess whether the available research evidence suggests that tests and treatments would do more good than harm *from the individual's point of view*. For example, doctors who are considering the applicability of evidence about a diagnostic test are told that 'the ultimate question to ask about using any diagnostic test is whether its consequences . . . will help your patient achieve their goals of therapy' (Sackett *et al.* 1997, p.163). Doctors who are considering whether valid and important evidence about a treatment can be applied in the care of a particular patient are encouraged to ask whether their patient's values and preferences would be satisfied by the treatment regimen and its consequences (Sackett *et al.* 1997, p.170).

The descriptions of evidence-based health care that we have drawn on have been prepared by health care professionals to encourage their colleagues to adopt evidence-based approaches in their encounters with individual patients. Health care professionals, policy makers, health service managers, academic commentators, and consumers who write from different perspectives have envisaged different roles for the public in attempts to ensure that the health care given to individuals and populations is based upon the best available research evidence (Haines and Jones 1994; Oliver *et al.* 1998). For the moment, we continue to focus on roles for individual patients within the context of discussions and decisions about their own health care. At the end of the chapter we will explore other possibilities for *consumers* (people with experience of living with particular conditions and of using health care services) to contribute more broadly to the production and use of research evidence.

Roles for patients in evidence-based health care: other possibilities

The basic steps of an evidence-based approach for health care professionals considering how to treat or manage an individual person are usually outlined as:

1. Formulate a precise question;
2. Search the medical literature for research evidence that addresses this question;
3. Critically appraise the research evidence to assess its validity and relevance to the question, person, and situation concerned;
4. Use the best available evidence to make decisions about health care; and
5. Reflect on performance.

Within this framework, patients could contribute in a variety of ways, although their willingness and ability to do so will vary according to their health status, personal characteristics, and the nature of the decision(s) they face. The roles that patients might play in question formulation, literature searching, critical appraisal of the literature, and the use of research evidence to make decisions are summarized in Table 3.1 and considered in a little more detail below.

Formulating questions

The first step of an evidence-based approach requires the formulation of a question that specifies the relevant health status and personal characteristics of the individual, the intervention option(s) to be considered, and the outcomes of interest. These questions tend to take the form: for a person with these particular characteristics, what are the effects of these particular tests or treatments (or of doing nothing) on these particular outcomes?

There are strong general arguments for encouraging patients to contribute to this step. The formulation of questions sets the parameters of which problems will be treated as relevant, which concerns will be addressed, which

Table 3.1 Roles for patients in the key steps of evidence-based health care

Step	Roles for patients	Importance of patient's input at this stage
Formulate question	Help to determine which health problems and interventions are considered and which possible outcomes are regarded as important.	High
Search research literature	Optional. May bring additional information to consultations.	Low
Critically appraise research literature	Optional. May contribute to discussions about relevance. Some patients may be interested and able to contribute to assessments of validity.	Low if their hopes and concerns were thoroughly explored during question formulation and no new possibilities emerge from the research literature identified.
Use the best available research evidence to make decisions	Help to determine what the research evidence means to them and which health care interventions, if any, they want to help them achieve their goals.	High, particularly for decisions that are sensitive to individual preferences.

interventions will be explored, and by which criteria the effectiveness of these interventions will be judged. Health care professionals should not assume that they can formulate questions that reflect the views of the individuals they care for without seeking their input. Although for some health care problems there is a wide consensus about which interventions should be considered and which outcomes are most important, individuals do vary in their concerns and preferences. Also, patients will tend to formulate the required questions in different ways from health care professionals who have been trained to think within a biomedical framework.

For example, people may think of their current health status in terms of symptoms and functional limitations rather than clinical signs or physical or biochemical markers. They may want to know about a wider range of interventions than individual health care professionals think about or offer (including, for example, counselling and complementary therapies), and they may focus on a wider range of possible health care outcomes (Oliver 1997). This has implications for the type of research evidence that is needed to answer the questions concerned.

This is not an argument for leaving patients to formulate questions alone. People will not always know which of their personal characteristics and health problems might affect their health care outcomes. They will not always know which interventions are possible and what kinds of outcomes might result from them. People may need to be told what the possibilities are before they can comment on how important these are to them personally.

If health care is to respond to people's own needs and concerns, the question formed at this stage must reflect their views. Also, health care professionals who explore their patients' perceptions, concerns, and preferences to inform the formulation of questions are more likely to be able to offer appropriate information and health care in a sensitive way. Indeed, they may also be more likely to recognize that in some circumstances the interventions they can offer may be inappropriate.

Searching the literature

In most circumstances it will be inappropriate for health care professionals to hand over the task of seeking out relevant research-based information to their patients. Few people have the skills and resources required to carry out systematic searches of electronic databases of research literature. Also, patients' involvement is probably unnecessary at this stage because once the important questions have been formulated, the search for research to answer them is a skilled task that does not involve major value judgements.

However, an increasing amount of information about health and health care, including research-based information, is accessible to the general public and growing numbers of people are actively seeking it out. Health care professionals must accept that people will search for information about their health and health care for themselves. Most people's searches will not be as systematic as those advocated in guides to evidence-based health care. They will find information that is more or less relevant to their care, more or less research-based, and more or less valid. They may or may not discuss this information with their health care providers and it may or may not end up contributing to decisions about their care.

Critically appraising the literature

In most cases it will be inappropriate for health care professionals to expect their patients to critically appraise the relevance and validity of original research papers. If patients' views are thoroughly explored at the question formulation stage then it is probably not crucial that they actively contribute to the critical appraisal of research papers. This does not mean, however, that people are not interested in or cannot contribute to considerations of relevance and validity. Some people bring information to health professionals and seek help to appraise and interpret it. Some consumer groups and advocates are equipping themselves with critical appraisal skills (Milne and Oliver 1996) and members of the public can now learn from popular texts how to review and interpret information to help themselves make good decisions about their health care (Irwig *et al.* 1999).

Using research evidence to make a decision

There are strong arguments for actively engaging patients in the process of using research evidence to make important decisions about their individual health care. An evidence-based approach does not remove the need for preferences and value judgements in health care decision making. The different perspectives and concerns of health care professionals and patients mean that they might disagree about which factors should be most influential in decision making and which health care options are preferable. It is increasingly accepted that patients' preferences rather than those of health care professionals should dominate – although individual choices may need to be constrained by policy decisions designed to ensure that whole populations can access basic effective health care (Royce 1995).

Ethical norms in most cultures require that people should give informed consent to interventions given by health care professionals. This implies that people should understand and agree to any decisions that are made. There is, however, plenty of scope for people to have a more active say.

Once health care professionals have the best available relevant research evidence to hand with some sense of its validity and strengths, there are various possibilities in terms of:

- what information is shared with the patient, how it is framed and presented;
- the extent to which the patient understands the information and is able to seek and obtain clarification;
- the kinds of discussion that occur about the decision and who is involved in those discussions;
- the amount of influence that different parties seek and have over the decision;
- the ways in which research evidence and other information are 'taken into account' (the approaches to decision making that are used); and
- the ways in which possible disagreements between health care professionals and patients about the interpretation of research evidence and the selection of interventions are handled.

Different approaches will be more or less likely and appropriate in different circumstances. Chapter 14 (O'Connor and Edwards) explores different ways that this can be done and argues that the approach should be tailored to the individual's needs and the condition concerned.

Roles for patients in decisions influenced by clinical practice guidelines

In practice, for the vast majority of decisions that they face, health care professionals do not carry out searches of the research literature and critically appraise all the relevant research evidence. For some decisions, they can turn to evidence-based clinical practice guidelines. These are usually developed by multidisciplinary teams, which may include consumers (Bastian 1996), who review the available research evidence, decide how to interpret it and make suggestions about how it should be applied in practice. The guidelines vary in the extent to which they prescribe and proscribe particular interventions and hence they vary in the amount of leeway they give to health care professionals to allow individuals to influence decisions about their care.

Some guidelines explicitly state that patients should be offered information about key options and be given a say in decisions about their care (NHS Executive 1996). These recommendations are usually made for situations in which the outcomes of care are less certain, or several health care options and their associated outcomes are generally deemed acceptable. In other situations, clinical practice guidelines advocate standard procedures for all patients and thus tend to limit the extent to which individuals are offered and able to make choices. This may or may not be inappropriate, and depends on a number of factors. These include:

- the nature of the decisions;
- the nature of the research evidence about the effects of the recommended options and the possible alternatives;
- the extent to which patients would opt for the recommended options if they were allowed to choose among alternatives; and
- the wider contexts in which the guidelines were produced and implemented.

Choices within an evidence-based health care framework

An evidence-based approach to health care should make it relatively easy to inform people about, and perhaps give them a say in, decisions about their health care. As described in its classic texts, evidence-based health care should tend to make decision making explicit and the basis for decisions open. It insists on the formulation of clear questions and the application of standard literature searching and critical appraisal techniques to identify the best available research evidence. In some scenarios, as we have seen, evidence-based health care explicitly requires attention to individual patient preferences when using this research evidence to make health care decisions.

The amount of research evidence that is available and the similarities and differences that it reveals between treatment options varies across treatment decisions. For some decisions, one option might generally be superior on all the outcomes that most people consider important. For others, several options might offer different types of risks and benefits, with more being known about the possible advantages and disadvantages of some options than others. The varying strength and nature of research evidence raises different types of issues for individual choice in relation to evidence-based health care.

Individual choice *within* an evidence-based health care framework is perhaps most easily envisaged in the following situations:

- When several treatment options are basically effective (on average they do more good than harm), but they involve different processes and different types of benefit and harm with different probabilities so the decision between them is sensitive to individual preferences (Kassirer 1994).
- When the available research evidence is very limited and sheds little light on the relative effectiveness of the available options. (The offering of choice in these circumstances is, however, only likely if a health care professional personally accepts that uncertainty exists and is willing to disclose the uncertainty to the patient (McPherson 1994)).

Examples of decisions that are sensitive to individual preferences are given in Box 3.1.

In other circumstances, health care policy makers, managers, and individual health care professionals may interpret and use research evidence in ways that affect the options that are available to people, the choices that are actively offered, and the way that people who have unusual preferences are treated. For example, health care systems may tend to constrain choices when policy makers decide not to offer certain options because they are not sufficiently effective or cost-effective, or because alternatives perform substantially better on these criteria. Individual health care professionals may then fail to offer options if they strongly believe that one intervention is the 'most effective', perhaps because they focus on one outcome as the key criterion of success. On the other hand, an evidence-based approach to health care can also be envisaged as likely to *reduce* the tendency to restrict the options offered to patients. In practice, professionals may limit options being offered, but only on the basis of personal opinions that cannot be sustained in the light of the best available research evidence. This would be counteracted by an evidence-based approach to health care.

The influence of research and other information on the choices that people make

People who are offered choices about their health care will not necessarily make their decisions solely on the basis of research evidence about the effects

---

Box 3.1   **Examples of health care decisions that are widely offered as choices to patients**

The choice between mastectomy and lumpectomy plus radiotherapy for women with early stage breast cancer. The options offer similar chances of survival but the treatments make different demands on women, have different impacts on body image, and are associated with different types of risk of morbidity (NHS Centre for Reviews and Dissemination, 1996).

The choice between a wide range of contraceptive options that reduce the chances of pregnancy with differing rates of success but make different demands on women and couples, vary in the extent to which they disrupt sexual intercourse, and have different side-effects (Walsh et al., 1996).

The choice between various medical and surgical treatments for problematic heavy menstrual bleeding. Again, no one option is superior in all respects. The treatment processes differ dramatically. The options offer different chances of reducing the bleeding problems but also vary in their possible side-effects (NHS Centre for Reviews and Dissemination, 1995).

of the interventions offered. They may reject the research evidence or be more heavily influenced by other information. The available research evidence may not provide any useful information about the outcomes that are most important to people. Even if it does, people (consumers as well as health professionals!) sometimes rate other types of evidence and information as more credible or more important than 'conventional' research evidence. These types of evidence include their own experiences, the experiences or opinions of those close to them, or what is said in the media. Individual horror or miracle stories can be more powerful than the statistical averages of research evidence even if the incidents they relate to are very rare.

People might want to take other factors as well as research evidence about the health outcomes of an intervention into account in their decision making. Information about treatment processes and timescales might be important. For example, working women with children might prefer a treatment option that does not require lots of repeat visits to hospital. Religious beliefs or cultural norms might override research evidence about the health benefits and risks of interventions, as for example in the case of circumcision (Christensen-Szalanski *et al.* 1987).

The question of whether policy makers' or health care professionals' interpretation of research evidence should in some circumstances be used to override individual choices or whether those choices should always be respected raises difficult ethical issues. These are discussed further in Chapters 4 (Ashcroft *et al.*) and 9 (Edwards and Bastian).

Implications for information giving

In this section, we draw together some of the broad implications of the issues highlighted above for the provision of information to patients. We consider the difficulties of trying to base information on research evidence, the dilemmas of presenting information in situations of constrained choice, and the types of information that might be needed to meet people's information needs as they consider their health care options. Many of the issues that we touch upon will be discussed in more detail in subsequent chapters, particularly Chapter 9 on 'risk communication' (Edwards and Bastian) and Chapter 17 on information sources and quality (Eysenbach and Jadad).

Information should reflect the best available research evidence

Within an evidence-based approach to health care it seems obvious that any information that is given to people about the causes and courses of health problems and the possible benefits and harms of interventions should be based on the best available research evidence. What is less obvious is exactly what research evidence should be presented and how.

People who are facing choices about their health care need to know what the options are and how they compare, particularly in terms of the outcomes that are important to them. Most health care interventions have a range of effects, both positive and negative. The effects vary in their severity, reversibility, and likelihood of occurrence. Some effects are almost certain to occur with a particular intervention, some are quite common, some are rare, and the frequency of others is simply not known. The quality of the evidence that is available about the effects of particular interventions on particular outcomes varies quite considerably, but is often limited.

Information producers and providers who aim to provide research-based information and help people contribute to decisions about their care need to consider:

◆   which possible effects people should be told about;

◆   how the probabilities of their occurrence should be presented;

◆   how and to what extent uncertainty should be communicated; and

◆   the extent to which implications are drawn out of the research evidence and guidance or recommendations made about the selection of interventions.

Opinions will vary on these issues, although a certain amount of consensus is developing about what constitutes good practice (see Chapter 17, Eysenbach and Jadad). As far as possible, the provision and presentation of information should be informed by patients' preferences and by empirical evidence of the effects of giving different types and amounts of information in different ways.

Research evidence varies in the extent to which it 'favours' particular options. It is difficult to present it in an 'unbiased' way. Ideally there should be a simple presentation of the main effects associated with different interventions. This should be combined with relevant context information and guidance about key points to consider when assessing its applicability. This would be less likely to attract accusations of bias than a presentation that makes assumptions about what the research findings suggest to be the best treatment.

Information providers must consider how to present constraints on choice

The options available to an individual might be limited for a number of reasons, although policy decisions to restrict the supply of particular interventions are usually based on considerations of research evidence about their relative effectiveness, costs, and available resources.

If options are limited, the question of whether people should be told about all available options or all possible options is a difficult one. If people are told about options that they cannot access within their current health care system, they may be dissatisfied because they are being denied these options. Having been made aware of their existence, however, they might try to seek them elsewhere. Information that explains the *reasons* for constraints on availability, particularly if these include research evidence about lack of effectiveness, should minimize both dissatisfaction and the chances of people making ill informed efforts to seek the options elsewhere.

Information needs will not be met by evidence of health care effectiveness alone

The information that health care providers give, whether verbally or in written or other recorded forms, should be geared to meet patients' information needs. People need information for a variety of purposes, including to help them understand and make decisions about their health care (Coulter *et al.* 1998). They also use information from a wide variety of sources.

An evidence-based approach to health care suggests that the information that is most needed to inform decisions about tests and treatments is research evidence about the outcomes that might result from the different options and the likelihood of those outcomes occurring. As we have argued above, however, people might also base their decisions on other types of information. Information providers need to recognize that people might have additional information needs when facing decisions about their care.

For example, before they can decide how strongly they want to achieve or avoid a particular health state, they might need to find out what it is like to experience that health state. They might therefore value information about what people who have that condition (or previous experience of it) think about it. People might also want to know about the procedures involved in particular tests and treatments, and what they would be expected to do over what timescale in order to derive the maximum possible benefit from them. Again, they might want to hear from people who have already experienced the procedures about what they felt like and how they coped. For some decisions in some health care systems, including, for example, decisions about dental care in the UK, people might need to know about the costs that they would incur for each of the different options.

Roles for consumers in the generation of research evidence and provision of information

The amount and quality of research evidence that is available about the effects of particular interventions on particular outcomes is determined by what research has been done. Partly because funds for research are limited and partly because researchers have not always addressed the questions that are most important to patients, there are some key gaps in the research evidence. The available research often fails to answer patients' own questions because it has not addressed them in the first place (Oliver 1997).

Even for topics on which research evidence exists, it is not always available in forms that are accessible to patients. Many of the information materials that are given to patients are not designed to support them in decision making, do not reflect the best available research evidence, and do not meet patients' own information needs (Coulter *et al.* 1998).

There is increasing interest in the potential for consumers to help to improve both the relevance and quality of the research evidence that is generated and the information materials that are given to people. People who have experience of living with health problems and being on the receiving end of health care can offer important expertise and insights that complement those of health care professionals. Their input into research and information development may help to ensure that these are better geared to meet patients' needs. People who additionally work in organizations that provide listening, information, support, or campaigning services for others with similar health problems and experiences can bring still greater expertise. They can present the views of a wider group of people and contribute political weight to research and information initiatives.

Consumers can influence the production, dissemination, and use of research in many ways, either as members or leaders of project teams or in occasional advisory capacities (Oliver 1995; Entwistle *et al.* 1998a; Goodare and Lockwood 1999). They may, for example, contribute to decisions about the design and conduct of clinical trials and influence judgements about the importance of the various outcomes that might be assessed. They may help to shape the way in which systematic reviews of the effectiveness of interventions are undertaken, either by helping to carry out those reviews, by commenting on review protocols or drafts, or by helping to interpret review findings (Bastian *et al.* 1999).

In the production of information materials, consumers may again serve as members or leaders of project teams or in occasional advisory capacities. Again, there is scope for them to make valuable contributions at all stages. These include the identification of patients' information needs, prioritization of topics, decisions about how information should be structured and presented, and review of drafts and piloting (Entwistle *et al.* 1998b).

Conclusion

The potential of evidence-based approaches to improve the quality of health care decisions will be enhanced if patients are appropriately involved in identifying the questions that need to be asked and in considering the implications of the available research evidence for their own health care choices.

Attempts to involve patients in these ways, however, are likely to highlight shortcomings in both the available research evidence and the available consumer health information materials. The involvement of consumers in the generation of research evidence and production of information materials should help to improve this situation and thus enhance the potential of evidence-based health care.

Patients may wish to go beyond simply contributing to a process of ensuring that better quality evidence is available and used in health care. They may also wish to assume greater roles in the decision making about their treatment or care than has hitherto been usual in the implementation of evidence-based health care. The paradigm of evidence-based health care is being developed in the direction of 'evidence-based patient choice'. Some of the theoretical background to this development will be discussed in the immediately ensuing chapters. Attention will then focus on the practical implementation of EBPC.

References

Bastian H (1996). Raising the standard: practice guidelines and consumer participation. *International Journal for Quality in Health Care* **8**: 485–90.

Bastian H, Broclain D, Buchan H, Entwistle V, Jadad A and Rio P (1999). Cochrane consumers and communication group: consumer participation. *The Cochrane Library*, Issue 1.

Christensen-Szalanski JJJ, Boyce T, Harrell H and Gardner MM (1987). Circumcision and informed consent: is more information always better? *Medical Care* **25**: 857–67.

Coulter A, Entwistle V and Gilbert D (1998). *Informing patients: an assessment of the quality of patient information materials*. London, King's Fund.

Entwistle VA, Renfrew M, Yearley S, Forrester J and Lamont L (1998a). Incorporating lay perspectives: advantages for research. *British Medical Journal* **316**: 463–6.

Entwistle VA, Watt IS, Davis H, Dickson R, Pickard D and Rosser J (1998b). Developing information materials to present the findings of technology assessments to consumers: the experience of the NHS Centre for Reviews and Dissemination. *International Journal of Technology Assessment in Health Care* **14**: 47–70.

Evidence-Based Medicine Working Group (1992). Evidence-based medicine: a new approach to teaching the practice of medicine. *Journal of the American Medical Association* **268**: 2420–5.

Goodare H and Lockwood S (1999). Involving patients in clinical research. *British Medical Journal* **319**: 724–5.

Haines A and Jones R (1994). Implementing the findings of research. *British Medical Journal* **308**: 1488–92.

Irwig J, Irwig L and Sweet M (1999). *Smart health choices: how to make informed health decisions*. New South Wales, Australia, Allen and Unwin.

Kassirer JP (1994). Incorporating patients' preferences into medical decisions. *New England Journal of Medicine* **320**: 1895–6.

McPherson K (1994). The Cochrane Lecture. The best and the enemy of the good: randomized controlled trials, uncertainty and assessing the role of patient choice in medical decision making. *Journal of Epidemiology and Community Health* **48**: 6–15.

Milne R and Oliver S (1996). Evidence-based consumer health information: developing teaching in critical appraisal skills. *International Journal for Quality in Health Care* **8**: 439–445.

NHS Centre for Reviews and Dissemination (1995). The management of menorrhagia. *Effective Health Care* **1**(9): 1–14.

NHS Centre for Reviews and Dissemination (1996). The management of primary breast cancer. *Effective Health Care* **2**(6): 1–16.

NHS Executive (1996). *Guidance for purchasers: improving outcomes in breast cancer: the manual*. Leeds, NHS Executive.

Oliver SR (1995). How can health service users contribute to the NHS research and development programme. *British Medical Journal* **310**: 1318–20.

Oliver S (1997). Lay perspectives on questions of effectiveness. In: *Non-random reflections on health services research* (ed. A Maynard and I Chalmers). London, BMJ Publishing, 272–91.

Oliver S, Entwistle V and Hodnett E (1998). Roles for lay people in the implementation of health care research. In: *Getting research findings into practice* (ed. A Haines and A Donald). London, BMJ Publishing, 43–51.

Rosenberg W and Donald A (1995). Evidence-based medicine: an approach to clinical problem-solving. *British Medical Journal* **310**: 1122–6.

Royce RG (1995). Observations on the NHS internal market: will the dodo get the last laugh? *British Medical Journal* **311**: 431–3.

Sackett DL, Richardson W, Rosenberg W and Haynes RB (1997). *Evidence-based medicine: how to practice and teach EBM*. London, Churchill Livingstone.

Walsh J, Lythgoe H and Peckham S (1996). *Contraceptive choices: supporting effective use of methods*. London: Family Planning Association.

Section 2
Theoretical perspectives on evidence-based patient choice

4 Ethical issues and evidence-based patient choice

Richard Ashcroft, Tony Hope, and Michael Parker

Introduction

The concept of 'evidence-based patient choice' (EBPC) brings together two important movements in modern medicine. The first of these, 'evidence-based medicine', has been described as a 'paradigm shift' in medical practice (Hope 1996). It is an approach to medicine based on the claim that clinical interventions are to be justified on the existence of evidence for the effectiveness of the intervention rather than on other grounds such as, for example, the authority of the clinician or of tradition. 'Patient-centred medicine' too has arisen out of a concern with and a critical response to traditional medical practice and the traditional overemphasis on the authority of the health care professional. Advocates of patient-centred medicine argue that the best protection for patients from excessive paternalism is to be gained by emphasizing the point that patients should play a central role in decision making about their clinical care. Like evidence-based medicine, patient-centred medicine has been described as marking a fundamental shift in medical practice, a 'Copernican revolution' (Battista 1993).

Taken together, these two ideas, which have a natural affinity, mark a significant shift in thinking about the relationship between the health care professions and their patients. Taken seriously, evidence-based patient choice has the potential to enhance the power of patients and aid the development of an increasingly effective patient-centred health care (Hope 1996).

While evidence-based patient choice can be justified on many grounds (such as 'veracity' (Elwyn and Edwards 2000) or the duty to inform or to tell the truth), it might be said to rest primarily upon two key principles in medical ethics: patient autonomy and patient benefit. The paradigm of autonomy is relevant because the patient is making choices about their own health care on the basis of good quality information. The better the relevant evidence concerning different management options, the more reliable the decisions about what will benefit patients most. It is in this sense for example that respect for autonomy can be said to bring with it an emphasis on the importance of 'veracity'. And in this sense too that respect for autonomy and for patient benefit are intimately related and concordant. An analysis of the ethical issues of EBPC should start with a general endorsement of its core values (Hope 1995).

However, EBPC is complex, and it is no surprise to find that ethical tensions emerge at many of the stages of its implementation. Two broad questions arise: how should EBPC be implemented; and are there situations in which promoting EBPC is not the right thing to do? Both these questions will be addressed, in various contexts, in this chapter. We will start by considering the generation of evidence in the first place, and then proceed to examine ethical issues which arise within a consultation between a health professional and a patient. Finally, we will go on to consider some of the broader ethical implications of evidence-based patient choice.

The generation of evidence

Evidence-based patient choice requires two sorts of evidence. First, patients need evidence which they will find useful and relevant in making their choices of treatment and care. Second, health care managers and professionals need evidence about the ways patients actively make choices, and about the most effective means for facilitating the participation of patients in those choices.

For EBPC to be successful, it is our view that a broad conception of 'good evidence' which is methodologically pluralist, must be adopted, while at the same time requiring high standards of methodological rigour in the generation of this diversity of forms of evidence. In the world of clinical medicine, it is widely agreed that the most reliable kind of evidence for the effectiveness of an intervention is the randomized controlled trial (RCT) (Chalmers 1989). Alongside this doctrine is the notion of a 'hierarchy of evidence' (Guyatt *et al.* 1995), which gives an ordinal ranking of different kinds of evidence in terms of reliability and generalizability.

Some interventions can be evaluated, using RCTs, relatively easily to produce evidence of effectiveness. In other domains, the RCT is less easily used, either for ethical reasons, or because recruitment is very difficult, or because 'objective' comparisons may be meaningless. For instance, RCT evaluations of treatments using patient preference endpoints may be considered meaningless, if the view is taken that patient preferences are not static or objective 'outcomes for comparison'. An RCT of two different ways of breaking bad news to patients may lack external validity over time, as cultural changes affect attitudes to truth-telling in diagnosis; this is unlikely to be a problem in an RCT of two pharmaceutical agents using 'hard' endpoints, such as survival.

Insistence on RCT evidence as the only standard in EBPC would be unrealistic. Other sorts of evidence can prove more accessible and on occasion more reliable or informative. The rise of qualitative research in medicine has generated a more useful understanding of the reasons why patients may not choose the apparently 'best' option (e.g. by not adhering to treatment plans) than was possible with quantitative survey or RCT evidence alone (Featherstone and Donovan 1998; Fineman 1991; Nettleton 1995). It is still too early to say how far this new family of methodologies will take us in generating good evidence for EBPC, but it is certainly as important to find out from patients *why* they do things as it is to find out the frequency with which they do them. Moreover, both patients and indeed doctors may find narrative evidence more valuable than statistical evidence from the point of view of meaning or indeed of utility for decision making (Greenhalgh 1998). We refer readers to Chapter 13 (Greenhalgh) for a fuller discourse on this topic.

Priorities in evidence generation

Most evidence generation (research) is not driven by the requirements of EBPC. Much of the evidence 'out there' is not generated with clinical practice in mind at all. The evidence-producer and evidence-consumer communities overlap only partially; and the consumers of evidence are a diverse group. They include the sponsors of research, academic or industry colleagues of the producers, clinical users of evidence, and patients – and on occasion the media, and political and pressure groups. We must therefore ask how research is prioritized, and how it should be prioritized in order to improve EBPC.

In the 1990s the health care professions, management, the public, politicians, and ethicists began to debate 'health care rationing' in the UK and abroad (New 1997; Daniels 1996; Seedhouse 1995). Much less attention has been paid to the way priorities are (and should be) set in research. Since from the viewpoint of EBM and EBPC, best practice in medicine is reviewed in the light of good evidence, and since to some extent purchasing of health care should also be based on best evidence of cost-effectiveness, areas where evidence is plentiful should, *prima facie*, take precedence over areas where the evidence is scarce. Therefore, decisions about research funding are likely to have a large influence 'downstream' on future purchasing and planning of health services.

Evidence-based patient choice must include a consideration of the priorities in evidence generation. In particular, patient involvement in priority setting within research could be extended considerably, following the lead of citizen involvement in priority setting in health care, in public inquiries in the energy industry, and in planning and environmental policy making

(Irwin 1995; Wynne 1982). Such involvement must be informed by good evidence about not only what preferences are expressed by the public, but also the reasons for those preferences (absence of the latter evidence has been one of the major weaknesses of public health care priority setting exercises to date).

Ethical dilemmas that arise from an EBPC paradigm

The danger that evidence-based medicine may reduce patient choice

The hope, encapsulated in EBPC, is that better evidence and better ways of presenting such evidence to patients will inform and assist the patient in the process of deliberation and choice. It may expand the range of choices, or place existing options in clearer light; it may explain why some apparently attractive options are not advisable or viable.

The reality and indeed the significance, however, of most conclusive RCTs is that they *reduce* the number of options, rather than expand them. If two treatments are compared, then the hope, usually, is that the trial will determine definitively which of the two is more effective. In the light of such evidence, the rational person would choose only the more effective of those two treatments. Tough-minded evidence-based purchasers would perhaps then de-list the less effective treatment and no longer offer it for prescription to patients. In this way, evidence could possibly be used to restrict patients' choices, rather than to assist them.

What price patient choice?

To restrict choice on this basis however would be to rest on too narrow an understanding of rational choice. Rational choice should involve, we believe, a consideration not only of the most effective means to our fixed ends, but also of the nature of those ends, and of what we hope to achieve as a result of our choices. A patient may disagree with the clinician, not because he or she disagrees with the evidence of effectiveness to some particular end, but because of a disagreement about the importance of that end *vis-à-vis* other subsidiary ends. English law gives adult competent patients a power of veto – the power to refuse a treatment which is on offer. It does not give patients a right to any treatment of their choice (Montgomery 1997).

In practice, there are three main reasons why a patient may be refused their treatment of choice:

1. That the treatment is regarded by the doctor as worse than no treatment. Doctors are not obliged to give treatments which they think are harmful to their patients.

2. That what the patient wants is futile – the treatment is ineffective.

3. That what the patient wants, whilst being effective, is not 'cost-effective'.

An interesting question which arises within the context of evidence-based patient choice is whether EBPC implies that, at least in this third case, patients should be given their choice despite the fact that it is considered not to be 'cost-effective'? Let us suppose that there is a new and expensive drug for a particular condition. It has some clear advantages over the cheaper current normal treatment. For example, the unwanted effects (side-effects) are less common, or the benefit from the treatment is more likely. This situation arises in some cancer treatments where new expensive drugs increase slightly the chance of patients' long-term survival. Whilst the expensive treatment may be effective, it may be considered not to be cost-effective. The cost, for example, per year of life saved may far exceed what the health service can normally afford. The health authority, or other purchasing organization may, quite reasonably, make the decision not to purchase this drug at all, or only to do so in a specified group of patients for whom the drug is more cost-effective (Hope *et al.* 1998).

Consider a patient who wishes to have this drug where it is not normally purchased for such patients. If the patient were paying for the drug him or herself there may be no good reason to refuse such treatment. But where the cost of the drug comes out of taxes, or out of an insurance scheme, then by giving this patient what he or she wants, we will be denying another patient a quality of treatment that would otherwise be possible. This patient's choice is another patient's lack of choice. The demands of justice require that patients should not have such choices.

Consider a different situation. Suppose that the treatment the patient wants is cheaper than the treatment on offer but considerably less effective and therefore less cost-effective. Giving the patient what he or she wants, rather than standard treatment would save money but it would lead to less overall benefit. The extreme of this situation is where a patient is choosing a futile but cheap treatment. This situation, again, raises an issue of justice. If the treatment which the patient wants is not normally purchased on the grounds that it is less cost-effective than what the health service normally provides, then by allowing the patient to choose the money is being used to less effect than if that money were used for another patient.

Evidence-based medicine and the notion of cost-effectiveness will need to take into account reasonable variation in how patients value outcomes, including side-effects, if it is to avoid undue restriction of choice. This again points to the need for qualitative research in medical ethics (Greenhalgh 1998).

Evidence-based guidelines and patient choice

Guidelines are another type of output from EBM which can affect patient choice. Evidence-based recommendations can be a benefit to patients because they can improve medical practice. But, specific recommendations can reduce patient choice if they are used in such a way that patients are offered only the one recommended choice (Hope 1996). In their paper, for example, Guyatt *et al.*, worked through the question of whether ranitidine should be administered to critically ill patients as prophylaxis for gastro-intestinal bleeding (Guyatt *et al.* 1995). The outcome of the recommendation was that such prophylaxis should only be recommended for patients who are not only critically ill but also have a clotting disorder. The calculation involved value judgements, in particular the weighing up of different risks. At root the recommendations are based on the view that those without a clotting disorder are at such low risk of bleeding that it is not worth risking the side-effects of ranitidine. The perspective of patient choice however, would emphasize that patients and their families should themselves be given the opportunity to weigh up these different risks and decide how they wish to balance them. In this way the development of evidence-based guidelines could be used to enhance patient choice if the implementation of those guidelines specifically includes taking account of the patient's perspective. The analysis which has to be undertaken helps to highlight exactly where value judgements come in, and the analysis could look at the sensitivity of the outcome to different values. A constructive combination of evidence-based guidelines and patient choice could lead to guidelines which really do enhance patient choice by helping patients to come to the best decision, given their particular values.

Patients who are making the 'wrong' choice

Another ethical challenge for EBPC arises when a well-informed patient makes what seems to the doctor (or relevant other) to be the wrong choice. EBPC implies a shift towards a model which respects each patient's autonomy. Patients have the right to contribute to or make their own choice if they wish (see Chapter 8 (Elwyn and Charles) for discussion of models of the doctor–patient relationship).

The concept of autonomy is, of course, complex. However, even a most basic concept would emphasize the value, in reaching an autonomous decision, of testing our views against counter-examples and other people's views. A patient may make a decision, let us say, to choose a treatment which is less invasive but also less certain of success, than an alternative. But such a choice could be mistaken, depending on the patient's actual values. For example the patient may value highly the maximizing of the chance of successful treatment and yet choose the less invasive (and less effective) treatment because of focusing excessively on the short-term. In such a situation, we believe that respecting patient autonomy would require the doctor explicitly to clarify with the patient what his or her values are and, where the decision seems to be in conflict with these values, to point this out.

Furthermore, a distinction, though not always clear cut, can be made between two types of situations in which this problem arises. In one situation the professional believes that the patient is making the wrong decision, given the patient's own values. In the second situation the doctor thinks that the wrong decision results from wrong values. An example of this second situation might arise when a Jehovah's Witness refuses blood transfusion. The question then arises as to whether, and to what extent, the doctor should challenge these values. It is our view that whereas the professional should normally challenge a patient's decision when this appears to be in conflict with the patient's own values, one needs to tread much more warily in challenging patients' values themselves.

Patients who want the doctor to choose

Consider three clinical scenarios.

Scenario 1

A patient has acute abdominal pain. Appendicitis is suspected. The patient says: 'I don't want to know the ins and outs. Do what you think right doctor'.

Scenario 2

A post menopausal woman in her fifties, raises the question of whether she should take HRT. She asks her doctor to decide: 'I don't want to know the ins and outs. You decide'.

Scenario 3

A patient has a benign condition (e.g. a hernia) which might benefit from surgery. However, there is a small chance of a serious side-effect (e.g. death or a stroke) from the surgery. Again, the patient says: 'You decide doctor'.

These situations raise the questions:

1.   What is the right thing to do? And,
2.   What is the thing to do which is most concordant with EBPC?

On one interpretation of respecting patient autonomy the doctor should do exactly what the patient says. For the patients' statements are unambiguous. On this view, the doctor should make the decision without involving the patient.

However, the three scenarios are different in two important respects.

1. Whether the patient's condition makes it difficult to take part in the decision.
2. Whether what is in the best interests of the patient is clear cut. It will most likely be clear cut where the patient is unlikely to hold a set of values that would radically alter the decision as to what is in their best interests.

In scenario 1, her condition makes it difficult to take part, and the patient's best interests are clear cut. In scenarios 2 and 3 the patient's condition does not interfere with the ability to make a decision. In scenario 3, the low level of risk would be worth taking, for most people, if the hernia caused discomfort. However this would not be true for everyone. But in scenario 2, the balance of risks and benefits depends so much on the patient's values that few professionals would feel comfortable in taking the decision themselves.

The most obvious interpretation of EBPC implies that the patient should play a significant role in the choice of management, and that is on the basis of good quality information. However, an alternative understanding of EBPC is that the 'choice' refers to the choice about what *role* to take in management decisions. Respecting patient choice implies, in this view, respecting her choice *not* to be involved in the treatment decisions. In this interpretation a doctor who made the management decisions on the basis of good quality information, in a situation where the patient clearly delegates decision making to the doctor, is an example of EBPC. We find this second interpretation of EBPC far-fetched. It is not, in our view, in the spirit of EBPC for a doctor, single-handedly, to make the decision even if this is clearly at the patient's request.

The 'patient choice', we believe, which is implied in EBPC refers to the choices about treatment. However, this does not decide the issue of what it is right to do in situations where the patient delegates treatment choices to the doctor. The three scenarios above suggest to us that the answer depends on the situation.

In scenario 1, for the reasons given, it would normally be right, we believe, for the doctor to decide to operate, and simply seek the patient's consent for this. This is an example where the right thing for the doctor to do is not an example of EBPC. EBPC is inappropriate in this situation. Scenario 2 is an example where EBPC would seem to us the right model. Scenario 3 is the most difficult. EBPC implies, to our minds, that the doctor would discuss the small, but serious risks of operation, and want the patient to play a part in the decision. However, whether this is the right thing to do, given the patient's clear wish not to be involved in making the decision, and the remoteness of the serious side-effect, is much less clear.

Broader implications of EBPC

How much information should patients be given in the context of EBPC?

In many clinical situations, patients neither ask for information nor do they specifically say they don't want information. Consider the following clinical case.

Dr A sees patient B in the outpatient department. B is suffering from depression of a type likely to be helped with anti-depressants. There are several slightly different anti-depressants available. Dr A advises B to take a particular anti-depressant (drug X) – the one with which he is most familiar and which is suitable for B. Dr A informs B about the likely benefits and the side-effects of drug X. However, he says nothing about the other anti-depressants which might be prescribed.

The concept of EBPC suggests that B should be given information relevant to choosing a drug treatment, and not simply information about the drug which the doctor chooses. Such a standard of informing is more akin to that demanded in therapeutic clinical trials than is routine in clinical practice. The 'double standard' between the level of information provision in clinical practice, and in the research setting, to which several authors have drawn attention (Chalmers and Lindley 2000) would be reduced by a clinical practice norm which is concordant with EBPC. Our view is that EBPC implies a high standard of informing unless the patient specifically requests not to receive much information (see discussion above).

The implications of the 'framing effect' for EBPC

The way in which information is presented makes a difference to what people actually choose (see e.g. Marteau 1989; O'Connor 1989; Mazur and Hickam 1990), a fact well known to the advertising industry and known as the 'framing effect' – see also Chapter 9 (Edwards and Bastian). This framing effect has been observed not only in the context of providing the basic information, but also in the context of helping patients to think through this information (P Salkovskis, personal communication).

An abstract view of perfect patient choice would be that the patient is free to make a choice without bias or coercion from others. There are three aspects of avoiding bias:

1. The provision of all relevant facts. The idea of relevance in a patient-centred model means relevant to the patient's values and interests;

2. The presentation of these facts in an unbiased manner; and

3. Helping the patient to relate these facts to his or her own situation.

The problem with the framing effect is that it seems to make 2 and 3 impossible. Although there is no clear and satisfactory way of dealing with the framing effect, it is important not to use this effect as an excuse for throwing up one's hands and saying that since there is no totally unbiased way of informing patients, it doesn't matter how patients are informed. There do seem to us to be a number of principles to be followed in presenting information to patients in the context of EBPC:

(a) There should be no intention to manipulate the patient (including through use of the framing effect) to come to a particular decision.

(b) All relevant information should be provided.

(c) The mode of presentation of the information should be as fair as possible – and certainly the information should not be presented in a way to exaggerate some particular aspect (e.g. by presenting relative risks in isolation).

(d) The same information might be presented in different ways in order to reduce the framing effect.

Developing the ethical perspectives on EPBC

Some limitations on 'autonomy'

Just as information can never be completely free of the framing effect, individual patient choices can never be totally free of social influences, including those arising from the relationship between the patient and health care professional. There are two quite different ways in which this might be said to have implications for patient autonomy. Firstly, in some situations, social pressures, including the influence of the health care professional, can mean that a patient's choice is not in fact an autonomous one because it has been coerced or unduly influenced. Secondly, if one takes a more positive view of the patient's embeddedness in networks of social relationships, it may be the case that to put too much emphasis on individual 'autonomy' may lead a professional (or a health care system) to undervalue or even to undermine the social values and relationships within which patients live their own lives and make their own choices.

In this second sense, it might be argued that we should not regard reasoned, individual autonomous choice as the primary goal of any ethical professional–patient encounter. Doing this would have the potential to lead to a view of people, in this case in their role as patients, as entities whose interests, wishes, desires, and values can be separated from those of others (including their family and friends) and can be accessed only by a process of 'individual reflection' on the part of the patient. From this perspective, the prioritization of individual choice might be said to depend upon a one-dimensional view of the human world. It would overlook the fact that we are all inevitably 'socially embedded' – such social embeddedness being not simply a contingent fact about us but *constitutive* of our identity. It is what makes us who we are and this includes, importantly, the values, desires, and interests that inform our choices.

From this perspective it might appear that to view people as individuals and to give priority to individual choice is not in all circumstances to empower patients. On the contrary, it may sometimes be to emaciate them and to make them vulnerable in new ways. Nevertheless, whilst attacks of this kind on the potentially harmful 'individualism' of EBPC and on its over-emphasis on individual choice are important, they can perhaps be avoided by adopting a broader view of patient-centredness. This view should see patients as socially located and recognizes the importance of the patient's social relationships, including those with health care professionals.

It is important to be aware however that the *prioritization* of social values and relationships over those of individual choice is not itself without significant dangers and risks. Evidence-based patient choice usefully reminds us that any moral theory, and indeed any moral society, must be capable of upholding the choices of individuals against the communal, the powerful, and the traditional. Any approach to medical ethics, and indeed to medicine itself, which is more broadly based on a prioritization of social values would find it difficult to explain just why it is that individual choices ought to be both recognized and upheld against the interests of families, communities, and so on.

Such considerations mean that, despite its weaknesses, the wholesale rejection of patient-centredness is not an option. Any ethical, and indeed any effective, approach to health care practice must be capable of recognizing the moral status of the choices of individual patients. Indeed this recognition must be central to such practice. The goal of good health care under any reasonable interpretation must include a concern with the promotion of the well-being of patients and their families and of their ability to live out their lives in the way they choose. The important point for practical ethics here is that patient choice will not be best served by simply giving the patient 'the evidence' and allowing her or him to get on with making his or her 'individual choice'. As in the question of 'framing', the interdependence between ethics and communication will continue to be of paramount importance.

The perspective of patient choice has implications for how evidence-based medicine should be developed. But respecting patient choice itself can pose ethical problems – several of which have been explored in this chapter. Neither is it always clear how such respect is to be interpreted.

References

Battista R (1993). Practice guidelines for preventative care: the Canadian experience. *British Journal of General Practice* **43**: 301–4.

Chalmers I (1989). Evaluating the effects of care during pregnancy and childbirth. In: *Effective care in pregnancy and childbirth* (ed. I Chalmers, M Enkin and M Keirse) **1**: 3–38.

Chalmers I and Lindley R (2000). Double standards in informed consent to treatment. In: *Informed consent: respecting patients' rights in research teaching and practice* (ed. L Doyal and JS Tobias). London, British Medical Journal Books.

Daniels N (1996). Rationing fairly: Programmatic considerations. In: *Justice and Justification: Reflective equilibrium in theory and practice* (ed. N Daniels). Cambridge, Cambridge University Press.

Elwyn G and Edwards A (2000). Informing patients and explaining risks. *Medicine* (in Press).

Featherstone K and Donovan J (1998). Random allocation or allocation at random? Patients' perspectives of participation in a randomized controlled trial. *British Medical Journal*, **317**: 1177–80.

Fineman N (1991). The social construction of noncompliance: A study of health care and social service providers in everyday practice. *Sociology of Health and Illness* **13**: 355–74.

Greenhalgh T (1998). Narrative-based medicine in an evidence-based world. In: *Narrative-Based Medicine: Dialogue and discourse in clinical practice* (ed. T Greenhalgh and B Hurwitz). London, British Medical Journal Books.

Guyatt G, Sackett D, Sinclair J, Hayward R, Cook D and Cook R (1995). A new method for grading health care recommendations. *Journal of the American Medical Association*, **274**(22): 1800–4.

Hope T (1995). Evidence-based medicine and ethics. *Journal of Medical Ethics* – Editorial, **21**: 259–60.

Hope T (1996). Evidence-based patient choice – a report to the Anglia and Oxford Regional Health Authority into the use of evidence-based information for enhancing patient choice. King's Fund Publications.

Hope T, Hicks N, Reynolds DJM, Crisp R and Griffiths S (1998). Rationing and the Health Authority. *British Medical Journal* 317: 1067–9.

Irwin A (1995). *Citizen science*. London, Routledge.

Marteau T (1989). Framing of information: its influence upon decisions of doctors and patients. *British Journal of Social Psychology* **28**: 89–94.

Mazur D and Hickam D (1990). Treatment preferences of patients and physicians: influences of summary data when framing effects are controlled. *Medical Decision Making* **10**: 2–5.

Montgomery J (1997). *Health Care Law*, p. 532. Oxford, Oxford University Press.

Nettleton S (1995). *The sociology of health and illness*. Cambridge, Polity Press.

New, B (1997). Rationing: talk and action in health care. Bill (ed). British Medical Journal/King's Fund Publications. p. 261.

O'Connor A (1989). Effects of framing and level of probability on patients' preferences for cancer chemotherapy. *Journal of Clinical Epidemiology*, **42**: 119–26.

Seedhouse D (ed.) (1995). *Reforming health care: the philosophy and practice of international health reform*. John Wiley and Sons, Chichester.

Wynne B. (1982) Rationality and Ritual: The Windscale inquiry and nuclear decisions in Britain. Chalfont St Giles, British Society for the History of Science.

5 Health economics and patient choice

Anthony Scott

Introduction

Economics is fundamentally concerned with choice and decision making, and seeks to encourage and influence choices to maximize consumers' (and therefore society's) objectives from the limited resources available. Much of economic theory and empirical work is concerned with measuring consumers' preferences, the influences on decision making, and analysis of the informational asymmetries between economic 'actors' (Gravelle and Rees 1992). In health care, this includes examining the choices made by health care consumers and providers. Economics therefore has much to say about information, choice, and decision making in health care.

In the economists' stylized model of the 'perfect market', patients (the consumers) are sovereign: that is, they are the best judges of their own welfare. They can make choices and express their preferences. They have full information, knowledge, and certainty about the products they are buying, and their 'rational' method of decision making is based on relative costs and benefits. This means that their utility or satisfaction is maximized from the resources they have available to them (this also rests on other assumptions about the behaviour of producers of goods and services). In this model they also bear the costs of goods and services from their own incomes. Although consumer sovereignty is regarded by economists as the 'gold standard' in terms of consumer choice, many economists recognize that the perfect market model does not represent most real world markets, where there often exists market failure. In health care, market failure is acute as nearly all of the assumptions of the economists' model do not apply (Donaldson and Gerard 1993). Many readers may now be thinking, 'then what use is economics?'

However, economists use their model of the 'ideal' perfect market by comparing the real world to it. By so doing, research agendas are generated that, as well as being based in theory and used to improve theory, are concerned with how policies can be used to help replicate some of the desirable properties and outcomes of the perfect market. One such property is consumer sovereignty.

The aim of this chapter is to examine the economic issues in trying to improve the extent of consumer sovereignty in health care. For the purposes of this chapter, this is defined as the provision of information and involvement in decision making, the principal cornerstones of 'evidence-based patient choice'. The first part of the chapter examines one of the main sources of market failure in health care, an asymmetry of information between professional and patient, and how this forms the basic framework for the economist's analysis of choice and involvement in decision making. Since patients' preferences cannot be observed easily in health care, the second part of the chapter outlines the various quantitative economic techniques that can be used to elicit patients' preferences over the different sources of 'utility' in health care. The results of such research can then be fed back to decision makers. The final section examines the main issues concerned with examining the costs and consequences of patient choice and involvement in decision making in health care. Areas needing further research are also then identified.

Agency and patient choice

One of the main reasons why health care markets are said to fail is asymmetry of information between professional and patient. In the perfect market, buyers and sellers have the same amount of information about the product in question. In health care, the professional acts as the patient's agent since the professional has more information than the patient about the effect of health care on the patient's health status (Evans 1984; Gafni *et al.* 1998). This puts the professional in a potentially powerful position and, since professionals have their own objectives to meet, may lead to supplier-induced demand (SID). This is where the professional induces the patient to receive more (or less) care than the patient would have demanded, if the patient had the same information and expertise as the professional (Evans 1984). It is however impossible to test whether a professional is a 'perfect agent' using this definition, since patients will never have the same information and knowledge as professionals. Furthermore, Evans suggests that it will be impossible to achieve perfect agency:

> If the agency relationship were complete, the professional would take on entirely the patient's point of view and act as if she were the patient ... The 'perfect agent' would need a split brain, one half advising the patient solely in the patient's interest, the other half reacting ... in a self-interested, own-welfare maximising way.

It is, however, more helpful to examine the potential sources of *imperfect* agency and departures from consumer sovereignty, and how these can be improved upon. The first of these is the extent to which professionals act in consumers' 'best interests'. Central to this is defining what consumers' best interests are. Imperfect agency can arise when the professional has an incorrect perception of the patients' best interests. There are two aspects to this misperception, both of which can be viewed as additional sources of information asymmetry. The first is that patients have more information than the professional about what is important to them (Evans 1984; Mooney and Ryan 1993). The second is that only patients possess information about the relative importance they attach to these factors. Professionals may therefore advise patients on the basis of what the professional would do, if the professional had the patient's illness. Imperfect agency arises where there is a difference between the professional's perception of, and the patient's actual best interests, and of the relative importance of those interests (Gafni *et al.* 1998).

The second main source of imperfect agency is the usual source of asymmetry of information; that the professional has more information and knowledge about the effect of health care on health status. Mooney and Ryan (1993) note that in searching for a definition of 'perfect agency', Williams sees the imbalance of information as being rectified by the professional giving the patient information so the patient can choose (Williams 1988). Two issues are important here, information transfer and choice.

With regard to the transfer of information, McGuire *et al.* (1988) have pointed out that it is important to distinguish between information and knowledge. The former concerns the quantity of information a patient receives and the latter concerns its quality – whether it is understood. The value placed on information may depend on whether it is understood or not.

With regard to choice, it has been suggested that, as in the standard economic theory of agency, it should be the professional agent who chooses the action and not the patient (Evans 1984), as Williams (1988) suggests. However, given the emphasis on co-operation and information transfer in the professional–patient relationship, the potential for the patient to be involved in decision making exists. If the patient is involved in decision making then he or she can use his or her own values in the decision making process, rather than rely on the values of the professional. Thus, information transfer and choice are clearly seen as important in assessing the effectiveness of the agency relationship.

Some of the above arguments implicitly assume that patients prefer more information to less, and prefer to be involved in decision making (Williams 1988) while others assume that patients prefer the professional to choose (Evans 1984; Culyer 1989). However, these should be regarded as testable hypotheses. If patients do not want information or choice then they are still maximizing their utility and, in their view, professionals are acting as perfect agents. This implies a broader definition of 'perfect' agency, suggested by

Labelle *et al.* (1994): '... whether the physician adopts a role that is congruent with the patient's wishes.'

The issue of whether patients want to be involved in decision making is therefore important and has been discussed by Shackley and Ryan (1994) and Jensen and Mooney (1990). They question whether patient involvement in decision making is a 'good thing' when patients may prefer their professional to choose. Using several philosophical definitions of autonomy, Jensen and Mooney (1990) emphasize that patient autonomy is not about patients choosing, but about patients deciding whether they want to choose or not. Autonomy can be defined as: '... the right not only to make consumption choices but also the right not to make consumption choices' (Mooney 1994).

Shackley and Ryan (1994) extend this by arguing that the process of decision making does not have a neutral effect on utility. Patients may actively prefer professionals to choose on their behalf. This may be because of patients not wanting to assume responsibility for that choice, and the potential regret experienced if a wrong choice is made. Such a scenario is consistent with patient autonomy and 'perfect agency' as outlined above. Elsewhere in this book it is debated whether it falls within the concept (Chapter 4, Ashcroft *et al.*). But it implies that in some circumstances at least, patient choice may *not* be a desirable goal (at least from the patient's perspective).

Nevertheless, a closer examination of the theory of agency in health care suggests several factors that influence the degree of imperfect agency in the professional–patient relationship.

(1) The extent to which information is transferred from patient to professional about the patient's objectives and valuation of health and non-health outcomes.

(2) The extent to which information is transferred from professional to patient about the effects of different courses of action on health status. Patients may also want information about the nature of the health problem. Also of importance is whether the information is understood by the patient.

(3) Who chooses the treatment or, more accurately, the extent to which the patient is involved in decision making.

The main policy responses to agency have been concerned with the 'protection' of patients, including the licensing and regulation of the medical profession, and more recently the role of medical accreditation and revalidation. Only recently have economists begun to focus on the source of the agency problem: information, communication, and patient choice in the professional–patient relationship. Although there have been many empirical studies conducted outside of economics about patient involvement in decision making, few have been conducted within economics (Guadagnoli and Ward 1998).

One study has examined these issues from an economics perspective in the context of patients with low back pain choosing a family doctor (Scott and Vick 1998). This used a discrete choice experiment (Ryan 1999). Vignettes were presented to patients registered with general practices, each giving the patient a choice between different types of consultation. Each consultation differed with respect to: the extent of involvement in decision making, information transferred from professional to patient, information transferred from patient to professional (whether the professional seemed to listen), clarity of explanations, and waiting time for an appointment.

Scott and Vick's study found that overall patients *preferred their doctor to choose*. However, being involved in decision making was the least important of the characteristics; the doctor listening was most important, followed by clarity of explanations, information, and waiting time. Thus, for low back pain, as long as the doctor seemed to listen and explained things clearly, then patients were happy to devolve decision making to the professional.

These are highly significant findings in the context of increasing advocacy of evidence-based patient choice or 'shared decision making' (Charles *et al.* 1997; Elwyn *et al.* 1999). They require replication in other settings and for a range of health problems. Patients may have different preferences for involvement for more serious or more chronic conditions. There may also be strong desire for involvement in higher levels of decision making such as when communities decide how best to provide local health care services (Mooney 1998). The need for more evidence at all levels of decision making is clear (Coulter 1997). The crucial issue is firstly whether and secondly how patients want to be involved.

Economic approaches to involving consumers in decision making

Since patients do not usually make treatment choices on their own in health care, their preferences are not observed easily. Health economics has developed a set of quantitative techniques and methods (that are beginning to be combined with qualitative methods), that are used to elicit patients' preferences for the different types of decisions that can be made in health care. These techniques are also being used to elicit the preferences of general populations, that is non-users of health care, as well as patients. Individuals are also being asked about their preferences for others', as well as their own health care. This introduces the idea that people have preferences as 'citizens' that are different to their preferences for their own health care consumption (Mooney 1998). A brief summary of different methods of evaluating patient preferences in health care will now be presented.

All economic techniques ask for stated preferences and provide respondents with information about the health treatment and its alternatives as part of the elicitation task. The techniques not only attempt to measure preferences in terms of 'I prefer option A over option B', but also attempt to elicit *strength* of preferences over options and their characteristics, as in, 'I prefer option A five times as much as option B'. This is the unique contribution of economic analysis and is the reason it is sometimes regarded as being controversial, since it attempts to quantify individuals' values. This controversy is explained further in Chapter 10 (Elwyn *et al.*) in terms of the issues arising from trying to capture preferences as quantified numbers (Elwyn *et al.* 1999).

The other unique fact about economic methods is that they elicit preferences using the explicit comparison of alternatives – the methods are choice-based. This is unlike usual health services research methods such as patient satisfaction studies, which rely on rating and ranking exercises, and where the comparator is always implicit. The use of explicit choices are preferred by economists because individuals are more used to making choices rather than rating or ranking options. Choice-based methods also introduce the notion of scarcity into the method, since patients in health care cannot always have their ideal choice because of resource constraints. Making choices therefore forces people to make trade-offs, and it is these trade-offs that are used to quantify strength of preference. Economic analysis combined with decision analytic approaches also incorporates uncertainty into the analysis, with individuals expressing preferences over probabilistic alternatives (Drummond *et al.* 1997). Economic methods are also based on economic theory. This is crucial, since it helps to interpret and analyse empirical data in a consistent way.

QALYs

Health economic research has been dominated by the Quality Adjusted Life Year (QALY). The QALY approach recognizes that health outcomes should be defined much more broadly than narrow clinical measures of effectiveness (such as reduction in blood pressure from anti-hypertensive therapy). Both mortality and morbidity are relevant to measuring health outcomes, and individuals' preferences for these outcomes are then important. The approach attempts to combine mortality and morbidity into a single composite measure. The QALY approach attaches weights to improvements in mortality (years of survival or life expectancy), with weights reflecting the respondent's valuation (or utility) of the quality of the additional years of life in a particular health state. Thus, if 1 is perfect health and 0 is death, then one extra year of survival in less than perfect health is given a weight between 0 and 1. It is the construction of the weights that has dominated research by health economists as it is these weights that are based on the preferences of patients (Drummond *et al.* 1997; Dolan, 2000). The two methods that have been most widely used to generate values (or weights) are standard gamble (SG) and the time trade-off method (TTO) (Drummond *et al.* 1997; Torrance *et al.* 1972; Von Neuman and Morgenstern 1944).

The entities to be valued using such weights are 'health states' that individuals can experience, conditioned by the length of time they spend in a particular health state. Health states have been formulated to be specific to diseases (such as stroke), or to be generic and applied to a range of health problems. Both disease-specific and generic measures of quality of life have defined health in terms of several attributes reflecting physical, social, and emotional functioning. For example, levels of disability and distress were used by Rosser and Kind (1978) and levels of mobility, self-care, usual activities, pain or discomfort, and anxiety or depression have been used by the EuroQoL Group (1990). Each attribute has a number of levels, and the respondent chooses which level best describes the health state (or their own health). Generic measures such as EuroQoL that compute a single index score from the various attribute scores are regarded as the most suitable for resource allocation decisions across different health care interventions.

Willingness to pay

The application of the willingness to pay (WTP) method to health and health care has grown rapidly during the 1990s. Its origin lies firmly in welfare economic theory, where maximum WTP is a measure of an individual's strength of preference (demand) for a commodity. Although this is initially regarded as problematic to apply in health care systems where people do not have to pay for health care, it is still regarded by economists as the theoretical gold standard of preference measurement. Willingness to pay asks individuals (either through interviews or self-completion questionnaires) their maximum WTP for a particular commodity. Values can be elicited using several techniques. These include:

- 'open-ended' approaches (where respondents are simply asked to state their maximum WTP);
- payment cards (where respondents are presented with a range of values and asked to choose their maximum WTP from each);
- and bidding techniques (where the respondent is presented with a value and asked whether or not they are willing to pay that value).

For example, several studies have examined the use of WTP for information from health care services, such as ultrasound and antenatal screening (Berwick and Weinstein 1985; Lange *et al.* 1990; Donaldson *et al.* 1997).

As well as growth in the number of studies, there has been growth in the range of methodological issues addressed (Diener *et al.* 1998). This includes the methods by which WTP is elicited, and validity and reliability. This research has been paralleled in environmental and transport economics.

Discrete choice experiments

Discrete choice experiments are a form of 'Conjoint Analysis'. They originated in mathematical psychology and have been used heavily in marketing, before being used by economists in transport economics. Conjoint analysis is also being used in environmental economics and its use in health care continues to grow (Ryan 1999; Ryan and Farrar 2000). Discrete choice experiments value the different attributes or characteristics of a good or service by asking individuals to make choices between different scenarios. A scenario comprises several attributes, each of which has several levels that are varied across scenarios. Attributes can therefore represent health, non-health, and process factors. An example is shown in Box 5.1.

Factorial experimental designs are used to compare successive pairs of scenarios, with the attributes varied from one to the next choice. The respondent's choices indicate the importance attached to the various attributes. Regression techniques are used to estimate the effect on utility of increasing or decreasing an attribute (i.e. marginal utility). The regression coefficients can then be used to establish which attributes influence choice, the extent

---

Box 5.1   **Example of a choice of attributes of a consultation for Conjoint Analysis**

◆ **CHOICE 1**	Visit A	Visit B
Who chooses your treatment	Both	Doctor
Information about risk associated with each treatment option are explained clearly	Not at all explained	Fully explained
Being able to talk to the doctor	Doctor does not seem to listen	Doctor seems to listen
Information about health problem	A lot	A little
Length of consultation	More than 10 minutes	Less than 10 minutes
	Prefer visit A	Prefer visit B
What kind of visit would you prefer? **(tick one box only)**	☐	or ☐

of trade-offs between attributes, and utility scores for different combinations of attribute levels. Methodological issues currently being addressed include issues of validity, reliability, and framing effects, and also testing the assumptions of the underlying economic model (e.g. completeness, stability, and continuity of preferences) (Ryan 1999).

Economic evaluation of evidence-based patient choice: assessing the provision of information and choice in health care

In health care, there are many different levels that patients can potentially be involved in decision making. These include government policies, health authority decisions about whether to provide certain services or not, whether to expand or contract services, whether to change the location or provider of services, and decisions about clinical treatment options.

At each of these levels, there are a range of strategies and interventions that could be used to increase patient information or increase the involvement of patients in health care decision making. This ranges from the provision of written information to patients, interventions that are administered in the medical consultation (such as educating professionals in communication skills and the use of decision aids), through to government policy, media campaigns, and the use of focus groups and citizens juries for priority setting. In primary care, further strategies that ensure continuity of care and frequency of contact between patients and the same professional may also be considered.

The resources used in these interventions are, however, scarce and therefore have opportunity costs. That is, they may have generated greater benefit to patients if used elsewhere. It is therefore important to examine the changes in costs as well as changes in benefits from providing information and involving patients in health care decision making. These interventions and how their effectiveness should be judged are considered in other chapters in this book and in other papers (Entwistle *et al.* 1998). However, effectiveness is also relevant from an economic perspective, since it is important to find out what it is that patients value about information and involvement in decision making. This will be related to the process of decision making (e.g. autonomy, information locus of control) and also to the effects on their health status, quality of life, and length of life. The economic techniques reviewed in the previous section can be used to examine some of these benefits.

However, there has been little research examining the *relative* costs of such interventions. A recent systematic review about informed decision making did not mention the relative costs of different strategies, although this was probably related to the fact that many primary studies did not examine costs (Bekker *et al.* 1999). For interventions at a clinical decision making level, the resources used will include the costs of the intervention itself (time of health professionals, information technology, and other sources of information such as leaflets). They will also include the costs to the health service and to patients of behaviour change as a result of the intervention (such as changes in visits to health professionals and changes in referrals and prescribing). These should be examined using standard methods of economic evaluation that involve the identification, measurement, and then valuation of resource use (Drummond *et al.* 1997).

For example, there is much evidence suggesting that professionals who have been trained in communication skills leave patients more satisfied, more adherent to treatment recommendations, and in better health (Ong *et al.* 1995; Kaplan *et al.* 1989; Wartman *et al.* 1983; Stewart 1995). However, these studies have not examined the opportunity costs of 'better' communication (Howie *et al.* 1991). In particular, the length of medical consultations is likely to increase and there may come a point in each consultation when the opportunity costs become greater than the benefits for the patient. It is possible that the time spent could have generated greater benefits if used to see another patient and this requires evaluation.

Conclusion

Economics and its gold standard of consumer sovereignty has much to offer in terms of a framework and research methods to analyse patient information and decision making in health care. Examining the agency relationship in health care is an important starting-point. Economics also offers a set of research methods and techniques that can be used to elicit patients' and populations' preferences for health care services and treatments. These are unique in that they attempt to examine individuals' strengths of preference. There are many different ways that patients can be more involved in decisions about health care, and many different types of decision in which they can be involved. However, there is very little evidence about the relative costs and benefits of these interventions. From an economics perspective many questions arise in relation to implementing evidence-based patient choice, and there is much research still to be undertaken in this important area.

References

Bekker H, Thornton JG, Airey CM, Connelly JB, Hewison J, *et al.*, (1999). Informed decision making: an annotated bibliography and systematic review. *Health Technology Assessment* **3**(1).

Charles C, Gafni A and Whelan T (1997). Shared decision making in the medical encounter: what does it mean? (Or it takes at least two to tango). *Social Science and Medicine* **44**: 681–92.

Coulter A (1997). Partnerships with patients: the pros and cons of shared clinical decision making. *Journal of Health Services Research and Policy* **2**: 112–21.

Culyer AJ (1989). The normative economics of health care finance and provision. *Oxford Review of Economics and Policy* **5**: 34–58.

Diener A, O'Brien B and Gafni A (1998). Health care contingent valuation studies: a review and classification of the literature. *Health Economics* **7**: 313–26.

Dolan P (2000). The measurement of health outcomes. In: *Handbook of Health Economics* (ed. J Newhouse and AJ Culyer). Amsterdam, North Holland, (forthcoming).

Donaldson C and Gerard K (1993). *The economics of health care financing. The visible hand*. Basingstoke, Macmillan.

Drummond MF, O'Brien B, Stoddart GL and Torrance G (1997). Methods for the economic evaluation of health care programmes (2nd edn). Oxford, Oxford Medical Publications, Oxford University Press.

Elwyn GJ, Edwards AGK and Kinnersley P (1999). Shared decision making in primary care: the neglected second half of the consultation. *British Journal of General Practice* **49**: 477–82.

Entwistle VA, Sowden AJ and Watt IS (1998). Evaluating interventions to promote patient involvement in decision making: by what criteria should effectiveness be judged. *Journal of Health Services Research and Policy* **3**: 100–7.

EuroQoL Group (1990). EuroQol – a new facility for the measurement of health related quality of life. *Health Policy* **16**: 199–208.

Evans RG (1984). *Strained mercy: the economics of Canadian health care*. Toronto, Butterworths.

Gafni A, Charles C and Whelan T (1998). The patient physician encounter: the physician as a perfect agent for the patient versus the informed treatment decision making model. *Social Science and Medicine* **47**: 347–54.

Gravelle H and Rees R (1992). *Microeconomics*. Essex: Longman.

Guadagnoli E and Ward P (1998). Patient participation in decision making. *Social Science and Medicine* **47**: 329–39.

Howie JGR, Porter AMD, Heaney DJ and Hopton JL (1991). Long to short consultation ratio: a proxy measure of quality of care for general practice. *British Journal of General Practice* **41**: 48–54.

Jensen UJ and Mooney GH (1990). *Changing values in medical and health care decision making*. London: Wiley.

Kaplan SH, Greenfield S and Ware JE (1989). Impact of the doctor–patient relationship on the outcomes of chronic disease. In: *Communicating with medical patients* (ed. M Stewart and D Roter). Newbury Park, Sage.

Labelle R, Stoddart G and Rice T (1994). A re-examination of the meaning and importance of supplier induced demand. *Journal of Health Economics* **13**: 347–68.

McGuire A, Henderson J and Mooney G (1988). *The economics of health care. An introductory text*. London, Routledge and Kegan Paul.

Mooney G and Ryan M (1993). Agency in health care: getting beyond first principles. *Journal of Health Economics* **12**: 125–238.

Mooney G (1994). *Key issues in health economics*. Hemel Hempstead: Prentice Hall/Harvester Wheatsheaf.

Mooney G (1998). 'Communitarian claims' as an ethical basis for allocating health care resources. *Social Science and Medicine* **47**: 1171–80.

Ong LM, Haes JC, Hoos AM and Lammes FB (1995). Doctor–patient communication: a review of the literature. *Social Science and Medicine* **40**: 903–18.

Rosser R and Kind P (1978). A scale of valuations of states of illness: is there a social consensus? *International Journal of Epidemiology* **7**: 347–58.

Ryan M and Farrar S (2000). Using conjoint analysis to elicit preferences for health care. *British Medical Journal* **320**: 1530–3.

Ryan M (1999). Measuring benefits in health care: the role of discrete choice conjoint analysis. Paper presented to the 2nd International Health Economics Association Conference, Rotterdam.

Scott A and Vick S (1998). Patients, doctors and contracts: an application of principal–agent theory to the doctor–patient relationship. *Scottish Journal of Political Economy* **46**.

Shackley P and Ryan M (1994). What is the role of the consumer in health care? *Journal of Social Policy* **23**: 517–41.

Stewart MA (1995). Effective physician communication and health outcomes: a review. *Canadian Medical Association Journal* **152**: 1423–33.

Torrance GW, Thomas W and Sackett D (1972). A utility maximization model for evaluation of health care programmes. *Health Services Research* **7**: 118–33.

Von Neuman J and Morgenstern O (1944). *Theory of games and economic behaviour*. Princeton, NJ, Princeton University Press.

Wartman SA, Morlock LL, Malitz FE, *et al.* (1983) Patient understanding and satisfaction as predictors of compliance. *Medical Care* **21**: 886–91.

Williams A (1988). Priority setting in public and private health care. A guide through the methodological jungle. *Journal of Health Economics* **7**: 173–83.

6 Evidence and risk: the sociology of health care grappling with knowledge and uncertainty

Paul Bellaby

Introduction

Evidence-based health care is iconoclastic. It seeks to shake professionals from paradigms of practice that are not proved to be of benefit to patients or that carry unacceptable risks. For example, in the inter-war and post-war period it was common to remove tonsils and adenoids in young children who presented with tonsillitis. That practice would probably have been swept away by evidence-based health care because the benefits were unproved. An instance before the First World War of what evidence-based health care would now consider an unacceptable risk was the use of highly toxic mercury in the treatment of syphilis. In retrospect these clinical practices seem mere fashions of the day. In its place, evidence-based health care seems designed to make medicine an applied science, no longer an art or craft founded on experience.

Of course, medicine continues to have an element of art or craft. This is because it is inherently practical. Medical *science* deals with aggregate data and what is known. Professionals act in the individual case, facing the uncertain future. They make judgements that are based on experience as well as knowledge. In doing this, professionals have to take risks and are no different from anyone else, except that they are far more likely to be responsible for other people's lives and well-being. Risk and our attitudes to it are a fundamental background to discussion of evidence and patient choice.

Recent policy has urged that patients should receive the evidence to make informed choices about their treatment (Hope 1996; Herxheimer *et al.* 2000). Like professionals, patients face a mix of knowledge and uncertainty. Moreover, their everyday lives and what is relevant to them are likely to differ considerably from the professional world of health care. Not least, ill health itself tends to be viewed from differing angles by health professionals and patients: by the former, as a biological or psychobiological process, often called 'disease'; by the latter, within personal experience and under the influence of popular culture, as 'illness'. At first sight, the concept of *evidence-based patient choice* seems to imply not only that science can be applied with no residue of uncertainty in the individual case, but also that the expert knowledge of the professional can be reproduced within the lay knowledge of the patient. This may be unrealistic. It may also be undesirable, for professionals have much to learn from patients as well as vice versa.

In what follows, I shall argue that risk cannot be fully understood in the abstract – in the manner of science – but must be placed in the social and cultural contexts of everyday life. This involves discussing the sociological perspective on how risks are accommodated in everyday life, by both the public and professionals involved in health care. I shall highlight the relevance this perspective has for the advocacy of evidence-based patient choice.

What is 'risk'?

At first sight, 'risk' has two faces: those of science and everyday life. In science, risk is the product of the financial or human cost of a hazard and the likelihood of people or property being exposed to the hazard. Yet, with even a cursory look at the issues, it is clear that neither the hazard nor its probability is wholly independent of social relations. In human populations, any hazard, say arising from an infection, is the greater the larger and more densely distributed the population that could be exposed. The likelihood of being exposed depends on the biological relation between the infection and the human host, but also on the lifestyles of the people at risk. Thus John Snow's finding that the source of the 1844 cholera outbreak in London was the water drawn from the Broad Street pump, implied a concentration of population and a lifestyle that enabled the epidemic to take off, as well as the contaminated water that caused the internal damage to human organisms.

Public perception of risk

The statistical concept of risk in which scientists (and particularly epidemiologists) deal gives rise to misunderstanding by the public. For instance, because neither zero risk nor certainty is meaningful, scientific statements made about the low probability of cross-species transmission of BSE have been widely interpreted as implying that beef is 'unsafe to eat'. The public tends to exaggerate risks when the hazard is great and exceptional, but the probability of exposure low. In contrast it also tends to depreciate risks when the hazard is small and familiar, but the probability is high. For instance, fear of plane crashes deters many from flying, even though air travel is safer than making the many journeys by car that people take for granted. Similar misunderstandings arise in health care too, especially when scientific knowledge is applied to regulate clinical practice. This has implications for the way policy is determined for health care delivery to populations. More particularly, there are implications for the way professionals may attempt to integrate evidence into their usual practice in dealing with individual patients.

Statistical risk, epidemiology, and clinical practice

Epidemiology makes statistical estimates of disease in human populations and seeks to identify the risk factors. The limitations of the method are understood among epidemiologists. Terms like 'predict' and 'cause' are avoided, because statistical associations based on current knowledge cannot prove what will happen or even why it happens now. On the other hand, risks are assessed not for the sake of pure knowledge, but to benefit health. Here the aim is not to predict and explain, but to control.

Health care practice applies epidemiological knowledge to try to control disease in individuals. It relies on statistical associations and uses them as if they were covering laws of nature that enable rational decisions on diagnosis and therapy. This is 'reasonable' in the legal sense of what the man on the Clapham omnibus would do, but it is problematic in the higher court of logic.

Risk assessments project from the known past into an uncertain future, and in so doing conjecture that all parameters are known and no known parameter will change. They venture where probability theory cannot provide support (Edwards *et al.* 1997). Furthermore, estimates are based on aggregates, and, in a heterogeneous population, each reflects the mean of a range of individual values. In principle, one could narrow down estimates to smaller groups, but eventually the groups will become too small for the parameters to be inferred reliably. This implies that a 'probability' (say, of death following smoking) is not necessarily valid at an individual level.

What makes it reasonable to project from past to future and to extend mean probabilities to individual cases is not any correspondence between reality and theory, because we cannot evaluate that. It is the practical consideration – similar to civil law – that outcomes judged on the weight of evidence to have been satisfactory in the past justify how we proceed now. It is with this justification that risk information is used in individual cases and in routine health care.

Assessing risk and practical action

In all spheres, bar the hypothetical one of pure science, assessing risk is linked with practical action that seeks benefits for self or others. In commerce, it engages with decisions about investment and its hoped for returns; in international relations, with what seems *realpolitik* and gaining an advantage for the nation state; in personal consumption, with wants and their satisfaction. Like businessmen, diplomats, and consumers, health care professionals meet risk in the course of practical action, for example in determining which drug to use and in what dose, in order to improve or stabilize the patient's condition.

However, when a risk is so encountered, it is seldom on its own, and trying to avert one risk may incur another. For instance, the overprotected child may become incapable of defending itself. This applies to indiscriminate use of antibiotics as much as it does to fussy parenting. Again, it is more the rule than the exception to pursue benefits that would be lost by averting the risks attached to them. Thus, all drugs that are therapeutic are likely to have adverse side-effects. Moreover, the patient may be dead before an investigation is finished that is thorough enough to cover all the risks.

The touchstones of practical action are as much in the future as the past, and typically involve conjecture about change for the better or worse, not about conditions remaining unchanged. So, for example, activists urged that AZT (azidothymidine) be used in the treatment of AIDS (auto-immune deficiency syndrome) in the developed world, well before clinical trials were completed, because of the urgency of prolonging lives currently affected by the condition (Treichler 1999).

Finally, everyday practice is based not only on assessment of the facts, but also on values and rules of conduct. Hence, *realpolitik* often appears unethical, and consumer wants and investment decisions often seem like greed. Similarly, what obstetricians perceive to be the risk of giving birth to a deformed baby can, from another angle, be seen as a threat to the rights to life of disabled people (Shakespeare 1998). It is often taken for granted among health care professionals that health is a prime value, so much so that it may be hard to take seriously that many members of the public consider 'healthy eating' to be losing weight for the sake of body image. In short, 'risk' is a moral category, and likely to be contested by parties with different values and interests (Furedi 1997). The influence of different values from professionals and different groups of patients on treatment or health care decisions is explored further in Chapters 12 (Rosenberg) and 14 (O'Connor and Edwards).

Risk aversion

Just as significant as any difference in principle between science and practice is a division between two forms of institutionalized practice in the modern context: entrepreneurial and administrative. In Autumn 1999, the UK government proposed tax concessions on share options as a reward to senior managers who (allegedly) *take* risks. This coincides with increasing pressure from all sides for those who minister to the needs of others – including doctors – to *avert* risks. Examples of the latter include hospitalization of childbirth and the reliance on double-blind randomized control trials as the touchstone for evidence-based practice.

Hospitalization of childbirth is premised on the idea that in childbirth nothing should be left to chance. To make that aim achievable, the range of potential targets is reduced. The immediate physical well-being of baby and mother are prioritized. What is placed beyond the planning horizon has, at least until recently, included the social relation between baby and mother and (connected to it) their respective psychobiological adjustments after birth.

Risk (whether to the baby or the mother) can never be eliminated. Attending to the immediate bodily risk of mother and baby in childbirth has a logic that is compelling, even obsessive. It starts with removing the birth from home to hospital and ends by removing the woman's control of her body in childbirth, and anaesthetizing her (Tew 1998). Such a logical pursuit of narrowly conceived risks is *irrational* in the final analysis, for not including benefits in the planning, such as the formative relationship between mother and baby after birth.

In general, the horizon of professional clinical practice must be practical. It must be neither immediate (and thus misleadingly secure) nor so long-term as to be lost in increasing uncertainty. The medium-term benefits are inevitably less tangible than the immediate risks. The benefits are likely to include the preferences of mothers, for they must cope with the baby in the months after birth. They are also likely to involve what seems from a biomedical viewpoint to be the 'softer' sciences of psychology and sociology. However, to confine attention only to what appears to be the hard evidence may well cause more harm than it averts.

The *double-blind* RCT has become the acid test of evidence-based practice. Two series are compared: the experimental and the placebo. Cases are randomly allocated to each. The drugs, surgery, or other therapy administered and the placebos are administered 'blind'. Neither doctor nor patient is aware which of the two is involved in the particular case.

The RCT is insufficient to identify the risks that treatments carry, and, just as significant, it tends to give a one-sided 'physicalist' view of the process of treatment. The samples used in RCTs are not representative but characterized ('biased') by the fact that recipients are patients with a diagnosed condition. Moreover, the risks of experimental treatments are observed *ex post facto*, not manipulated in the trial. Thus, they may provide a suggestive indication of the risks attached to treating that condition with that therapy, but not a reliable test of the risks of that treatment in all circumstances. An example can be seen in the debate over anti-coagulation with warfarin for atrial fibrillation. It is often advocated for all patients, but on the basis of the results from largely hospital-based trials or those with highly selected samples of patients taking part (Jacobson *et al.* 1997). Perhaps of more relevance to other conditions, the RCT tests for only one confounding factor, the placebo effect, and not for others that may be critical, for example a tendency for the progress of a disease to enter spontaneous remission. They may, as a result, misrepresent the efficacy of the treatment.

Moreover, the comparison with the placebo effect assumes that the treatment has an effect independent of the expectation of the patient and the way doctor and patient relate, not that the treatment interacts with these factors. If there is an interaction, it may be necessary to administer the treatment in a socio-culturally specific way to achieve its effect (as Kleinman 1980, Chapter 8 suggests to be the case in temple-cult healing of mental illness in Taiwan). This gives the lie to the dualist metaphysics that underpins the RCT. Only the physical effect is considered 'real', while that of the social relation of doctor and patient and the expectation of the patient is treated as if illusory. Both effects, however, may be material for recovery.

The experimental treatment is grounded in the science of statistical risk assessment. However, the 'placebo' effect that the RCT seeks to control for, concerns how cost and benefit are encountered in the course of practical action. These effects may be very important in health care, and should play a particular role in discussions about how to implement evidence-based patient choice.

Risk perception revisited

Statistical risks are a source of confusion for those who are not adept at statistics, but, as we have seen, the application of risk assessment in health care is not always securely grounded in logic either. Rather, expert approaches to risk tend to rest on assumptions that are practically useful and so rarely questioned, but not logical: that the past is a reliable guide to the future, and that aggregated frequencies are informative about risks in individual cases. Evidence-based practice, the scourge of unquestioning beliefs, has already acquired one of its own, the RCT. As above, there may be reason to doubt the reliability of the RCT in assessing the benefits and risks of treatment.

It would be rash indeed, then, to jump to the conclusion that experts are rational and lay people are irrational about risks. Only if 'rationality' were defined as knowingly doing what is known to be cost free, could the most expert person be deemed rational and others irrational. However, where 'risk' is concerned, one cannot speak of perfect knowledge and perfect control. Risks are risks because known effects cannot be controlled or because effects are uncertain.

Fortunately, it is possible to approach 'rationality' in a less unrealistic way, which allows for the facts that beliefs and controls are often flawed and that things often turn out in ways that were not intended. Then, with Simon (1954), one thinks of rationality in the world of practical action as 'bounded'. In Simon's view, also, risks are not just matters of fact, but matters of value.

Another issue is the relation between reason and the emotions. Elster (1999) rightly argues against seeing them as antithetic, suggesting that cognition often triggers emotions and vice versa. Stock markets are susceptible to swings in confidence that are 'bullish' or 'bearish' following on calculations of probable gains and losses. Notoriously, emotion may affect cognitions too, where commitment to victory in war makes much higher risks acceptable than would be the case in peace. So far as health care is concerned, we might contrast the euphemistically titled 'heroic' age of surgery that preceded anaesthetics and antiseptics, in which, by today's standards, considerable risks were taken with patients' lives, with our own risk-averse age. In the latter, any death or injury under treatment is likely to be treated as a scandal and professional indemnity premiums are unprecedentedly high. The attitude of patients to the risks of their conditions and treatments has become an overriding context for health care. Discussions about how evidence-based patient choice can be realized must take account of it.

Risk society and risk culture

Several examples already discussed suggest that risk perception has to be understood in the contexts of social relations and culture in everyday life. What applies to lay risk perception applies no less to risk perception in science and medicine.

Science and its application has been the core of what sociologists often call 'modernity'. Science has been dedicated to the identification and removal of the risks of the human condition. Neither modernity nor science has ever been without critics. However, it is only very recently, in the most technologically developed countries, that mistrust of science appears to have become widespread. So far from reducing risk, science appears now to the public both to *identify* risks hitherto unknown and to *be* a major risk in its own right. An illustration of this is the recent public reaction to genetically modified (GM) foods. Science has produced GM crops to reduce the need for pesticides, and science has also identified the risks GM crops might pose to genetic variability. But GM science is also seen as a risk. Thus public reaction extends beyond being unwilling to eat GM foods and as far as resisting scientific experiments to assess the risks of GM crops. Moreover, science itself is visibly divided here, not only on matters of fact, but by opposing values between those allied with 'progress' and those allied with 'conservation'.

The risk society

The term 'risk society' was coined by the German sociologist Ulrich Beck (1992, but in the original German 1986). Where we stand, relatively few forces of nature appear unpredictable and beyond control. Earthquakes are at this moment one risk that is beyond either prediction or control. They are the typical *risk* of modernity, apparently awaiting reduction by scientific progress. Many other risks arise as unintended consequences of human actions, and these are numerous in the *late* modern risk society.

As the consequences of individual actions become the less predictable and controllable, the longer the chains formed by actors who have an effect on each other, and the more different or specialized their identities. The chains are made longer and the identities more different, when they are spread worldwide. The globalization of markets has multiplied these effects. Admittedly, telecommunications have closed what used to be wide, often unbridged, gaps of space and time between parts of the world, but they do not necessarily reduce the likelihood that individual acts will have far-reaching unintended consequences. This is clear from the GM episode, for neither the massive Monsanto corporation, the prime producer, nor the UK government could avert the public reaction that seems to have put a block on the development. Nor do the consumer and even supermarket chains find it easy to realize their intentions, because it is difficult to identify and elim- inate GM traces from food that comes from all over the world and is combined in the final product on the shelf. Thus, in Beck's terms, the risks of *late* modernity have ceased to be as local and under control as hitherto. They are now distant in source and remote from control.

There have long been attempts to order these otherwise anarchic human chains of cause and effect. Formal organizations, such as the hospital, the business firm, the welfare state, and the United Nations, seek to generate hierarchies in which superiors supervise subordinates. They aim to co- ordinate the different identities assumed by human actors, say managers, doctors, and nurses, making of them complementary not competing roles. Overall, they try to minimize uncertainty (Crozier 1964). Bureaucracy of this kind is best suited to relatively stable conditions (Perrow 1978). The buoy- ancy of developed economies in the post-war period favoured 'full employment' (of white adult males, under retirement age), underpinned mass production for a mass market, and produced a tax surplus that funded social security and health, welfare, and education provision by the state. When the boom faltered, the stability that favoured large formal organizations faltered too. Sociologists (Lash and Urry 1987; Offe 1985) have characterized the economic and social order that they believe to be emerging as 'disorganised capitalism'. Uncertainty made both business and political decisions seem more perilous.

Then the commitments that employers and the state had made to the futures of employees began to seem unsupportable. Employment became relatively insecure and underemployment relatively common, especially among women, the young, and non-white, but increasingly among adult white males (Brown 1997, pp.69–86). Associated with this (not necessarily caused by it) was a trend towards shorter sexual partnerships than had been the case since early widowhood had been prevalent. Partnerships were being dissolved voluntarily at an increasing rate, though also re-made at an increasing rate, with effects on the financial security of members of reconstituted households. As a result, in both the public sphere of the economy and the state and the private sphere of interpersonal relations, less can be taken for granted. More seems at risk, and some have begun to ask whether British society, at least, can be sustained (George and Wilding 1999).

Risks in late modernity are thus products of far-reaching and as yet unfinished change in social relations. Of course the starting-points of these changes differed from country to country. The change in what was West Germany at the time Beck was writing would have seemed less extreme to someone in Britain or the USA than to Beck, because his country's business, labour markets, and pension provision remained highly regulated and gave an impression of stability.

According to Beck, the implications of the risk society are as far-reaching for sociological analysis as for science, for social differences, hitherto based on class, gender, and ethnicity, are being reconfigured into 'at risk' groups which cut across the old divisions. For example, whether one has secure employment, is insecurely employed, or is underemployed is becoming almost as much a source of difference in life chances as occupation and hierarchical position was in the past (Ferrie *et al.* 1995, 1998; Bellaby and Bellaby 1999).

Risk and culture

Yet risks may not, as Beck assumes, be just 'real', they may also be *constructed*. The implication then would be that risks are forged in the medium of culture. They are not just a consequence of the vagaries of nature or even of social structure and its change or disintegration. If science too is viewed as cultural, its role then is not to *identify* risks that await discovery, but rather to *represent* aspects of the lived world as risky.

An example close to health care is the redefinition of 'accidents' as 'risks' (Green 1997). In lay discourse, there are vestiges of fatalism still. The gambler believes in a 'law of averages' which makes the chances of a win greater after a string of losses. In motoring, it is still common to speak of road traffic *accidents*, as if they were twists of fate. However, bookmakers and insurance companies believe that there are causal patterns, and calculate the odds of losses or injuries associated with them, in order to quote prices to punters or set premiums for clients. It is not coincidental that bookmakers and insurance companies make money out of their businesses and punters and motorists finance them, for, behind the change of definition that makes 'accidents' into 'risks', lies a relationship of power.

From this point of view, health care has ascended to a position of prominence. What once seemed the course of nature has been redefined as the object of surveillance, prediction, and control. As Lock (1993) has observed in commenting on the heavy investment of recent years in HRT in North America, ageing is a natural process, which – in the case of women and the menopause – has been redefined as undesirable and an object of medical control. Childbirth is another example in which natural processes have been redefined as health problems. These changes reflect how biomedicine has gained power.

Thus, many of the *risks* with which medicine deals are its own constructs. This is not the same thing as saying that the biological processes we call 'diseases' and 'normal development', are *merely* constructs of the mind (Hacking 1999). They tend to be real and socially constructed on different levels at the same time. As above, it is important to be aware of this perspective on risk, when coming to explore further how evidence, health care, and consumer choice can come closer together.

Risk, contemporary culture, and the body

Two hundred years ago, medicine began to view the body and disease in a new light (Foucault 1973). The new idea was that disease lay hidden from view, but could be deciphered in the living body through signs. It could be traced, at least after death, to a specific lesion within the body. It supplanted the prevailing practice of classifying diseases by clusters of symptoms that might appear anywhere on the surface of the body, and were taken to represent imbalances of the 'humours'.

Where the older approach was holistic, the newer one focused on the hidden site of the disease, and so analysed and fragmented the body into 'systems'. In the older approach, the 'sick person' had been a participant in the course of their condition, which (in acute disease) was held to progress through crisis to either death or recovery. The doctor had held the role of umpire rather than engineer of the outcome. The newer approach relegated the sick person to a spectator, accompanied by his body as the object of medical intervention. It also elevated the doctor to master of the disease process.

Its legacy is that biomedicine tends to think that risk to the body is first and foremost internal and to be understood biologically. It has been widely assumed that only professionals can define what the patient needs to manage such risks. A paternalistic paradigm has become dominant. A further consequence of this construction of roles for professionals and patients and the understanding of disease has been that the point of decision about the allocation of resource to the individual case has become the consultation. Most resource deployment in health care is now the aggregate outcome of many such individual clinical decisions.

However, in *late* modernity the hitherto authoritative role of the individual doctor has begun to be challenged from several directions at once, as is discussed in many other chapters in this book. How might perception of risk be changing in medicine? How much has this to do with the changing social organization of health care?

Changing culture of risk and the changing social organization in health services

A significant contributor to the general sociological debate about risk is the social anthropologist, Mary Douglas. I shall use her ideas to analyse how, first, evidence-based health care and, second, evidence-based patient choice have emerged since the end of the post-war period of the UK NHS. The same concepts will enable me to speculate about the prospects for each approach. The analysis serves to illustrate the general idea that the culture of risk – that is, the shared perception of risk – is changing in association with changes in social organization (Bellaby 1990).

Douglas developed a 'grid/group analysis' for cultures of risk, which she describes as follows:

> a way of checking characteristics of social organization with features of the beliefs and values of the people who are keeping the form of organization alive. *Group* means the outside boundary that people have erected between themselves and the outside world. *Grid* means all the other social distinctions and delegations of authority that they use to limit how people behave to one another.
> *(Douglas and Wildavksy 1982, p.138)*

In different forms of social organization, group varies from a high to low integration, while grid varies from high to low difference within the particular collective.

Cross-tabulating the extremes of the two dimensions, grid and group, generates four cells (see Fig. 6.1). High group and high grid corresponds to a society or group with strong boundaries and equally strong internal lines, which is 'hierarchical'. Its opposite, where group and grid are both low, has weak boundaries and little internal differentiation. It is 'individualist'. The remaining cells are also of distinctive types. Strong boundaries and lack of internal lines suggest an 'egalitarian' society or group. Weak boundaries and strong internal lines suggest a 'fragmented' society or group, lacking a common identity.

I have added, in italics, an indication of which culture of risk prevails in each type of social organization. In the hierarchical group (for example, a well-ordered administration), knowledge almost eliminates uncertainty and risk seems under control. Its members may be said to be 'complacent' about risk. In the individualist group, however (for example, the free market),

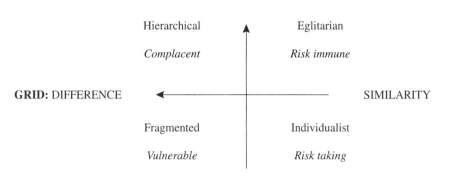

GROUP

Hierarchical   Eglitarian

Complacent   *Risk immune*

GRID: DIFFERENCE ←—————————————→ SIMILARITY

Fragmented   Individualist

Vulnerable   *Risk taking*

PERSON

Fig. 6.1 Grid and group distractions in professional groups.

knowledge gives way to uncertainty and risks seem like opportunities that must be taken, albeit with no guarantee of success. In the egalitarian group, there are risks to be sure, but solidarity is seen to protect its members from the worst effects. Thus, members consider themselves to be 'risk-immune'. Finally, in the fragmented group, risks abound. Each sharply differentiated stratum feels threatened by those above and below. There is an overriding 'vulnerability'.

These variations in risk culture can be illustrated with findings from a comparative study of smoking tobacco and drinking alcohol among employees of a health authority and a large food-processing firm in the same locality (Bellaby 1999, Chapter 7). First, the prevalence of smoking was much lower among employees of the UK NHS. This might appear to be expected, but in fact it occurred despite the fact that smoking was banned in work with food. Smoking rates also varied sharply by occupation and division within the NHS. Medical and scientific staff smoked only exceptionally, while ambulance staff and psychiatric nurses frequently did so. Second, drinking was more common in the NHS than in food-processing. Variations between the workplaces in use of alcohol reflected differences in their social composition, and thus individual social status in the wider community – gender, age, and class. However, variations in smoking reflected differences between the 'missions' of the organizations themselves and also differences in the way work was organized in different parts of the NHS.

There were identifiable low grid/high group categories in the form of ambulance staff and psychiatric nurses. Workers in these categories engaged with threats at the margin of health service work – accidents on the streets and people who deviated from the taken-for-granted rules of everyday behaviour. These professionals probably felt that they became immune to risk themselves by so often confronting it to save others from harm. In contrast, senior medical staff might be placed in the strong group and grid or hierarchical cell.

Senior doctors have been at the centre of power. From this position, they could afford to be quite complacent about the risks associated with their work. Yet, the common boundary of the NHS has come under threat in recent years. This arises from pressure of numbers on what are seen to be inadequate resources and a rising tendency for the public to initiate lawsuits for alleged negligence. Consultants are also having to defend their line within the NHS from a management that sees an opportunity to raise its stature by responding positively to external pressure. Management thus increasingly favours accountability, through audit, formal rationing, and open complaints procedures.

At the boundary and the line, the defence rests on medicine's *moral authority* as curer. It also depends on doctors' claims to be uniquely able to resolve indeterminate questions of diagnosis and treatment. This leads them to try and keep collegiate control of audits of practice and disciplinary actions. Evidence-based *health care* belongs here and has rested easily in this paradigm. It provides a means by which health care can develop and progress but in which a core group of health care professionals and scientists retain control of the direction. It represents a further specialization of health care, with yet another layer of technicality. As a result, the opportunity for patients or consumers to contribute to personal or societal decisions may have become even more remote. Even within the health care system only a minority of professionals and scientists have the expertise to shape the nature and context of health care provision; so influence and authority are further restricted to an 'elite'.

A further way in which the authority of professionals is reinforced is by deflecting the external threat. This is done by and going on the offensive against what they see as body abuse by the population (self-inflicted illness). Smoking is for several reasons an appropriate focus: the outcome seems unequivocally adverse; there is a 'famous discovery' (Doll 1976) to serve as its sanction; finally, doctors themselves made an 'heroic response' to that discovery, by remedying what used to be a widespread smoking habit among themselves. The moral crusade can be renewed by assaults on tobacco advertising, sales to children, secondary smoking effects, and so on. In sociological terms, this increasing tendency towards identification of risk factors and risk groups, and then the placing of blame on the individuals concerned has been encapsulated in the concept of 'privatization of risk' (Wright Mills 1970 Chapter 1; Beck 1992; Edwards *et al.* 1997).

As the market became the pattern *preferred* to hierarchy in the 1980s, individualism eclipsed the collectivism of the welfare state, and risk to health and safety came to be perceived as a private trouble not a public issue. At the same time, egalitarianism, with its work-based culture of mutual protection and sense of immunity to risk, declined with the loss of working-class community and trade union solidarity.

However, the *actual* society that has emerged is best characterized as 'fragmented' rather than individualist. If anything, lines between strata have sharpened (for instance, inequalities in income and wealth have widened, while the consensus and sense of shared 'British' identity that prevailed in the post-war period have been steadily undermined by globalization). The lay person feels vulnerable to risks that are remote and out of control and, increasingly, so too does the health professional. For most people risks are not so much opportunities as threats, and individuals blame higher or lower strata for their vulnerability.

It is not surprising that 'patient choice' should be emphasized in this climate, or that it should coincide with a hierarchical approach to health care that bases practice on scientific knowledge. However, the combination is unstable. Without the trust in the doctor that was typical of the paternalism of post-war collectivism, patients are less likely to 'understand' and accept treatments, even when they are grounded in evidence. Other health professionals are now more likely to contest the authority of medical knowledge and to seek space for their own claims to truth. The general public is more likely to perceive itself vulnerable to threats which health professionals consider spurious. In such a climate, patients (however well informed), may choose treatments that evidence-based practice suggests are ineffective and unnecessary.

To make evidence-based patient choice a solution to the dilemmas that contemporary health services confront, there would have to be a partial return to the post-war ethos. What we need to recover is the sense that risks are localized rather than remote and can be controlled by co-operatively applying knowledge that everyone values. For instance, we need to be able to locate health and safety risks in the workplace, at home, or on the roads and develop a shared understanding of how they are caused and how they can be prevented. However, many risks to health and safety are indeed remote in origin rather than localized. They include uncertain labour markets, transcontinental pollution, and maybe the products of global agri-business. Controlling these often demands co-operation on an international scale.

Two factors are present today and are necessary to EBPC. First, more people than in the past, though far from all, have a sense of autonomy and self-determination and the education to realize it. Second, health care practice (medicine above all) is more accountable, both to governance within the particular health system and to the public. It was the lack of these that held back the development of EBPC in the post-war NHS in Britain.

To succeed, evidence-based *patient choice* must deviate from the post-war paradigm of medical authority. Control and direction must shift from lying completely with the professionals and scientists to a middle ground in which patients have both more authority and greater responsibility. At the same time, the public must have education in science and respect for conscientious professional practice. If both these sets of conditions are fulfilled, health itself will benefit. This will occur both when patients contribute to decisions about their personal health care and consumers contribute to societal decisions about the distribution of resources for further research and health care provision. These issues are examined further in Chapter 3 (Entwistle and O'Donnell).

Conclusion

Evidence-based health care represented a moment in the ever-shifting dialectic of control between health carers, public, and the state. Undoubtedly, it was a significant step for the health care professions in putting their own house in order. However, it may also have served to reinforce the authority of a small elite of professionals. While it was not intended to eliminate the need for judgement based on experience with individual patients, it may have been viewed (by the public as much as professionals) as one step along the road towards eliminating risk. Paradoxically, the credibility of evidence-based health care may have suffered from highlighting the great areas of uncertainty in health care that it could not hope to eliminate.

Evidence-based patient choice represents a significant development of the evidence-based health care paradigm. It can be seen as a way in which patients are given greater authority in decision making about their treatment or care, but also a greater share of the responsibility for continuing risks. I have speculated about the perils that may lie in its path and considered what might need to be done to ensure its success.

Risk has become almost an obsession in late modern society. We must find ways of accommodating risk rather than attempting to eliminate it, for risks are opportunities to be taken as well as threats to be averted. We must also try to understand the shapes that risk cultures take and the forms of social organization that give rise to them, for 'risk' is as much a social construct as it is a reality.

References

Beck U (1992). *Risk society: towards a new modernity*. London, Sage.
Bellaby P (1990). To risk or not to risk? Uses and limitations of Mary Douglas on risk-acceptability for understanding health and safety at work and road accidents. *The Sociological Review* **38**: 465–83.

Bellaby P (1999). *Sick from work: the body in employment*. Aldershot, Ashgate.

Bellaby P and Bellaby FNW (1999). Unemployment and ill health: local labour markets and ill health in Britain 1984–1991. *Work, Employment and Society* **13.3**: 461–82.

Brown RK (1997) 'Flexibility and security: contradictions in the contemporary labour market'. In: *The Changing Shape of Work*. Editor: Brown RK. Basingstoke: Macmillan Press.

Crozier M (1964) *The bureaucratic phenomenon*. Chicago, University of Chicago Press.

Doll R (1976). Mortality in relation to smoking: 20 years of observations on male British doctors. *British Medical Journal*, 25 December: 1525–36.

Douglas M and Wildavsky A (1982). *Risk and culture*. Berkeley, University of California Press.

Edwards AGK, Prior L and University of Wales College of Medicine Department of General Practice (1997). Communication about risk – dilemmas for general practitioners. *British Journal of General Practice* **47**: 739–42.

Elster J (1999). *Alchemies of the mind: rationality and the emotions*. Cambridge, Cambridge University Press.

Ferrie JE, Shipley MJ, Marmot MG, Stansfeld S and Smith GD (1995). Health effects of anticipation of job-change and non-employment: longitudinal data from the Whitehall II study, *British Medical Journal*, **311**(7015): 1264–9.

Ferrie JE, Shipley MJ, Marmot MG, Stansfeld S and Smith GD (1998). The health effects of major organizational change and job insecurity. *Social Science and Medicine* **46**(2): 243–54.

Foucault M (1973). *The birth of the clinic*. London, Tavistock Publications.

Furedi F (1997). *Culture of fear: risk-taking and the morality of low expectation*. London, Cassell.

George V and Wilding P (1999). *British society and social welfare: towards a sustainable society*. Basingstoke, Macmillan.

Green J (1997). *Risk and misfortune*. London, UCL Press.

Hacking I (1999). *The social construction of what?* Cambridge, Mass., Harvard University Press.

Herxheimer A, McPherson A, Miller R, Shepperd S, Yaphe J and Ziebland S (2000). Database of patients' experiences (DIPEx): a multimedia approach to sharing experiences and information. *The Lancet* **355**: 1540–3.

Hope RA (1996), *Evidence-based patient choice*. London, King's Fund.

Jacobson LD, Edwards AGK, Granier SK and Butler CC (1997). Evidence-based medicine and general practice. *British Journal of General Practice* **47**: 449–52.

Kleinman A (1980). *Patients and healers in a context of culture*. Berkeley, University of California Press.

Lash S and Urry J (1987). *The end of organized capitalism.* Cambridge, Polity.

Lock M (1993) *Encounters with ageing: mythologies of the menopause in Japan and North America.* Berkeley, University of California Press.

Offe C (1985). *Disorganized capitalism: contemporary transformations of work and politics.* Cambridge, Polity.

Perrow C (1978). *Complex organizations: a critical essay.* (2nd edn). Glenview, Illinois, Scott, Foreman.

Shakespeare T (1998). Choices and rights: eugenics, genetics and disability equality. *Disability and Society* **13**: 665–81.

Simon H (1954). A behavioural theory of rational choice. *Quarterly Journal of Economics* **69**: 99–118.

Tew M (1998) *Safer childbirth? A critical history of maternal care.* (2nd edn). London, Free Association Press.

Treichler PA (1999). *Chapter 9: how to have theory in an epidemic.* London, Duke University Press.

Wright Mills C (1970). The Sociological Imagination. Harmondsworth, Penguin.

Section 3
Conceptual development for clinical practice

7 Patient-centredness in medicine

Moira Stewart and Judith Belle Brown

Introduction and background

This chapter will present the patient-centred clinical method of which one component is particularly congruent with the concepts of shared decision making and patient choice – the component of finding common ground. The chapter begins with an account of concepts which have influenced the need for and articulation of the patient-centred clinical method. Next, the method itself is described. This is followed by a literature review of the studies of health benefits accruing from patient-centred approaches. Finally, emerging research issues are covered.

At the outset, this book mentions that patients often desire information and involvement in decision making. Our contention based on Beisecker and Beisecker (1990) is that the need for information and involvement varies from patient to patient. Thus, the health care professional's task is to ascertain the degree of information and involvement required by each patient. The most appropriate and effective means to achieve this task is the patient-centred method.

The Cochrane Collaboration have decided to use the term 'consumer'. However, this chapter, focusing on the patient-centred approach declines the corporate imagery implied in the term 'consumer' and instead uses the term 'patient'. The origin of the word patient is 'to suffer' and it implies that caregivers respond to the patient's pain in a compassionate and caring manner. The term 'consumer' does not capture the illness experience of patients and the suffering they endure. Medicine is more than an exchange of commodities or products. Rather it involves a caring human interaction.

The patient-centred model of care requires a shift in the mind-set of the clinician. The historical, hierarchical notion of the professional being in charge and the patient being passive is no longer valid. To be patient-centred, the health care professional must enable the patient to share the power in the relationship. This means renouncing the control which has traditionally been in the hands of the professional. This is the moral imperative of patient-centred practice. In making this shift in values, the health care professional experiences a new direction that the relationship can take when power is relinquished and shared.

Evolution of patient-centred thinking

As evolution towards patient-centred practice is occurring in all health professions, researchers and academics have defined the knowledge, skills, and attitudes of the effective clinician. Yet there have been limited descriptions, in practical terms, of a method of clinical practice. As health care professionals, we need to explain clearly and pragmatically, the essential clinical tasks (White 1988). Models of practice are valuable in that they:

- guide us by directing our attention to specific features of practice;
- provide a framework for understanding what is going on – both the process and content; and
- guide our actions by delineating what is relevant and critical.

A model of clinical practice may simplify dealing with the complexity of the patient's problems. It focuses our attention on aspects of a situation that are most important for understanding and effective action.

The patient-centred clinical method described later in this chapter is medicine's attempt to describe the clinical tasks. The patient-centred clinical method has much in common with other therapeutic models developed in other disciplines such as the psychotherapeutic concept of client-centred therapy (Rogers 1951), Newman and Young's (1972) total person approach to patient problems in nursing, and with the two-body practice in occupational therapy (Mattingly and Fleming 1994). The following brief history of the evolution of thinking refers to a context which applies to the health professions generally, but is written from the perspective of medicine in particular.

The dominant model in medical practice has been labelled the 'conventional medical model'. It has its roots in the work of Descartes who provided the method for modern science and in doing so succeeded in the separation of mind and matter. Through the separation of subject and object, complex phenomena could be reduced to their simplest components. But as the medical model became more abstract and focused, it also became dramatically removed from the experience of the patient. The focus was on diagnosis with an emphasis on physical pathology. The method was analytical and impersonal. Thus the feelings and the life experiences of the patient were not relevant. Given the model's Cartesian origins, it divided psyche and soma, which only came joined again through illnesses such as 'conversion reactions' or 'psychosomatic disease'. This dichotomy between the mental and the physical further separated patients and their experience from the disease process.

The language and terminology which has evolved during the establishment of the 'conventional medical model' has further entrenched this dualistic thinking. It separates the patient into parts and promotes 'silo' thinking. These ways of thinking and communicating are contrary to the goals of the patient-centred method. Thus, we must seek new terminology that reflects the whole person, both psyche and soma, and includes all aspects of the patient's experience.

The influence of the conventional medical model has been widespread, but in the last two decades of the twentieth century, it has been challenged as oversimplifying the problems of sickness (Odegaard 1986; White 1988). As Engel (1977) noted, the conventional medical model 'leaves no room within its framework for the social, psychological, and behavioural dimensions of illness'.

In response to this challenge several alternative conceptual frameworks have been articulated (Carmichael and Carmichael 1981; Cohen-Cole 1991; Foss and Rothenberg 1987; Kleinman *et al.* 1978; Pendleton *et al.* 1984). For example, the seminal work of Engel's (1980) biopsychosocial model used systems theory as a basis for understanding human sickness. The patient was conceptualized as being composed of systems (tissues, cells, molecules) and, in turn, as being part of several larger systems (dyads, families, communities, nations). Engel's model alerts us always to be cognizant of the biological, psychological, and social dimensions of the patient's illness experience. However, what Engel's model lacked was an understanding of the dynamic interaction of these multiple aspects of the person.

All of these conceptual models have been informative, have moved the practice of medicine forward, and have served as antecedents to the patient-centred model. In particular, authors have pointed out the importance of acknowledging a distinction between the clinician's theoretical understanding of the patient's disease and the patient's personal experience of illness (Cassell 1985, 1991; Fabrega 1974; Levenstein 1984; Levenstein *et al.* 1986 1989; McWhinney 1989; Mishler 1984; Reiser and Schroder 1980; Stephens 1982; Stetten 1981). This distinction highlights patients' need for more than a scientific formulation and treatment of their problems and concerns. Patients generally want to feel understood and valued. They may want to be involved in making sense of their health problems and be participants in resolving those problems. This may include involvement in decisions about management. Being patient-centred means attending to the patients' experience and values as well as exploring with them the degree to which they prefer to be involved in the management decisions.

Clinicians and researchers are recognizing the many benefits to the patient of a more compassionate caring approach which integrates attention to the person in their social context and physical environment. The biological basis for the observed benefits is shown in the psychoneuroimmunology literature as well as in several key studies in the primary care literature (Kaplan *et al.* 1989) which will be discussed in detail later in this chapter. However, an effective model of practice needs to be explicit about when and how to go beyond the conventional medical model.

The patient-centred clinical method

Balint *et al.* (1970) first introduced the term 'patient-centred medicine' and contrasted it with 'disease-centred medicine'. They described an under-standing of the patient's complaints, based on patient-centred thinking, as the 'overall diagnosis,' while an understanding based on disease-centred thinking was called 'traditional diagnosis.' The work of Stevens (1974), Tait (1979), and Wright and MacAdam (1979) further elaborated the patient-centred clinical method. Similarly, Byrne and Long (1976) developed a method for categorizing consultations as either doctor-centred or patient-centred. In their analysis of 1,850 general practice consultations, Byrne and Long (1976) suggested that many physicians develop a relatively static style of consulting that tends to be doctor-centred: 'The problem is that the doctor-centred style is extremely seductive.'

Clinical teaching in medical schools has historically emphasized a doctor-centred approach (or disease-centred, as we prefer). According to this model, physicians ascertain the patient's complaints and seek information that will enable them to interpret the patient's illness solely within the physician's frame of reference. This involves diagnosing the patient's disease and prescribing an appropriate management. One criterion of success is a precise diagnosis, such as kidney failure, stroke, lung cancer, diabetes, elder abuse, or depression. In pursuit of this goal, physicians use a method designed to obtain objective information from the patient. In contrast, the patient-centred clinical method seeks both a diagnosis as well as an understanding of the patient's experience of being ill. Disease and illness are intertwined and therefore cannot be artificially separated.

The patient-centred model and method was developed by Levenstein (1984) based on observation of 1,000 clinical encounters in his own family practice and further developed at The University of Western Ontario, London, Canada (Stewart *et al.* 1995; Levenstein *et al.* 1986; McCracken *et al.* 1983). The method consists of six interconnecting components:

- exploring both the disease and the illness experience;
- understanding the whole person;
- finding common ground;
- incorporating prevention and health promotion;
- enhancing the patient–doctor relationship; and
- being realistic.

These six components, although arising out of family medical practice, are highly relevant to all health professions. All six are described below because they are inextricably interwoven. However, particular emphasis will be placed on the third component, finding common ground, as it is most pertinent to the principal thesis of this book.

1   Exploring both the disease and the illness experience

The first component involves the health care professionals' understanding two conceptualizations of ill health: disease and illness (Levenstein 1984; Levenstein *et al.* 1986, 1989; Stewart *et al.* 1995). As noted previously, disease is a theoretical construct, or abstraction, by which clinicians seek to describe patients' symptoms or concerns in terms of abnormalities of structure or function of body organs and systems. It includes both physical and mental disorders. Illness refers to patients' personal experiences of being unwell. The ultimate diagnosis defines what each individual with a disease shares as a common experience with others with the same symptoms. The illness experience for each person remains unique and defined by their personal experience.

Thus effective patient care requires attending to both patients' personal experiences of illnesses and to their diseases or diagnoses. The identification of disease is established by using the conventional medical model, but understanding illnesses requires an additional approach. A patient-centred method focuses both on disease and on four key dimensions of patients' illness experiences: (a) their *feelings*, especially fears about being ill; (b) their *ideas* about what is wrong with them; (c) the impact of their problems on *functioning*; and (d) their *expectations* about what should be done (*FIFE*). Central to the patient-centred approach is attention to patients' cues related to these dimensions. The main objective is to follow patients' leads and to understand patients' experiences from their own perspective.

To appreciate and understand the patient's illness experience requires specific interviewing skills. Historically these have not been a priority in health care education and practice. How do health care professionals 'enter into the patient's world,' and understand the illness from the patient's point of view? Often this is straightforward, but at other times the provider must be alert for cues to the patient's feelings, ideas, effect on function, or expectations. Patients may prompt a professional if he or she misses cues. This can be through the patient's repeated reference to a specific event or expression of worry or concern. Sometimes, it is only at the end of an interview that a crucial comment is made. These 'door handle' remarks may indicate that the health care professional has missed earlier cues or that the patient finally gathered enough courage to raise a fearful or embarrassing issue.

2 Understanding the whole person

The second component is an integrated understanding of the whole person. Over many encounters, clinicians gather a great deal of information about their patients. They begin to know the whole person. In doing so, they come to understand not only the patient's disease but also their experience of illness in the context of his or her life setting and stage of personal development. Knowledge of the person may include their family, work, faith, and struggles with various life crises.

Of particular importance is the role of the family or significant support systems in the ill person's experience. By understanding the impact of these relationships and their concomitant roles, the health care professional can gain knowledge of how these interactions ameliorate, aggravate, or even cause illness. Of equal importance are the patient's cultural beliefs and attitudes which also influence his or her care. Finally, understanding the whole person can deepen the health care professional's knowledge of the human condition, especially the nature of suffering and the responses of individuals to sickness.

3 Finding common ground

The third component of the method is the mutual finding of common ground. Developing an effective management plan requires that both clinician and patient reach an agreement in three key areas: (a) the nature of the problems and priorities, (b) the goals of treatment or management, and (c) the roles of both the health care professional and the patient. Often, clinicians and patients have widely divergent views in each of these areas. The process of finding a satisfactory resolution is not so much one of bargaining or negotiating, but rather of moving towards a meeting of minds or finding common ground. This framework reminds health care professionals to incorporate patients' feelings, ideas, function, and expectations into treatment planning. It also requires that health care professionals be clear in their description of the problems, actively engage patients in clarification, and, in the decision making process, encourage patient participation as appropriate. We will expand how this is implemented in the following section.

4 Incorporating prevention and health promotion

The fourth component is perhaps particularly relevant to primary care and incorporates discussion of issues of prevention and health promotion during the patient–professional encounter. Disease prevention and health promotion require a collaborative, ongoing effort on the part of patient and clinician. Thus, the multiple opportunities for disease prevention and health promotion become an important component of every visit. Application of the patient-centred approach throughout this process constitutes active engagement of the patient in both relevant prevention activities (such as blood pressure, cervical smear screening) and health promotion (exercise, stress management).

Together, health care professionals and patients can monitor areas in patients' lives that need strengthening to enhance both emotional and physical health. Health care professionals also need to monitor recognized problems and to screen for unrecognized disease. Finally, health care professionals need to collaborate with other members of the health care team to implement programmes of health promotion and screening in practice.

Fundamental to this component of patient-centred method is that continuing and comprehensive care is an underlying philosophy of practice. This carries the expectation that a protocol for screening and health promotion, as well as a medical record system supporting the protocol (problem list, flow sheets, computer reminder systems), be implemented.

5   Enhancing the patient–health care professional relationship

The core foundation of the patient-centred clinical method is the relationship. Continuity of care and the long-term nature of many patient–professional relationships enhances the interaction with time. By seeing the same patients over time, often with a variety of problems, clinicians acquire considerable personal knowledge about the patient that may be helpful in managing subsequent problems. The ultimate goal is to develop an effective working relationship with each patient and build on its healing potential. In order to fully attend to patients and their needs, clinicians use personal self-awareness and the qualities of effective relationships: positive regard, empathy, and genuineness. Health care professionals need to recognize that different patients require different approaches. They must respond in a variety of ways to meet patients' needs. These include sensing a patient who has unquenchable need for support and is vulnerable to abandonment, or recognizing and accommodating an assertive patient. Clinicians, at the very least, must be able to empathize with their patients and, at most, use themselves and their relationship to mobilize the strengths of patients for a healing purpose.

6   Being realistic

The sixth component of the patient-centred clinical method involves being realistic. It addresses several key concepts that challenge traditional medical practice. First we must recognize that health care professionals frequently have competing demands for their time and energy. They must learn to manage their time efficiently for the maximum benefit of their patients. They must also develop skills of priority setting, resource allocation, and team-work. Many clinicians in primary care, as they are the providers of first entry into the health care system, must also be wise stewards of the community's resources. In doing so they are often challenged with decisions of what is for the good of the patient versus the needs of society. Economic pressures resulting from escalating health care expenditures often place enormous deci-sion burdens on these clinicians in their gatekeeper role. When does patient benefit outweigh society's needs? These questions, we feel, must be answered on an individual basis and cannot be subject to stringent rules and regula-tions. At the same time primary care clinicians, charged with the responsi-bility of being the wise stewards of the health care system, must assume this task backed by evidence and tempered by humanity.

Finally, all health care professionals must respect their own limits of emotional energy and not expect too much of themselves. This includes recognizing the boundaries that must separate one's personal and profes-sional life. Our commitment to be caring and compassionate must also include ourselves as caregivers. The concept of interdisciplinary care is now – more than ever – a critical component of patient care. However, team care, while not new, remains an untested means of practice in primary care.

Although the six components of the patient-centred clinical method have been presented as separate and discrete, in reality the components are intri-cately intertwined and hence continuously interact with one another. Thus the skilled clinician moves effortlessly back and forth, following the patients' cues, among the six components and in doing so is enacting the patient-centred clinical method. As mentioned at the beginning of this chapter, the third component of 'finding common ground' is the one most closely aligned to the issues and principles of EBPC. We will now examine how this is imple-mented in more depth.

How to find common ground

To reach a mutual understanding or to find common ground often requires that two potentially divergent viewpoints be brought together in a reason-able management plan. Once agreement is reached on the nature of the problem, the goals and priorities of treatment must be determined. Important factors here concern the extent to which the patient will be involved in the treatment plan, and how realistic the plan is in terms of the patient's percep-tions of the illness. It is also important to understand the patient's wishes and ability to cope and, finally, how each of the parties – patient and profes-sional – defines his or her role in this interaction.

Many authors describe the clinical encounter as a process in which the health care professional and patient negotiate to define what is important and what should be done (Anstett 1981; Heaton 1981; Quill 1983). We prefer to describe this process as a mutual effort of finding common ground between the patient and the clinician in three key areas: (a) defining the problem; (b) establishing the goals of treatment or management; and (c) identifying the roles to be assumed by the patient and the clinician. We can see that these bear at least a passing resemblance to the competences of shared decision making (SDM) now being proposed (see Chapter 8, Elwyn and Charles). We will describe the understanding of these stages as they have been interpreted in medicine. Chapter 8 will describe them further and their development and application to shared decision making and evidence-based patient choice.

The work of Fisher and Ury (1983) is relevant to the issue of finding common ground and overcoming differences. They describe two common and erroneous approaches to negotiating differences. The first they call 'hard bargaining': participants are viewed as adversaries, and the goal is victory. This approach generates tension and mistrust. The second approach they call 'soft bargaining': the emphasis here is on building and maintaining the relationship, and the goal is agreement. The risk of this approach is an unclear and vague agreement. Fisher and Ury recommend an alternative, which they call 'principled negotiation'. Four basic tactics make up this approach: separate the people from the problem; focus on interests, not positions; generate a variety of possibilities before deciding what to do; and use objective criteria to judge the solution, rather than pit one personal opinion against another. We will now use this understanding of negotiating differences in examining further the three key areas of finding common ground.

1 Defining the problem

It is a universal human characteristic to seek an explanation for what is happening to the individual – whether mental or physical. By labelling the experience of illness it gives people a sense of control over the often terrifying experience. Most patients want a 'name' for their illness, or at least an explanation of their problem that makes sense to them (Cassell 1991; Kleinman 1988; McWhinney 1989). Without some agreement about the nature of what is wrong, it is difficult for the health care professional and patient to agree on a plan of management acceptable to both of them. It is not essential for the clinician actually to believe that the nature of the problem is as the patient sees it, but the clinician's explanation and recommended treatment must be at least congruent with the patient's perception of the problem and make sense in the patient's world. People may develop quite magical or irrational notions of what is happening to them when they become ill. Some explanation of the problem – regardless of how obscure or unscientific – may be more acceptable and readily available. Patients will even blame themselves for the problem, rather than see the illness as simply random or impersonal.

Problems develop when patient and health care professional have differing ideas of the cause of the problems. For example:

♦ A patient says he is disabled by a back problem, and the health care professional thinks he is malingering.

♦ The doctor has diagnosed hypertension, but the patient insists his blood pressure is probably only elevated because he is nervous in the doctor's office and refuses to see it as a problem.

♦ The parent of a 6-year-old thinks something is seriously wrong because the child has frequent colds: six per year. The health care professional thinks that this number is within normal limits and that the parent is overly protective of the child.

Health care professionals often get into difficulty in defining patients' problems by inappropriate use of the conventional medical model. In using this model, there is the risk of applying improper treatment for problems that do not fit the model. For example, tranquillizers have, in the last several decades, become the answer to 'problems of living' and many of the new generation of anti-depressants are forging a similar promise to 'cure' the common problems of daily living.

2 Defining the goals

When a health care professional and a patient meet, each has expectations and feelings about the encounter. If these are at odds or inappropriate, difficulties may arise. For example:

♦ The patient has a sore throat and expects to receive an antibiotic but instead is urged to use throat lozenges.

♦ The patient is concerned about palpitations but is found to have high blood pressure. The health care professional launches into a treatment of the hypertension without explaining to the patient the benign nature of the cardiac symptoms.

♦ The patient demands muscle relaxants for chronic muscular pain, but the health care professional wants to use relaxation therapy to address the problem.

If health care professionals ignore their patients' expectations, they risk not understanding their patients, who, in turn, will be angry or hurt by this perceived lack of interest or concern. Some patients will become more demanding in a desperate attempt to be heard. Others will be resentful and potentially hostile towards the health care system. Patients may be reluctant to listen to their health care professionals unless they believe they first have been listened to themselves. The distress articulated by patients' may often challenge health care professionals. Thus, they must use their intuition and feelings to enter into their patients' inner lives, to experience empathetically their patients' pain, confusion, hopes, and fears. But we must recognize that this experience may be both threatening and emotionally draining for health care professionals.

New and inexperienced health care professionals are often uncomfortable with the conventional biomedical responsibilities of making the correct diagnosis. They are hesitant to add another dimension to a task that already seems difficult enough. Health care professionals are concerned, on many occasions, that a patient may ask for something they disagree with because they are not comfortable with confrontation. To avoid the prospect of facing a confrontation they may in fact avoid the issue altogether. By not addressing the patient's request the health care professional may hope that the patient will view it as unimportant and not worthy of further discussion.

Timing is key. If the professional asks for a patient's expectations too early in the encounter, the patient may think the clinician is evading making a diagnosis and therefore the patient may be reluctant to offer much detail. If the health care professional waits until the end of the interview, however, time may be wasted on issues of little interest to the patient. Clinicians may even make suggestions or recommendations that need to be retracted. Health care professionals must express questions in a clear and sincere manner such as, 'Can you help me understand how I may help you today?' It is important that neither the professional's words nor tone of voice suggest any accusation that the patient is wasting time on something trivial or insignificant. Often, it is helpful to pick up on a patient's comments that suggest or hint at his or her ideas, expectations, or feelings – for example, 'I have had this leg pain for 3 weeks now and none of those medications you gave me has relieved the pain'. The health care professional should avoid becoming defensive in trying to justify previous advice. Instead, it is more useful to address the patient's frustration and the expectation that something must be done – 'You sound fed up with the length of time this problem has persisted. Are you wondering if it is something serious? Are you wanting something in particular to make it better?'

Thus, the goals of treatment must take into account the expectations and feelings of both the professional and the patient. If the agendas of both are not acknowledged, it may be difficult to reach agreement. What clinicians often call 'patient non-compliance' may in fact be a patient's expression of disagreement about treatment goals. Hence, the patient's adherence to the treatment plan is often contingent on finding common ground.

3   Defining the roles of patient and doctor

Sometimes there is profound disagreement about the nature of the problem or the goals and priorities for treatment. When such an impasse occurs, it is important to look at the relationship between the health care professional and patient and at their perception of each other's roles. Clinicians, as in the example of the cancer patient, may see themselves wanting to bring about remission and may expect the patient to assume the role of a passive recipient of treatment. Patients, however, may be seeking a professional who expresses concern and interest in their well-being, and who is prepared to treat them in the least invasive manner, viewing them as autonomous individuals with a right to have a voice in deciding among various forms of treatment. This is not such a dilemma for professionals when the various forms of treatment are equally effective, but professionals are understandably concerned when the patient chooses a treatment they consider harmful or less effective.

The clinician's commitment is to 'hang in' with the patient to the end. Patients need to know they can count on their health care professionals to be there when they need them. If there are difficulties in their relationship or differing expectations of their roles, they will have problems in working together effectively. For example:

♦   if the patient is looking for an authority who will tell him or her what is wrong and what to do; the health care professional, however, wants a more egalitarian relationship in which the decision making is a shared experience.

♦   if the patient longs for a deep and meaningful relationship with a parental figure who will fill the patient's earlier losses in his or her family; the health care professional's focus is on the biomedical aspect of the patient's problem.

♦   if the health care professional endorses a holistic approach to patient care and wants to learn about all aspects of the patient's life; the patient seeks only technical assistance from the clinician.

Commonly, health care professionals react in one of two ways to problems in their relationships with patients. First, they tend to blame the patient, who often is viewed as 'malingering'. This response often is chosen to justify ignoring complaints that are not viewed as 'legitimate', that is organic in nature. Patients can be rejected in a variety of ways: they may be subjected to unnecessary and sometimes dangerous or punitive investigations; they may be given medication instead of time; and they may be referred inappropriately to a variety of specialists. As a result patients become dissatisfied with their health care providers and may continue to present numerous unresolving complaints. In addition, they may not adhere to the prescribed treatment plan, and instead actively seek alternative health care opportunities.

Second, it is common for health care professionals to blame themselves. They believe they must have done something wrong – 'if only they knew more' or were more skilled at interviewing or therapy. The rescue fantasy that led many health care professionals into the field of health care is severely tested by demanding, needy patients. Many professionals take courses to improve their patient management skills, hoping to find 'The Answer'. Only after repeated failure with a variety of approaches are they able to come to terms with their limitations.

A more effective and satisfying reaction is to realize that the problem is not one-sided. On realizing this, professionals can give up their need to be perfect and instead be prepared to do their best, to be 'good enough,' to be real persons to their patients, rather than needing to find someone to blame for the limitations of medicine.

4 The process of finding common ground

The process of finding common ground begins with the health care professional clearly describing his or her definition of the three key areas: problem, management goals, and potential roles in the ensuing care.

Subsequent discussion of each area would proceed with the patient having an opportunity to ask questions and raise concerns or issues, and a mutual discussion of these questions, concerns, and issues. There should also be an explicit expression by both patient and professional on their agreement with the problem definition or management goal being discussed. In the event of a lack of agreement between health care professional and patient, a flexible response by the clinician would enhance the finding of common ground.

Having provided a detailed description of the content and process of finding common ground, we now turn to a different perspective, the perspective of the research evidence. What do we know about potential benefits of finding common ground in particular and being patient-centred in general?

Evidence of the benefit of patient-centred approaches in relation to patient outcomes

A literature review published on this topic in 1995 found 21 studies relevant to patient-centred communication (both exploring the disease and illness experience and finding common ground) and patient health outcomes (Stewart 1995). An update of this review using the same Medline search strategy for the years 1993 to 1998, uncovered one new relevant paper (The

Writing Group for the SUPPORT Investigators 1995). This paper, added to the studies included in the published paper, leads to the following summary.

With regard to exploring the disease and the illness experience (component 1 of the patient-centred approach), four randomized trials and four analytic studies were reviewed, of which seven obtained significant positive findings. Those aspects of exploring the disease and the illness experience that were found to have a significant association with patient outcomes are summarized in Table 7.1. In general, the important aspects seem to be the professional asking questions about the patient's illness experience, the professional showing support, and the patient fully expressing him or herself.

In the studies that examined finding common ground, seven of the eight randomized controlled trials and six of the eight analytic studies found significant correlations between communication interventions or variables, and patient health outcomes. The aspects of care relevant to finding common ground that were found to significantly influence health outcomes are summarized in Table 7.2. These focus on information sharing, mutual decision making, and patient–provider agreement.

Table 7.1 Elements of exploring the disease and the illness experience

Element	Patient Outcomes Affected
Health Care Professional	
Asks many questions about the patient's understanding of the problem, concerns and expectations, and about his or her perception of the impact of the problem on function	Patient anxiety (Evans et al. 1987) and symptom resolution (Haezen-Klemens and Lapinska 1984)
Asks the patient about his or her feelings	Psychologic distress (Roter and Hall 1991)
Shows support and empathy	Psychologic distress (Roter and Hall 1991) and symptom resolution (Haezen-Klemens and Lapinska 1984)
Patient	
Expresses himself or herself fully, especially with regard to conveying feelings, opinions and information	Role limitation and physical limitation (Greenfield et al. 1985); health status, functional status, and blood pressure (Kaplan et al. 1989, Orth et al. 1987)
Perceives that a full discussion of the problem has taken place	Symptom resolution (Headache Study Group of The University of Western Ontario 1986)

Table 7.2 Elements of effective discussion of the management plan

Element	Patient Outcomes Affected
Patient is encouraged to ask more	Anxiety (Thompson *et al.* 1990), role limitation, and physical limitation (Greenfield *et al.* 1985; Kaplan *et al.* 1989; Greenfield *et al.* 1988)
Patient is successful at obtaining information	Functional (Greenfield *et al.* 1985; Kaplan *et al.* 1989) and physiologic (Kaplan *et al.* 1989; Greenfield *et al.* 1988) status
Patient is provided with information programmes and packages	Pain (Egbert *et al.* 1964), function (Johnson *et al.* 1988), mood, and anxiety (Rainey 1985)
Health Care Professional gives clear information along with emotional support	Psychologic distress (Roter and Hall 1991), symptom resolution (Haezen-Klemens and Lapinska 1984), blood pressure (Orth *et al.* 1987)
Health Care Professional is willing to share decision making	Patient anxiety (Fallowfield *et al.* 1990)
Health Care Professional and patient agree about the nature of the problem and the need for follow-up	Problem (Starfield *et al.* 1981) and symptom (Bass *et al.* 1986) resolution

Five additional studies were relevant to other aspects of communication such as a positive style, (Thomas 1978, 1987), a directive style (Savage and Armstrong 1990), patient knowledge of instructions (Hulka *et al.* 1975), and multifaceted in-patient support and information (The Writing Group for the SUPPORT Investigators 1995). Of these, four studies showed no significant association between communication and the patient health outcome.

Therefore synthesizing Tables 7.1 and 7.2 leads to these broad dimensions which affect patients' health outcomes: health care professionals facilitating patients to fully describe their experience; empathy and support; clear information from professional to patient; and shared decision making leading to agreement on the course of action.

Four more recent studies raise the fundamental issue: what is patient-centredness? Levenstein (1984) and Stewart *et al.*'s (1995) concept of patient-centred care, upon which this chapter is based, arose empirically from observation of practice, supporting it as grounded theory. Recent results confirm the importance of these concepts to patient health outcomes and efficiency of care (Stewart *et al.*, in press). However, the evidence from the audio-tapes of this study was not directly related to patient outcomes and efficiency of care. Rather, the patient's perception that the visit with the health professional had been patient-centred was the key predictor of patient health outcomes and the efficiency of care (Stewart *et al.*, in press). These truly patient-centred results indicate the importance of the validation of research measures against the only real gold standard, the patient's point of view.

Mead and Bower (2000) have noted the similarities and differences among three other observation-based measures of communication in health care, none of which are theory-based or validated against patient perceptions of patient-centredness or health outcomes. The differences that Mead and Bower found among the three measures reinforce the need for researchers to take care in selecting measurement tools for their future projects.

As well, two recent studies have produced findings which illuminate the challenges to the implementation of patient-centredness (Kinmonth *et al.* 1998; Pill *et al.* 1998). Their interventions, which were designed to implement patient-centredness, were quite distinct from the integrated patient-centred clinical method that we have described in this chapter. In both of these studies, discussions with patients about the management plan for their diabetes care were separated from the usual clinical encounter and were conducted by a member of the clinical team who was not a doctor. This separation of medical and educational efforts in the clinical process may have been responsible for the findings that while patients' knowledge and satisfaction were higher in the intervention group than control group, the physiologic measures of health were not better in the intervention group than in the control group (Kinmonth *et al.* 1998). Perhaps the integrated clinical method will bridge such separations in the future.

In summary, the four recent papers just cited lead us to recommend measures and interventions which are grounded in the patients' perceptions of patient-centredness, and which integrate tasks into one clinical method which we call a patient-centred clinical method.

Trends in research

Research regarding patient-centred care and shared decision making has an opportunity to make important contributions in the near future. In keeping with the message in the previous section that integration in the clinical process will be essential to create positive outcomes across the whole continuum of outcomes from patient self-report of health to physiologic variables, the best up-and-coming research will integrate sound research methods and patient perspectives. Three examples will illustrate this.

First, we recommend studies which use both quantitative and qualitative methods to illuminate not only the outcomes of patient-centred clinical care (quantitative) but also the process of the interactions as well as the perspectives of both patients and health care professionals (qualitative). Second, we recommend that much more time and thought be given to the development of interventions designed to improve shared decision making or patient-centred care. These interventions should integrate the educational, medical, and decision making processes into a coherent whole (such as the patient-centred clinical method) in an effort to improve all the possible patient outcomes. Third, and similarly, the development of tools to aid health care professionals in these efforts, needs to be integrated into regular care so that clinical decision-support tools will be used to facilitate a full discussion between patient and provider, never in isolation. Furthermore, the evaluation of decision-support tools will take place in the context of the communication processes, which will be measured quantitatively and illuminated qualitatively. This will be examined further in Chapter 14 (O'Connor and Edwards).

A salient question for future research will be whether a patient-centred approach should be used only for some consultations or for all consultations. Such research will have to be able to distinguish between a patient-centred method which seeks to find common ground with patients about how much the decision making will be shared, and methods based on patient choice which assume the patients have a preference for choice. As well, our current research methods and designs, which tend to specify eligibility criteria for patients, should not muddy our thinking as clinicians and falsely force us into thinking that we may need patient-centredness only for certain types of consultations and not others. Our conviction at the outset is that clinicians need to attend to the process of finding common ground with all patients in all consultations. However, clinicians may not need to share decision making with all patients. The two stages are not the same. The former can be viewed as a cornerstone of clinical care. The latter represents a development and a philosophy which is still to be evaluated. This will be explored in the succeeding chapter (Elwyn and Charles).

Summary

The chapter began with an overview of the evolution of patient-centred ideas in health care. Next, after a brief description of the six interacting components of the patient-centred clinical method, we focused in more detail on the component most congruent with shared decision making and patient choice: finding common ground. Important literature was then cited supporting the hypothesis that finding common ground positively influences patients' health. The chapter closed with a brief commentary on recent research and future research ideas and challenges.

References

Anstett R (1981). Teaching negotiating skills in the family medicine centre. *Journal of Family Practice* **12**: 503–6.

Balint M, Hunt J, Joyce D, Marinker M and Woodcock J (1970). *Treatment or diagnosis: A study of repeat prescriptions in general practice.* Philadelphia, J.B. Lippincott.

Bass MJ, Buck C, Turner L, *et al.* (1986). The physician's actions and the outcome of illness in family practice. *Journal of Family Practice* **23**: 43–7.

Beisecker AE and Beisecker TD (1990). Patient information-seeking behaviours when communicating with doctors. *Medical Care* **28**(1): 19–28.

Byrne PS and Long BEL (1976). *Doctors talking to patients.* London, England, Her Majesty's Stationery Office.

Carmichael LP and Carmichael JS (1981). The relational model in family practice. *Marriage and Family Review* **4**(1,2): 123–33.

Cassell EJ (1991). *The nature of suffering and the goals of medicine.* New York: Oxford University Press.

Cassell EJ (1985). *Talking with patients: II. Clinical technique.* Cambridge, MIT Press.

Cohen-Cole S (1991). *The medical interview: The three function approach.* St. Louis, Mosby/Yearbook.

Egbert LD, Ballit GE, Welch CE, *et al.* (1964). Reduction of postoperative pain by encouragement and instruction of patients – a study of doctor–patient rapport. *New England Journal of Medicine*, **270**: 825–7.

Engel GL (1977). The need for a new medical model: A challenge for biomedicine. *Science* **196**: 129–36. Copyright 1977 by the American Association for the Advancement of Science.

Engel GL (1980). The clinical application of the biopsychosocial model. *American Journal of Psychiatry* **137**(5): 535–44.

Evans BJ, Kiellerup FD, Stanley RO, *et al.* (1987). A communication skills programme for increasing patients' satisfaction with general practice consultations. *British Journal of Medical Psychology* **60**: 373–8.

Fabrega H (1974). Disease and social behaviour: an interdisciplinary perspective. Cambridge, MA, MIT Press.

Fallowfield LJ, Hall A, Maguire CP, *et al.* (1990). Psychological outcomes of different treatment policies in women with early breast cancer outside a clinical trial. *British Medical Journal* **301**: 575–80.

Fisher R and Ury W (1983). *Getting to yes: negotiating agreement without giving in.* New York, Penguin.

Foss L and Rothenberg K (1987). *The second medical revolution – from biomedicine to infomedicine.* Boston: Shambhala.

Greenfield S, Kaplan S and Ware JE (1985). Expanding patient involvement in care – effects on patient outcomes. *Annals of Internal Medicine* **102**: 520–8.

Greenfield S, Kaplan SH, Ware Jr JE, Yano EM and Frank UJL (1988). Patient's participation in medical care: Effects on blood sugar control and quality of life in diabetes. *Journal of General Internal Medicine* **3**: 448–57.

Haezen-Klemens I and Lapinska E (1984). Doctor–patient interaction, patients' health behaviour and effects of treatment. *Social Science Medicine* **19**: 9–18.

Headache Study Group of The University of Western Ontario (1986). Predictions of outcome in headache patients presenting to family physicians – a one year prospective study. *Headache* **26**: 285–94.

Heaton PB (1981). Negotiation as an integral part of the physician's clinical reasoning. *Journal of Family Practice* **6**: 845–8.

Hulka, BA, Kupper LL, Cassel JC, *et al.*, (1975). Doctor–patient communication and outcomes among diabetic patients. *Journal of Community Health* **1**: 15–27.

Johnson JE, Nail LM, Lauver D, *et al.* (1988). Reducing the negative impact of radiation therapy on functional status. *Cancer* **61**: 46–51.

Kaplan SH, Greenfield S and Ware JE (1989). Assessing the effects of physician–patient interactions on the outcomes of chronic disease. *Medical Care* **275**: 5110–27.

Kinmonth AL, Woodcock A, Griffin S, *et al.* (1998). Randomized controlled trial of patient-centred care of diabetes in general practice: impact on current well-being and future disease risk. *British Medical Journal* **317**: 1202–8.

Kleinman AM, Eisenberg L and Good B (1978). Culture, illness, and care. *Annals of Internal Medicine* **88**: 251–8.

Kleinman A (1988). *The illness narratives: suffering, healing, and the human condition*. New York, Basic Books.

Levenstein JH (1984). The patient-centred general practice consultation. *South Africa Family Practice* **5**: 276–82.

Levenstein JH, McCracken EC, McWhinney IR, Stewart MA and Brown JB (1986). The patient-centred clinical method: I. A model for the doctor–patient interaction in family medicine. *Family Practice* **3**(1): 24–30.

Levenstein JH, Brown JB, Weston WW, Stewart M, McCracken EC and McWhinney I (1989). Patient-centred clinical interviewing. In: *Communicating with medical patients* (eds M Stewart and D Roter). Newbury Park, Sage.

McCracken EC, Stewart MA, Brown JB and McWhinney IR (1983). Patient-centred care: The family practice model. *Canadian Family Physician* **29**: 2313–16.

McWhinney IR (1989). *A textbook of family medicine*. New York, Oxford University Press.

Mattingly C and Fleming MH (1994). *Clinical reasoning. Forms of inquiry in a therapeutic practice*. Philadelphia, FA Davis.

Mead N and Bower P (2000). Measuring patient-centredness: a comparison of three observation-based instruments. *Patient Education and Counseling* **39**: 71–80.

Mishler EG (1984). *Discourse of medicine: dialectics of medical interviews*. Norwood, NJ, Ablex.

Newman B and Young RJ (1972). A model for teaching total person approach to patient problems. *Nursing Research* **21**: 264–9.

Odegaard CE (1986). *Dear doctor: a personal letter to a physician*. Menlo Park, CA, Henry J. Kaiser Family Foundation.

Orth JE, Stiles WB, Scherwitz L, *et al.*, (1987). Interviews and hypertensive patients' blood pressure control. *Health Psychology* **6**: 29–42.

Pendleton D, Schofield T, Tate P and Havelock P (1984). *The consultation: An approach to learning and teaching*. Oxford, Oxford University Press.

Pill R, Stott NCH, Rollnick SR, *et al.* (1998). A randomized controlled trial of an intervention designed to improve the care given in general practice to Type II diabetic patients: patient outcomes and professional ability to change behaviour. *Family Practice* **15**(3): 229–35.

Quill TE (1983). Partnerships in patient care: A contractual approach. *Annals of Internal Medicine* **87**: 228–34.

Rainey LC (1985). Effects of preparatory patient education for radiation oncology patients. *Cancer* **56**: 1056–61.

Reiser D and Schroder AK (1980). *Patient interviewing: The human dimension*. Baltimore, Williams and Wilkins.

Rogers C (1951). *Client-centered therapy: Its current practice implications and theory*. Cambridge, MA, Riverside.

Roter D and Hall J (1991). Improving psychosocial problem address in primary care: Is it possible and what difference does it make? [Lecture] International Consensus Conference on Doctor–Patient Communication. Toronto. November 14–16.

Savage R and Armstrong D (1990). Effects of a general practitioner's consulting style on patients' satisfaction: a controlled study. *British Medical Journal* **301**: 968–70.

Starfield B, Wray C, Hess K, *et al.* (1981). The influence of patient–practitioner agreement on outcome of care. *American Journal of Public Health* **71**: 127–31.

Stephens GG (1982). *The intellectual basis for family practice*. Tucson, AZ, Winter.

Stetten D, Jr. (1981). Coping with blindness. *New England Journal of Medicine* **305**: 458.

Stevens J (1974). Brief encounter. *Journal of the Royal College of General Practice* **24**: 5–22.

Stewart M (1995). Effective physician–patient communication and health outcomes: A review. *Canadian Medical Association Journal* **152**(9): 1423–33.

Stewart M, Brown JB, Donner A, *et al.* (2000). The impact of patient-centered care on patient outcomes. *Journal of Family Practice* **49**: 796-804

Stewart M, Weston WW, Brown JB, *et al.* (1995). *Patient-centered medicine.* Thousand Oaks, CA, Sage Publications.

Tait I (1979). The history and function of clinical records. Unpublished MD dissertation, University of Cambridge, England.

The Writing Group for the SUPPORT Investigators (1995). A controlled trial to improve care for seriously ill hospitalized patients. *Journal of the American Medical Association* **274**(20): 1591–8.

Thomas BK (1978). The consultation and the therapeutic illusion. *British Medical Journal* **1**: 1327–8.

Thomas BK (1987). General practice consultations: Is there any point in being positive? *British Medical Journal* **294**: 1200–2.

Thompson SC, Nanni C and Schwankovsky L (1990). Patient-oriented interventions to improve communication in a medical office visit. *Health Psychology* **9**: 390–404.

White KL (1988). *The task of medicine: Dialogue at Wickenburg.* Menlo Park, CA, Henry J. Kaiser Family Foundation.

Wright HJ and MacAdam DB (1979). *Clinical thinking and practice: Diagnosis and decision in patient care.* Edinburgh, Scotland, Churchill Livingstone.

8 Shared decision making: the principles and the competences

Glyn Elwyn and Cathy Charles

The principles and theory

Identifying, describing, and comparing different approaches to treatment decision making is an issue of interest to a surprisingly diverse range of health related disciplines, including medicine, nursing, bio-ethics, medical sociology, and health economics (Brody *et al.* 1984; Mishler 1984; Beisecker and Beisecker 1990; Emanuel and Emanuel 1992; Llewelyn and Hopkins 1993; Deber 1994; Ong *et al.* 1995; Quill and Cassel 1995; Deber *et al.* 1996; Quill and Brody 1996; Charles *et al.* 1997 1998 1999; Coulter 1997; Williams and Calnan 1991; Degner *et al.* 1997; Lupton 1997; Gafni *et al.* 1998; Gwyn and Elwyn 1999). Each discipline explores the issue through its own conceptual lens. Health economists, for example, tend to view the treatment decision making process as requiring two components – technical information about available treatment alternatives, their benefits and risks, and information about patient preferences and values. Since the former resides with the professional and the latter with the patient, some way must be found to bring the two together in the same individual. This person then possesses both necessary components to make an informed choice that also respects the patient's values. One way to do so, while maintaining patient sovereignty, is to conceptualize the professional as the patient's agent who uses technical information to make a treatment decision that is identical to the decision that the patient would have made, had the patient possessed the professional's knowledge. Health economists recognize that a perfect agency relationship between professional and patient exists in theory only and in practice will be influenced by factors such as professional motivation and incentives in the health care system (Gafni *et al.* 1998; see also Chapter 5, Scott).

Medical sociologists, on the other hand, have increasingly conceptualized the professional–patient relationship in treatment decision making as one which has a high probability of conflict. This arises from the different agendas each party brings to the encounter, the different types of discourse used by each party to discuss health and health care concerns (Mishler 1984), and the role of the professional as gatekeeper to services wanted or needed by the patient. Many medical sociologists also argue that in addition, informational asymmetries exist, which result in professional dominance of the interaction (Waitzkin 1985). From this perspective, the way to maintain patient sovereignty in treatment decision making is to ensure that professionals provide patients with information on treatment alternatives (harms and benefits) to enable them to make informed choices that reflect their preferences rather than those of their professional.

In this chapter we focus on several conceptual and empirical issues related to treatment decision making. In part 1, we identify, describe, and compare characteristics of the three key treatment decision making models discussed in the academic literature: the paternalistic, the informed, and the shared models. In part 2, we explore the extent to which the communication and interpersonal skills necessary to practice shared treatment decision making can be taught to professionals. In part 3, we describe some of the recent work that has been undertaken to identify the communication and competency skills that will help professionals involve patients in treatment decision making and begin to identify some instruments that are being developed to assess this area in more depth.

Part 1   Treatment decision making framework

A conceptual framework developed by Charles *et al.* (1997) and updated in 1999 (Charles *et al.* 1999) identifies key characteristics of three well known approaches to treatment decision making: the paternalistic, the informed, and the shared decision making approaches (Table 8.1).

Different phases of the treatment decision making process are also identified and include: information exchange, deliberation (discussion) of treatment preferences, and deciding on the treatment to implement (Table 8.1). While these phases are analytically separate, in practice, they are often woven together in an iterative process. Comparing the role of the professional and the patient in each phase of each approach helps to clarify similarities and differences among them. Each of the treatment decision making approaches identified in Table 8.1 is presented as an ideal type or pure version of the approach, even though in practice the actual approach used by professionals is more likely to lie somewhere between these anchor points.

Treatment decision making phases: information exchange

Information exchange refers to the type and amount of information exchanged between professional and patient and whether the flow is one or

Table 8.1 Models of treatment decision making (φ)

Analytical stages	Models	Paternalistic	Shared	Informed
Information exchange	Flow Direction	One way (largely) Professional ∀ patient	Two way Professional ∆ patient	One way (largely) Professional ∀ patient
	Type	Medical	Medical and personal	Medical
	Amount*	Minimal legally required	All relevant for decision making	All relevant for decision making
Deliberation		Professional alone or with other professionals	Professional and patient (plus potential others)	Professional and patient (plus potential others)
Deciding on treatment to implement		Professional	Professional and patient	Patient

φ Illustration for an encounter focusing on the case of a (treating) professional–patient dyad.
* Minimum required.

two way (reciprocal). In the paternalistic model the exchange is largely one way, and the direction is from professional to patient. At a minimum, the professional must communicate to the patient legally required information about treatment. The professional must also obtain informed consent for the treatment recommended. Beyond this, it is the professional's prerogative to determine what other, if any, information will be given to the patient.

In the informed model, information exchange is again largely one way from professional to patient. The professional's responsibility is to communicate to the patient information about relevant treatment options and their harms and benefits so that patients are enabled to make informed decisions on their own. The professional's role as research transfer agent is the defining characteristic of this approach.

The defining characteristic of the shared model is its interactive nature. Both professional and patient share information with each other. At a minimum, the professional informs the patient of 'all' the information that is relevant to making the decision, for example, treatment options and their benefits and risks. The patient reveals personal information to the professional, for example, lifestyle, preferences for different health states, and issues of importance regarding quality of life. This enables both the professional and patient to evaluate the various treatment options within the context of the latter's specific situation, needs, and values.

Deliberation

The deliberation phase refers to the process of revealing treatment preferences, and expressing and assessing the harms and benefits in a particular clinical context. In the pure version of the paternalistic model, the professional deliberates alone or with colleagues about the preferred treatment while the patient's preferences are either not solicited or are overridden. In this approach professionals believe that they know which treatment is in the patient's best interest: hence patient input into this process is not regarded as necessary to select the best treatment.

In the informed approach, the patient deliberates about treatment options either alone or with family and friends. The professional functions as a research transfer agent, providing the patient with the most rigorous and current research findings on the harms and benefits of available treatments. In the pure version of this approach the professional does not express treatment preferences or opinions on the patient's treatment preference. This would be regarded as introducing an (illegitimate) professional bias into the decision making process rather than helping to support patient sovereignty. The treatment decision making process unfolds through a division of labour in which the professional and patient have specific but separate tasks. The professional provides information to patients so that they can make an informed choice, and the patients weigh the options and decide on the best treatment to implement.

In a shared approach to treatment decision making, both patients and professionals are assumed to have a legitimate investment in the treatment decision. Each discloses treatment preferences for this particular situation. If the professional's and patient's preferences are compatible, discussion will quickly build towards a consensus about the best treatment to implement. If they disagree, each participant may try to persuade the other of the merits of his or her favoured option. In this case, the process will become more of a negotiation and may escalate to a conflict if the negotiation does not produce a solution that both participants can support. In this situation, professionals will have to decide whether they can support the patient's position as part of a negotiated agreement in which the patient's view counts, even though they think another treatment is more appropriate.

Deciding on the treatment to implement

The last phase of the process is making a decision about the treatment to implement. In the pure version of the paternalistic and informed models, one person makes the treatment decision: in the first case, the professional and in the second, the patient. In the shared model the professional and patient work together to build a consensus on the preferred treatment. If they fail to reach consensus, the deliberation phase is still defined as shared but the outcome of that deliberation, the decision, is not.

A shared decision making approach incorporates patient and provider preferences as well as the principle of joint responsibility for determining the preferred treatment to implement. This model represents a middle option between the paternalistic and informed approaches to treatment decision making. It enables professionals to have some influence on the treatment decision without dominating the process altogether. It also fosters patient participation in treatment decision making to the level preferred by patients, without requiring them to bear total responsibility for the decision or fostering feelings of what Quill terms 'abandonment' by their professional (Quill and Cassel 1995).

Current practice

There is increasing pressure on professionals to practice the shared treatment decision making approach. This is especially so in certain clinical areas such as breast cancer where lobby and support groups, as well as professionals and patients, are advocating greater patient involvement. This approach is perhaps particularly important in clinical situations where the illness being treated is serious or life threatening, where there is no one best treatment available, where each treatment option has both benefits and risks requiring trade-offs to be made, and where preferences for different health states and quality of life are important factors in the decision making process.

Little is known about the extent to which professionals actually practice some form of shared decision making or the specific medical specialities in which this approach is likely to be most prevalent. Exploring this issue is difficult for several reasons. Firstly, there is conceptual confusion or disagreement about the defining characteristics of shared treatment decision making. Secondly, the likelihood is that professional behaviour does not conform exactly to one of the ideal type descriptions in Table 8.1, but rather reflects an in-between approach that may combine elements from different models at different stages of the decision making process. Thirdly, there are methodological challenges in measuring and classifying the professional approaches to decision making.

In beginning an attempt to learn more about the meaning of shared decision making to practising professionals, a Canadian study is currently underway to explore this issue among oncologists and surgeons in Ontario who treat women with early stage breast cancer. It also seeks to identify why professionals adopt a particular decision making approach. Key determinants may relate to innate personality characteristics, an ethical imperative, socialization in medical education, or peer and patient pressures once in practice. Some patients insist on being involved in decisions but the literature (and observed practice) supports the view that the power dynamic within consultations is such that 'involvement' is a facility typically granted (by the professional) rather than seized by the patient (Ainsworth-Vaughan 1998).

From an educational perspective, key issues regarding treatment decision making are the extent to which professionals can be taught to identify and practice communication and other related skills that will facilitate adoption of different approaches to treatment decision making and their limitations. From a public policy perspective, it is important that advocates of shared decision making are clear about the meaning of the concept, the goals which shared decision making is intended to achieve, and the types of incentives that may be needed to encourage this practice (Entwistle *et al.* 1998).

Part 2   Can professionals learn the communication skills necessary to involve patients in treatment decisions?

In the professional education literature, the extent to which interpersonal skills can be defined, deconstructed, and taught is a controversial issue. This controversy is relevant to the issue of shared decision making because the answer to the question will have a major impact on the feasibility of teaching the professional interpersonal skills necessary to involve patients in treatment decision making. Advocates such as Hargie and others argue that interpersonal skills can be defined, deconstructed, and taught (Argyle 1994; Hargie 1997; Hartley 1999) and consider them part of the galaxy of social skills that are implemented in human interactions. Stating an important starting position, Hargie defines a social skill as a 'process whereby the individual implements a set of goal-directed, interrelated, situationally appropriate social behaviours which are learned and controlled'. Those who want a fuller discussion should turn to his text. This discussion focuses on the final elements of his definition, 'behaviours which are learned and controlled'. These are in many ways the most critical components. The term 'controlled' here refers to our ability to use, and modify behaviours to achieve our selected goals. For example, in our context we may take time to describe options and to explore patient preferences by using clear descriptions on the one hand and open, facilitative questioning on the other. One of the most important controlled areas is our ability to formulate schemas. Schemas are cognitive structures which are developed after repeated exposure to the same situation, and contain 'scripts which have been learnt and are readily available for enactment when required'. Triggered by a concept known as inner speech, single words or events can trigger schemas and scripts. The phrase 'Well, it was nice to see you' can signal the end of a meeting and both parties usually engage schemas and scripts to deal with the task of 'doing' closure, saying farewell and so on. Think of the schema and script you engage as you enter a restaurant. One reason why new situations and events are so difficult is that we have not developed the relevant schemas with which we can operate smoothly and effectively. It is argued that only when individuals have a set of readily available schemas (such as 'now I'm going to share a decision') that learnt skills can make the transition from competence to performance.

Facilitating patient involvement in treatment decision making is only one aspect of a more comprehensive communication process between patient and professional in the medical encounter. Some argue that it is not appropriate to isolate and deconstruct one component of the interaction such as 'facilitating patient involvement' in decision making from the other components. They argue that this is a reductionist approach and decry the dissection of a complex activity (what Tannenbaum calls 'practical wisdom' (Tanenbaum 1993)) into a sequence of defined tasks (Eraut 1993; Barnett 1994). Greenhalgh warns of the danger of grafting the 'competences' model, extensively used for selection and development in the field of human resource (Anderson and Herriot 1994), onto the performance of health professionals (Greenhalgh and Macfarlane 1997). Their views can be summarized as saying that the 'whole is greater than the sum of the parts' and this standpoint rejects the notion that it is meaningful to isolate small segments of an overall sequence and to study them in isolation of the whole. Parts are not the same as the whole they argue, in the same way that three separate lines do not constitute a triangle.

Advocates of communication skills training would argue however that interpersonal skills (such as listening, questioning, clarifying, providing cues, back-channelling) are not broken down into identifiable behaviours merely to isolate them (Hargie 1997). Their interrelatedness is recognized, but at the same time they argue that it is important to focus on identifiable behaviours in order to gain greater understanding of their nature and their relation to other components in any given sequence. This emphasis on the development of a smooth and appropriate repertoire of skills is common to texts on communication skills training in the clinical context (Kurtz *et al.* 1998). To extend the metaphor, developers of such skills are examining the angles of the triangle.

Another argument in favour of 'deconstructing' interpersonal skills is the fact that it is perfectly possible to be skilled at interpersonal interactions without fully understanding the underlying processes. Most people drive a car without understanding how it operates at the mechanical level. If communication breaks down or becomes difficult (either because of content or process complexity) then the competence-based teaching model proposes that the most useful ways of 'homing in and honing up' is to identify the 'micro' (component) skills and work on the areas of weakness (Hargie 1997). This is not to suggest that a list of ideal 'behaviours' should be emulated slavishly, but rather be seen as providing a framework that informs educational procedures and strategies, and guides the assessment of learning.

Competence: the currency of effective performance

When considering work tasks and roles, the literature in management and occupational psychology increasingly speaks of evaluating 'competence' and 'competencies' (Boyatzis 1982; Barnett 1994). In lay language, these terms are often used interchangeably but it is useful to draw attention to the specific definitions they have attained, which we will do below. Given the myriad of definitions regarding competence and the confusing range of assumptions about their design and application, it is not surprising that their use can sometimes serve to confuse rather than clarify issues associated with defining, developing, and measuring poor, acceptable, and superior performance. In discussing how clinicians can most effectively involve patients in treatment decision making, why bother to use the language of competence? Why not simply use the language of schemas and scripts to describe performance within the context of shared decision making?

Schemas (or scripts) provide the basic building blocks for describing what should or could be said or enacted in response to a specific trigger. The assumptions associated with schemas (situational scripts) are that:

◆   they can be learned; and
◆   their production is linked to a specific situation or task rather than being triggered by an individual as a result of an intrinsic characteristic such as an individual trait or motive.

Scripts are in essence the building blocks for describing what should happen in a given situation if the person is performing acceptably. By deriving a list of scripts and schemas from individuals who are judged to be 'experts' by some predefined criterion, scripts can provide the bedrock of a description of acceptable performance.

Scripts share the same features as a *competence* model of effective performance but the language of competence draws an important distinction between characteristics that are personal attributes (*competencies*) and skills that can be learnt (*competences*). *Competences* are assumed to be situational and task linked. Both *competencies* and *competences* provide a means of evaluating performance. On their own they are not enough. *Competencies*, as defined by Boyatzis, describe aspects of a person that enable him or her to develop and learn competences and scripts (Boyatzis 1982). Consider the following 'stages' of involving patients in health care decisions:

◆   Define the clinical problem
◆   Explore the patient's ideas, fears and expectations of the possible treatments for the problem
◆   Portray options
◆   Portray clinical 'equipoise'
◆   Identify preferred format for, and provide tailored information

There are a number of scripts (verbal and non-verbal behaviours; *competences* essentially) possible for each of the above stages but according to Boyatzis a person's capacity to learn and use these effectively will be determined by their *competencies*. In other words, a person's inherent characteristics determine the extent to which they are able to demonstrate and integrate a set of specific actions (Boyatzis 1982).

The evidence that Boyatzis' *competencies* are operating in the consulting room comes from two observations:

- some professionals will choose one script over another in a given situation; and
- professionals will vary in the extent to which they demonstrate specific *competences*.

Two relevant features of the *competencies* and *competences* in use in the consulting room are that:

- the competencies have a broader application than the specific context of patient involvement (e.g. learning to learn useful skills in a number of contexts)
- the competences (scripts) are situation specific.

The scripts in Fig. 8.1 represent *competences* and the space in-between represents *competencies*. Where some texts talk of *inputs* and *outputs*, we

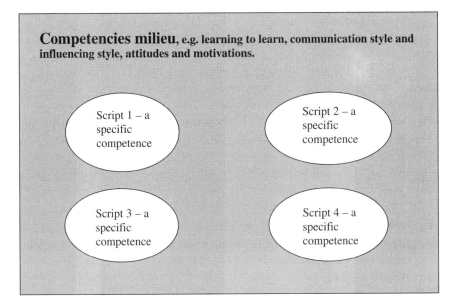

Fig. 8.1 Competencies and competences.

can now see that the outputs are the scripts and the inputs are the competencies that the professional brings to the consultation. Effective performance requires a person to know the scripts (competences) and also knows when and how to use them most effectively (competencies). In terms of learning theory, when a task is deconstructed into component parts it is widely viewed as helping with effective learning. It is relatively straightforward to deconstruct situation specific scripts. It is much harder to deconstruct competencies. As a consequence, *competences* are said to define and determine threshold or acceptable performances. *Competencies* are said to determine superior performance (Boyatzis 1982). Learning programmes need to pay attention to both.

How should 'competencies' and 'competences' be identified?

How should the absence and presence of a 'competence' be ascertained? Which 'competences' fit together to make a composite whole and fulfil an exemplar of high quality performance? Should these judgements be undertaken by peers (other professionals) or made by end-users (patients)? It is highly likely that because of the interactive nature of the dialogue and the different stance taken by the actors that *both* perspectives are required in order to build a complete picture. There is no disputing that the perception of 'involvement' is important. What is not clear to date is whether the linkage of that perception is to a process that contains accurate information conveyed skilfully or whether it is associated with other more elusive, relevant, and longitudinal factors, such as trust, empathy, and satisfaction.

The classic ways of identifying 'competencies' and 'competences' are techniques developed by those who have been interested in selection and development within human resource departments, and include the Critical Incident Technique, the Repertory Grid Analysis, and descriptive work that usually involves observational work, including interviewing key informants. Data derived using Critical Incident Technique more closely resembles a description of competences (scripts) and data derived from Repertory Grid Analysis more closely resembles a characterization of competencies.

The Critical Incident Technique was developed by Flanagan as a means of selecting and training pilots as quickly as possible for deployment in the Second World War (Flanagan 1954). He developed a method that asked pilots to recall 'critical incidents' which had shaped their flying skills (either effective or ineffective) and requested specific factual details about the context, their actions, and reasons why they felt their interventions had been successful or otherwise. By repeating this exercise using expert trainers, experienced pilots, and those in mid-training, Flanagan identified specific behaviours needed by pilots.

The Repertory Grid Analysis represents a psychological approach to analysing skill and attitudes. It was developed by Kelly as a way of measuring an individual's understanding of the world (Kelly 1955). It is suggested that by using a 'grid' to describe and, subsequently, agree tasks and processes, it is possible to predict the traits and personal characteristics that would produce a skilled performance (Fransella and Bannister 1977). Although they seem to have generic applicability, as far as we are aware, neither of these two approaches have been used to assess either the competences or competencies of shared decision making. The methods used to identify the skills and stages of shared decision making include observational research and interviews with key informants. Examples of this type of research are described briefly below.

Part 3 The identification and assessment of competency skills for shared decision making

This research area is still evolving and this section of the chapter describes work that is either recently published or in development. The authors have performed extensive searches of the literature (Elwyn *et al.* 1999a) but would welcome information of any work we have not included in this account.

Key informant interviews

Key informant interviews have been used to determine the stages and skills that family doctors in the UK think are both necessary and feasible for involving patients in 'shared decision making' (Elwyn *et al.* 2000a). The term 'key informants' originates from anthropological studies (Crabtree and Miller 1992) where 'informants' are used to obtain opinions 'grounded' in specific contexts (Gilchrist 1992). They are chosen because they have special knowledge, status, or skills and access to perspectives otherwise denied to a researcher (Goetz and Le Compte 1984). As key informants who answer questions and provide explanations, they inevitably become engaged in the research process (Schatzman and Strauss 1973). This straddling is important – theoretical constructs are thus tempered against field-based perceptions – and the relationship between informants and researchers contributes to a 'joint construction of reality' (Agar 1980). They are able to comment on the researcher's interpretations and expand, modify, and clarify views as the process unfolds.

In 1999, one of the authors of this chapter undertook a research project using the key informant method described (Elwyn *et al.* 2000a). The work was an exploratory study and general medical practitioners were selected in order to provide a bridge between 'theoretical' ideas about the process of involving patients in decision making and the practical problems met in actual practice. The sample taken fulfilled the following criteria:

♦   experienced general practitioners;

♦   with experience in assessing consulting skills competences; and

♦   educational involvement at undergraduate or postgraduate levels.

Six sequential focus groups were held over a time span of three months. The family doctors deconstructed 'shared decision making' and contributed to a process whereby a list of competences was proposed, discussed, and agreed (see Table 8.2).

The listing in Table 8.2 delineates a chronological sequence of the competences (and associated stages) that the key informants felt should be features of a consultation which aimed to involve patients in treatment decisions. Springing out of this work, other qualitative studies, and a systematic appraisal of instrumentation in this area (Elwyn *et al.* 2001), the research team have designed and are validating a tool to measure the extent to which clinicians 'involve' patients in decisions, named OPTION, short for Observing Patient Involvement in Treatment Choices (Elwyn *et al.* 2000b). Psychometric testing is being conducted within an explanatory randomized controlled trial of 'shared decision making' and 'risk communication', and the developers will be actively seeking opportunities to use the tool more widely over the next few years.

1.   Problem definition

It must be emphasized that the starting-point for this process needs to be a clear understanding of the problem and that a 'decision' is then required. Some aspects of clinical practice do not fulfil this criterion (such as exploring

Table 8.2   Stages and competences of involving patients in health care decisions

1	*Implicit* or *explicit* involvement of patients in decision making process
2	Agree and define problem that needs a decision process
3	Explore ideas, fears and expectations of the problem and possible treatments
4	Portrayal of equipoise and options
5	Identify preferred format and provide tailor-made information
6	Checking process: Understanding of information and reactions (e.g. ideas, fears, and expectations of possible options)
7	Checking process: Check that patients accept the process and decision making role preference i.e. involving the patient to the extent they desire to be involved.
8	Make, discuss or defer decisions
9	Arrange follow-up

(Elwyn, *et al.* 2000a)

an issue in detail or providing support and reassurance). The issue of whether some decisions are easier (or more appropriate) to 'share' with patients needs further elaboration. It is certainly true that where there are prior views about the 'best' outcome, for example where patients perceive the need for antibiotic therapy for what professionals diagnose as 'self-limiting viral problems', it is difficult to 'share' the decision – opposing views militate against an agreed resolution (Elwyn *et al.* 1999b; Gwyn and Elwyn 1999).

2. Involve patient (either implicitly or explicitly)

The key informants concluded that the best way to involve patients was to do it implicitly, rather than ask at the beginning of a consultation whether or not a patient 'wanted' to participate in the decision making process. This latter (explicit) approach was considered contrived and likely to confuse patients, unless it was, as Towle suggests (Towle and Godolphin 1999), explained in the context of establishing and explaining the preferred professional–patient relationship model. This process occurs more overtly in health care systems where patients change and often 'choose' professionals. Systems which encourage patients to remain on the 'lists' of named professionals (such as the NHS in the UK) are not as open to a negotiated consultation style.

3. Explore ideas, fears, and expectations of the problem and possible treatments

Patients often have preconceptions about illness and it is wise to explore their views so that their perspectives on the problem can be addressed in the discursive elements that follow. This aspect is covered in more depth in Chapter 7 (Stewart and Brown).

4. Portrayal of options

The identification of choices is a critical part of 'sharing' decisions. It is well known that the range of options provided by the clinician will fundamentally determine the discussion about the management decision. It may be that the choice to do nothing may not be presented, although it is recognized that patients often find conservative management presented as 'doing nothing' very difficult to consider. One way of circumventing this perception of inaction is to label conservative management with a term such as 'watchful waiting', so that the option (highly recommended in many circumstances) is seen in a more positive light. It is important as well to explore what options the patients feel may be available. Too often it seems, two or more choices are given from a biomedical menu, and little time is spent exploring what other strategies patients consider relevant.

5. Convey equipoise

This work did not directly observe professional behaviour and was there-fore offered as a theoretical model of practice. Further analysis of actual consultations has revealed that the practice (even among those who consider themselves as professionals who involve patients in decision making) is much more varied and pragmatic. Indeed it has to be in order to deal with the digressions and diverse concerns of patients. When we examined practice (10 consultations purposively selected in order to audio-tape clinicians who were intent on 'sharing' decisions with patients) a common feature was the pres-ence of a short but distinct statement of 'uncertainty' (Elwyn *et al.* 1999d). It may alternatively have been mentioned that there were two possible approaches to the treatment and each could be reasonably chosen. We have called this clinical 'equipoise', and define it to occur when the professional admits that there are two or more possible directions, that the clinician does not have a strong view towards any given option, and that the implicit sugges-tion underpinning the talk is that the patient's views are important within the decision making process. The insertion is short but important as it acts to legitimize the patient's involvement. The natural inclination of patients when invited to take part in decision making is to regard the offer as rhetorical, and retort by typically saying, 'you should decide, you're the doctor . . .'. Fig. 8.2 contains two examples from the sample collected.

6. Identify preferred format and provide tailor-made information

The practicalities of clinical work may mitigate against asking and providing each patient with information that is 'tailored' to their preferred format, and, even more difficult, that the risk information is specific to their individual-ized risk profile rather than a presentation of formulaic population level data (see also Chapter 9, Edwards and Bastian). Nevertheless, it is feasible for a clinician to have at hand a 'basket' so to speak of data formats, graphs, bar charts, tables, and so on that can be used to explain and illustrate the concepts of relative and absolute risks. The practicality of this type of information exchange is increasing dramatically as decision aids become available and desktop access to Web-based databases and graphics increases (for further discussion on this see Chapters 14 (O'Connor and Edwards) and 17 (Eysenbach and Jadad).

7. Checking process: understanding of information and reactions, for example, ideas, fears, and expectations of possible options

The ability of patients to comprehend the issues will vary and in many cases the process of involvement will need repeated consultations, opportunities to reflect, to consult with family and others. In this way the plethora of factors that play a part in any individual's decision making processes can be

---

Consultation 1 (Dr X)

111	D	um (.) I think (.) as you say you don't want to have a stroke (.)
112		there is a good case I would say to having some treatment (.)
113		the question is which <u>one</u>
114		and I think to be <u>honest</u>
115		um many (.) doctors would be divided as to the
116		best treatment to go for (.)
117		so it (.) it's probably a case of (.)
118		not just <u>me</u> deciding the treatment (.)
119		it's a <u>joint</u> decision I would say because
120		(.) I couldn't say (.) from the heart for <u>definite</u>
121		which one is the best one (.)

Consultation 2 (Dr X)

159	D	Sure. When um different people have been asked about
160		this choice many people go with warfarin
161		and many people go with aspirin alone,
162	Pt	Yes, mm:
163	D	so there's no clear-cut answer here.

(.) indicates a pause of less than 2 seconds duration; underlining indicates emphasis in speech.

Fig. 8.2 Equipoise: two examples of different clinicians when discussing treatment for atrial fibrillation.

brought to bear on it. Where patients are ready to receive probabilistic information, their comprehension will need to be reviewed.

8. Acceptance of process and preferred role in decision making

It has been argued that it is important to assess an individual's preferred role in the decision making process at the start of a consultation (Towle and Godolphin 1999). It may however be very difficult for patients to understand such a de-contextualized question if they do not have a grasp of the options they face, the associated risks, and uncertainties. Professionals in our key informant groups considered it more reasonable to ask patients about their preferred role in decision making *after* they have been informed about the available choices and have had a chance to think about their personal reactions to them.

9. Make, discuss, or defer decisions

In the absence of an urgent need to make a quick decision professionals should help their patients see that time can be used as a tool within the process. Patients often look for guidance regarding the 'best' decision in the 'shared decision making' approach, in stark contrast to the 'informed choice' model where there is a danger that patients feel 'abandoned' when no professional opinion is forthcoming (Quill and Cassel 1995). It is also important however to recognize that the time available for consultations is limited, and that clinicians have to be able to manage the interaction effectively. Striking a balance between limited time and making space for the information exchange and discursive nature of a decision making process is one of the greatest challenges facing medical practice, particularly in the primary care context.

10.   Arrange decision review

There is an accepted clinical need to review a patient's progress within most management plans. But an additional requirement is the explicit agreement that it will be acceptable to review any decisions made. Patients may wish to reconsider their choices after a time when they have had the benefit of discussing the problem with family members, or with other patients in similar predicaments, or they may have sought out further information from other sources.

A Canadian framework for 'informed shared decision making'

Using the results of a literature search, and semi-structured interviews with five family doctors, four patients, and three patient educators in British Columbia, Towle listed eight *competencies* [sic] by which she meant: 'knowledge, skills and attitudes that represent the instructional intents of a programme, stated as specific goals' (Towle and Godolphin 1999). The competencies (see Table 8.3) are presented as a 'framework for teaching, learning, practice, and investigation of what should be a coherent process and an accomplishment of any professional–patient encounter in which a substantive decision is made about treatment or investigation for which reasonable choices exist.' The authors recognize that they essentially describe communications skills, but suggest that they are pitched at a higher level than those typically taught in undergraduate and postgraduate education. This assertion can be contested, as perhaps it is not the skills themselves that are 'higher' or 'more difficult'. Rather, it is the notion that patients should be consulted and provided with information, not only about the harms and benefits but also about the extent of the uncertainty that exists over the 'evidence' that is novel and difficult (Elwyn *et al.* 1999c).

   Towle correctly warns against viewing the framework as a 'prescriptive check list of behaviours' and notes that the 'time and attention paid to the separate elements will vary with circumstances; they may occur over several encounters and will probably be iterative'.

Table 8.3
'Competences [sic] for professionals for informed shared decision making' (Towle and Godolphin 1999)

1	Develop a partnership with the patient.
2	Establish or review the patient's preferences for information (such as amount or format).
3	Establish or review the patient's preferences for role in decision making (such as risk taking and degree of involvement of self and others) and the existence and nature of any uncertainty about the course of action to take.
4	Ascertain and respond to patient's ideas, concerns, and expectations (such as about disease management options).
5	Identify choices (including ideas and information that the patient may have) and evaluate the research evidence in relation to the individual patient.
6	Present (or direct patient to) evidence, taking into account competencies 2 and 3, framing effects (how presentation of the information may influence decision making), etc. Help patient to reflect on and assess the impact of alternative decisions with regard to his or her values and lifestyle.
7	Make or negotiate a decision in partnership with the patient and resolve conflict.
8	Agree an action plan and complete arrangements for follow-up.

NB. Towle's use of the term 'competencies' does not accord with the definitions given here or in the wider literature (Boyatzis 1982; Greenhalgh and Macfarlane 1997; Towle *et al.* 1999).

Therapeutic alliance model

Dowell and Dowie have proposed a consultation method in order to achieve a 'concordant therapeutic alliance'. This draws on the concept of achieving 'concordance' about taking medication (an agreement between the patient and the professional) and was a reaction to the term 'compliance' (which was deemed to have coercive overtones) (Blenkinsopp 1997). The model was developed within 'ten half-day "Balint" style research meetings' (A Dowie 1999, personal communication), and starts with the 'perception of a problem' and requires a professional to signal a change in consultation style (see Fig. 8.3). The following terms are then used in sequence: identify, explore and address issues in terms of understanding, and accepting the experience of illness. This exploratory phase leads to the step of 'agreeing goals and negotiating control', and then an agreement on action and future appraisal. Further evaluations of this model are awaited from its proponents.

Finding common ground

The 'shared decision making' approach within consultations is situated within the broader paradigm of the 'patient-centred consultation' method that was promulgated from the late 1970s onwards by authors such as McWhinney

Therapeutic Alliance Model

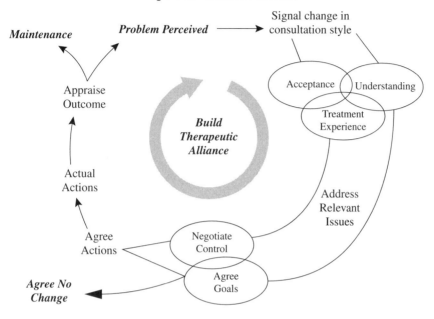

Fig. 8.3   Therapeutic alliance model.

(1972), Levenstein (1984), and Stewart *et al.* (1995a). Revisiting that model reveals that the 'management' aspect of the consultation was not considered at a detailed level (see also Chapter 7, Stewart and Brown). The focus of the 'patient-centred' approach was on information gathering and understanding the patient's perspective on the illness experience. The outcome measures devised by Stewart *et al.* (1995b) reflect this emphasis. More recent versions of the 'patient-centredness' measures do contain a scale that aims to assess the achievement of *common ground* between the professional and patient, but the construct is not extensively developed and relies on assessments of 'mutual discussions'. Stewart has however described an interesting elaboration of this concept using a 'professional–patient partnership paper' that provides a written log of mutually agreed questions and documents the 'evidence' which is obtained and discussed over a series of consultations (Stewart 1998). This approach provides a parallel to the role that Entwistle and O'Donnell suggest may be increasingly relevant to patients within consultations (Chapter 3).

Strengths and weaknesses of the work reviewed

Although the studies so far into the competences have had a large measure of professional 'face' validity, the narrow range of disciplines consulted and the limited sample of patients and their advocates included in the qualitative work points to the need to consider a much wider range of techniques, such as the critical incident and repertory grid techniques. These would enhance validity and enable assessments to occur as both formative and summative processes. Assessments of these attributes could be implemented at critical points in a professional's career and adjustments proposed. The confusion regarding 'competence' and 'competencies' also needs to be addressed and clarified and a suggested framework for this is illustrated in Table 8.4. The main criticism of a 'competency' approach to these skills is the argument against reductionism – that it is impossible to deconstruct and analyse a set of 'skills', without viewing patient involvement from the more logical standpoint of patient perceived 'outcomes'. How can 'shared decision making' be measured (objectively) from the patients' perspective or from a professional 'expertise' perspective? How informed is 'informed'? Should we insist that patients meet some arbitrary 'standard' of understanding what is 'good enough'? Is it acceptable to concede that measurements of observable 'involvement' interactions are unlikely to correlate with patient 'perceptions of involvement'? It is highly likely that both viewpoints are necessary in order to achieve a fuller understanding of this area.

Measurement of patient involvement in treatment decision making: the existing literature

Are there ways in which patient involvement can be observed, evaluated, and linked to the perceptions of patients that they have been involved appropriately in health care decisions? The short answer is that the concepts, the principles, and the competences are not yet well enough established for valid and reliable instruments to be designed. There are however tools being developed and literature reviews have informed their design.

A systematic search of the literature pertaining to decision making and the professional–patient relationship was undertaken (Elwyn *et al.* 2001). It included electronic searching, snowball sampling, and correspondence with field specialists, and aimed to identify whether valid and reliable research instruments exist which focus on measuring how, and to what extent, professionals involve patients in treatment and management decision making. The results revealed eight instruments that met the inclusion criteria – that they had to be research instruments assessing consultations by observational methods and include at least two of the core aspects of 'involving' patients 'in the process of decision making' (a portrayal of options and a decision making or decision deferring stage).

Two aimed to assess communication skills in a global sense – the MAAS-Global (van Thiel *et al.* 1992) and Calgary-Cambridge Observation Guides (Kurtz and Silverman 1996) – and two aimed to assess components

Table 8.4 A competency framework for involving patients in treatment decision making (assuming clinical competence)

Core competence	Competency training	Other requirements	Other requirements in the organization
Defines problems and liaises with patient to generate appropriate options	Listening skills. Interpersonal communications skills.	High levels of clinical competence and knowledge.	A culture of participation and patient-centredness, which understand that these processes are time-sensitive.
Evidence-based Practice v (Greenhalgh T and Macfarlane F 1997)	◆ How to formulate 'answerable' clinical questions. ◆ How to access evidence using latest technologies and sources of validated content e.g. Cochrane Databases. ◆ How to grade and appraise primary and secondary studies using critical appraisal and biostatistical techniques.	Motivation and acceptance that 'evidence' changes and requires reappraisal.	Access to electronic databases and journal archives.
Provides information about risk to patients in an accessible way	◆ Use of language and diagrams to exchange data with patients. ◆ Design of data formats. ◆ Interpersonal communications skills (see listed models, should include flexibility and creativity).	Ability to use decision aid, graphical or charting software.	Information and communication technology.
Engages patients in decision making according to their preferred role	◆ Listening skills. ◆ Interpersonal communications skills.	Provision of information, audio-cassettes, and other sources of data.	Time, flexibility of approach, and positive attitudes towards patient and consumer involvement in decision making.

v Greenhalgh's Competency Framework for Evidence-based Practice could be inserted at this point (Greenhalgh and Macfarlane 1997).

of *patient-centredness* (Patient Centredness (Stewart *et al.* 1995b) and Euro Communication instruments (Mead and Bower 2000)), and had items that contained aspects of patient involvement within *decision making*. Four of the instruments were more focused in nature, and are concerned respectively with *problem-solving* (Pridham and Hansen 1980), *exploration of patient concerns* (Marvel and Schilling 1994), assessment of patient *reliance* (Makoul *et al.* 1995), and *informed decision making* (Braddock *et al.* 1997). Overall, the results revealed that little attention has been given to a detailed assessment of the processes of patient involvement in decision making.

The involvement of patients in decision making is a 'construct' that has not been considered to any significant depth in clinical interaction assessments. The existing instrumentation only includes these concepts as subunits within broader assessments, and does not allow the construct of patient involvement to be measured accurately. Instruments developed to measure 'patient-centredness' are unable to provide enough focus on 'involvement' because of their attempt to cover so many dimensions. The concept of patient involvement (shared decision making; informed collaborative choice) is emerging in the literature and requires an accurate method of assessment.

Studies are currently assessing the psychometric properties of purposively designed instruments (Elwyn *et al.* 2000b), and a codification system using detailed transcripts of consultations has revealed the ability to portray consultations using a 'banding' method (Elwyn *et al.* 1999d). In the latter, the six categories are 'problem definition', 'option portrayal and the provision of risk information', 'equipoise', 'enabling clarification', 'decision making', and 'reviewing arrangements'. The amounts of time given to these issues within the consultation are summed and displayed in a radial format. This work needs further substantiation but may provide a way to compare communication styles within consultations and between differing disciplines in health care.

The empirical work has also demonstrated that although it may be possible to define the skills and sequences of shared decision making, there is inherent and necessary variability within actual performance, a feature that Curran calls 'equifinality' (Curran *et al.* 1984). It remains to be seen whether this matters to a significant degree. It may be that there is a minimum set of tasks and a rudimentary sequence that needs to be accomplished before 'involvement' is achieved. This would be the focus of training and formative feedback to professionals.

Conclusion

As other chapters in this book make clear, communication skills on their own cannot satisfy the full demands of evidence-based patient choice. A stripped down set of tasks or skills also fails to encompass the complexity of blending information with the degree of emotional support that is both necessary and a fundamental part of the clinical consultation. This is especially so when patients are ill, anxious, or lack the willingness, for whatever reason, to engage in 'rational' models of decision making, including those based overtly or covertly on decision analysis methods (Schneider 1998; Charles *et al.* 2000). But as more and more health care moves towards an anticipatory model, predicting and preventing problems *before* they occur, professionals will have to deal with consumers not patients. Paternalism will no longer satisfy an increasingly well informed client group. Professionals will need fast, transparent portals of information and options that can be displayed in ways people can understand. Or they will be left behind. The current technological push will help this process in many ways. It is highly likely that obtaining access, appraising, and explaining data using well-honed interpersonal skills to arrive at negotiated and comfortably accepted decisions will be the bedrock of future clinical practice. This chapter has followed the early steps taken towards such a framework.

References

Agar MH (1980). *The professional stranger: an informal introduction to ethnography*. Orlando, Academic Press.

Ainsworth-Vaughan N (1998). Claiming power in doctor–patient talk. Oxford, Oxford University Press.

Anderson N and Herriot P (ed.) (1994). *Assessment and selection in organizations. First update and supplement*. Chichester, John Wiley and Sons.

Argyle M (1994). *The psychology of interpersonal behaviour*. London, Penguin.

Barnett R (1994). *The limits of competence*. Buckingham, Open University Press.

Beisecker A and Beisecker J (1990). Patient information-seeking behaviors when communicating with doctors. *Medical Care* **28**: 19–28.

Blenkinsopp A (1997). *From compliance to concordance*. London, Royal Pharmaceutical Society of Great Britain.

Boyatzis RE (1982). *The competent manager. A model for effective performance*. New York, John Wiley and Sons.

Braddock CH, Fihn SD, Levinson W, Jonsen AR and Rearlman RA (1997). How doctors and patients discuss routine clinical decisions: informed decision making in the outpatient setting. *Journal of General Internal Medicine* **12**: 339–45.

Brody DS, Miller SM, Lerman CE, Smith DG and Caputo GC (1984). Patients' perception of involvement in medical care. *Journal of General Internal Medicine* **4**: 506–11.

Charles C, Gafni A and Whelan T (1997). Shared decision making in the medical encounter: what does it mean? (Or it takes at least two to tango). *Social Science and Medicine* **44**: 681–92.

Charles C, Gafni A and Whelan T (1999). Decision making in the professional–patient encounter: revisiting the shared treatment decision making model. *Social Science and Medicine* **49**: 651–61.

Charles C, Gafni A and Whelan T (2000). How to improve communication between doctors and patients. *British Medical Journal* **320**(7244): 1220–1.

Charles C, Redko C, Whelan T, Gafni A and Reyno L (1998). Doing nothing is no choice: lay constructions of treatment decision making among women with early-stage breast cancer. *Sociology of Health and Illness* **20**: 71–95.

Coulter A (1997). Partnerships with patients: the pros and cons of shared clinical decision making. *Journal of Health Services Research and Policy* **2**: 112–21.

Crabtree BF and Miller WL (ed.) (1992). *Doing qualitative research.* London, Sage.

Curran J, Farrell D and Greenberger A (1984). Social skills training: a critique and rapproachment. In: *Radical approaches to social skills training* (ed. P Trower) London, Croom Helm.

Deber RB (1994). Professionals in health care management: 7. The patient–professional partnership: changing roles and desire for information. *Canadian Medical Association Journal* **151**: 171–6.

Deber RB, Kraetschmer N and Irvine J (1996). What role do patients wish to play in treatment decision making? *Archives of Internal Medicine* **156**: 1414–20.

Degner LF, Kristjanson LJ, Bowman D, Sloan JA, Carriere KC, O'Neil J, *et al.* (1997). Information needs and decisional preferences in women with breast cancer. *Journal of the American Medical Association* **277**: 1485–92.

Elwyn G, Edwards A and Kinnersley P (1999*a*). Shared decision making: the neglected second half of the consultation. *British Journal of General Practice* **49**: 477–82.

Elwyn G, Gwyn R, Edwards AGK and Grol R (1999*b*). Is a 'shared decision' feasible in a consultation for a viral upper respiratory tract infection: assessing the influence of patient expectations for antibiotics using discourse analysis. *Health Expectations* **2**: 105–17.

Elwyn G, Edwards A, Gwyn R and Grol R (1999*c*). Towards a feasible model for shared decision making: a focus group study with general practice registrars. *British Medical Journal* **319**: 753–7.

Elwyn G, Edwards A, Wensing M, Hibbs R and Grol R (1999*d*). *Shared decision making observed: visual displays of communication sequence and* *patterns.* Cardiff, Division of General Practice: University of Wales College of Medicine.

Elwyn G, Edwards A, Kinnersley P and Grol R (2000*a*). Shared decision making and the concept of equipoise: defining the competences of involving patients in health care choices. *British Journal of General Practice* **50**: 892-899.

Elwyn G, Edwards A, Hood K, Smith C, Wensing M and Grol R (2000*b*). Observing patient involvement in treatment options (OPTION): the development of an instrument to measure patient–clinician decision making interactions. Internal Report, Division of General Practice: University of Wales College of Medicine.

Elwyn G, Edwards A, Mowle S, Wensing M, Wilkinson C, Kinnersley P and Grol R (2001). Measuring the involvement of patients in shared decision making: a systematic review of instruments. *Patient Education and Counseling*, in press.

Emanuel EJ and Emanuel LL (1992). Four models of the professional–patient relationship. *Journal of the American Medical Association* **267**: 2221.

Entwistle V, Sowden AJ and Watt IS (1998). Evaluating interventions to promote patient involvement in decision making: by what criteria should effectiveness be judged? *Journal of Health Services Research and Policy* **3**: 100–7.

Eraut M (1993). *Developing professional knowledge and competence.* London, Falmer Press.

Flanagan JC (1954). The critical incident technique. *Psychological Bulletin* **5**: 327–58.

Fransella F and Bannister D (1977). *A manual for repertory grid technique.* London, Academic Press.

Gafni A, Charles C and Whelan T (1998). The professional–patient encounter: the professional as a perfect agent for the patient *versus* the informed decision making model. *Social Science and Medicine* **47**: 347–54.

Gilchrist VJ (1992). Key informant interviews. In: *Doing qualitative research* (ed. BF Crabtree and WL Miller). London, Sage.

Goetz JP and LeCompte MD (1984). *Ethnography and qualitative design in educational research.* Orlando, Academic Press.

Greenhalgh T and Macfarlane FB (1997). Towards a competency grid for evidence-based practice. *Journal of Evaluation in Clinical Practice* **3**: 161–5.

Gwyn R and Elwyn G (1999). When is a shared decision not (quite) a shared decision? Negotiating preferences in a general practice encounter. *Social Science and Medicine* **49**: 437–47.

Hargie ODW (ed.) (1997). *The handbook of communication skills.* London, Routledge.

Hartley P (1999). *Interpersonal communication.* London, Routledge.

Kelly GA (1955). *The psychology of personal construct*. New York, Norton.

Kurtz S, Silverman J and Draper J (1998). *Teaching and learning communication skills in medicine*. Abingdon, Radcliffe Medical Press.

Kurtz SM and Silverman JD (1996). The Calgary-Cambridge referenced observation guides: an aid to defining the curriculum and organizing the teaching in communication training programmes. *Medical Education* **30**: 83–9.

Levenstein JH (1984). The patient-centred general practice consultation. *South African Family Practice* **5**: 276–82.

Llewelyn H and Hopkins A (1993). *Analysing how we reach clinical decisions*. London, Royal College of Physicians.

Lupton D (1997). Consumerism, reflexivity and the medical encounter. *Social Science and Medicine* **45**: 373–81.

McWhinney IR (1972). Beyond diagnosis: an approach to the integration of clinical medicine and behavioural science. *New England Journal of Medicine* **287**: 384–7.

Makoul G, Arntson P and Schofield T (1995). Health promotion in primary care: professional–patient communication and decision making about prescription medications. *Social Science and Medicine* **41**: 1241–54.

Marvel MK and Schilling R (1994). Levels of professional involvement with patients and their families: a model for teaching and research. *Journal of Family Practice* **39**: 535–44.

Mead N and Bower P (2000). Measuring patient-centredness: a comparison of three observation-based instruments. *Patient Education and Counselling* **39**: 71–80.

Mishler E (1984). *The discourse of medicine: dialectics of medical interviews*. Norwood, NJ, Ablex.

Ong LML, de Haes JCJM, Hoos AM and Lammes FB (1995). Doctor–patient communication: a review of the literature. *Social Science and Medicine* **40**: 903–18.

Pridham KF and Hansen MF (1980). An observation methodology for the study of interactive clinical problem-solving behaviour in primary care settings. *Medical Care* **18**: 360–75.

Quill TE and Brody H (1996). Professional recommendations and patient autonomy: Finding a balance between professional power and patient choice. *Annals of Internal Medicine* **125**: 763–9.

Quill TE and Cassel CK (1995). Non-abandonment: a central obligation for professionals. *Annals of Internal Medicine* **122**: 368–74.

Schatzman L and Strauss AL (1973). *Field research: strategies for a natural sociology*. Englewood Cliffs, NJ, Prentice Hall.

Schneider CE (1998). *The practice of autonomy: patients, doctors, and medical decisions*. New York, Oxford University Press.

Stewart M (1998). Teaching and learning with patients: the professional–patient partnership papers (PPPP). In: *Evidence-based family medicine* (ed. WWR Rosser and MS Shafir). Hamilton, B C Decker Inc.

Stewart M, Brown JB, Weston WW, McWhinney IR, McWilliam CL and Freeman TR (1995a). *Patient-centred medicine: Transforming the clinical method*. Thousand Oaks, CA, Sage Publications.

Stewart M, Brown JB, Donner A, McWhinney IR, Oates J and Weston W (1995b). The impact of patient-centred care on patient outcomes in family practice. London, Ontario, Centre for Studies in Family Medicine (final report).

Tanenbaum S (1993). What professionals know. *New England Journal of Medicine* **329**: 1268–71.

Towle A and Godolphin W (1999). Framework for teaching and learning informed shared decision making. *British Medical Journal* **319**: 766–9.

van Thiel J, van der Vleuten C and Kraan H (1992). Assessment of medical interviewing skills: generalizability of scores using successive MAAS-versions. Approaches to the assessment of Clinical Competence. Proceedings of the Fifth Ottowa Conference, Dundee, Scotland.

Waitzkin H (1985). Information giving in medical care. *Journal of Health and Social Behaviour* **26**: 81.

Williams SJ and Calnan M (1991). Key determinants of consumer satisfaction. *Family Practice* **8**: 237–42.

9 Risk communication – making evidence part of patient choices

Adrian Edwards and Hilda Bastian

This chapter examines the importance of discussing risk information when making choices about treatment or care that are informed or supported by evidence. The sharing of risk information is one of the key competences in involving patients in choices (Chapter 8, Elwyn and Charles). The content of 'effective' information and the context in which discussions are most effective are described. However, we discuss also that risk information is highly susceptible to errors of interpretation by professionals and patients and the danger of manipulation. This chapter summarizes the existing literature on these issues, and describes how steps can be made to ensure that the information of most value to patients can be presented and discussed, and in an accurate and balanced way.

The importance of risk communication

Over recent years the amount of literature on risk-related topics has risen exponentially (Skolbekken 1995). This reflects the emergence in the late twentieth century of the 'risk society' (Beck 1992), that is a society in which risk is increasingly the focus of attention. Many fields and aspects of life come to be interpreted by means of the attached risks. This can be seen in news stories, economics, litigation, domestic responsibilities, and environmental influences.

However, it is particularly evident in the fields of medicine and health where there is a huge volume of literature addressing aspects of risk. There are many different areas of this literature covering the assessment of risk, perception of risk, and the management of risk (usually interpreted as limitation of personal or corporate liabilities). The risk information itself can be used to identify individuals or populations who are at 'high risk' of developing disease. Health care professionals often then intervene to try to reduce these risks. It is in using this information that *risk communication* itself is important. Likewise, individuals may get access to information themselves and try to address their risks of future illness. Risk communication is also important in this 'individual-led' approach. This can be at initial stages when the risk information is made publicly available ('mass risk communication'), or when patients seek access to health care itself and discuss options for treatment or care with professionals.

Health care professionals spend much of their time discussing the risks and benefits of treatments or care with their patients (Makoul *et al.* 1995). This can take the form of describing the broad advantages or disadvantages of different options. Alternatively it may involve the specific use of numerical data about the potential outcomes of choosing one treatment or another (Jacoby *et al.* 1993). In reality data are rarely available to professionals when needed (Edwards *et al.* 1998d). In both the broad description and the specific discussion of risks the relevant information about risks may not be being used to maximum effect. Even when the information is available professionals are unclear about how best to discuss the risks and benefits of treatment most effectively with patients (Edwards *et al.* 1998d). There are certainly great risks of misleading patients depending on how the information is presented (Skolbekken 1998). Patients may also be unsure about the nature of the information they seek from the professionals. There is a need for greater understanding of how risk information can be most helpfully discussed between patients and professionals.

The understanding of risk communication

Theoretical models in the literature

The usual conceptual framework for this is derived from two main strands: cognitive psychology and decision making theory. Some theoretical models have been proposed and in general they seek to provide an understanding of how individuals perceive risk and how this influences behaviour. These models frequently attribute *consequences* in behaviour change to two underlying dimensions: an individual's perception of the *value* of an outcome presented in a health recommendation, and perceived *threat* presented by the outcomes in the recommendation.

The Health Belief Model (HBM), Theory of Reasoned Action, Theory of Social Behaviour, and Prospect Theory all emphasize the perceived value of a presented consequence (Becker 1990; Wilson *et al.* 1988). The Transtheoretical Model ('stages of change') is another model in which interpretation of the likelihood of behaviour change is understood in terms of an individual's *readiness* to change and interventions may be targeted accordingly (Prochaska and DiClemente 1992). Many of these models are indeed the basis for planning several risk communication interventions, as will be seen later.

These models are all, however, concerned with predicting changes in an individual's behaviour based on the understanding of specific determinants of behaviour. These would therefore appear to be one step removed from being models by which to understand risk *communication*. In the way it has been referred to so far, risk communication concerns contact between a professional and a patient and is therefore an interactive process. Specific models which address this interaction rather than focusing on the individual are not currently available. This may have limited progress in understanding risk communication to date.

The influence of risk information on patients

In distinction to this apparent void of theoretical work, some pragmatic work has been done on the influence of risk information on patients. The interpretation of risks varies greatly (Mazur 1990) with wide ranges in the meanings or numerical values attributed to verbal descriptions of risks ('rarely', 'sometimes', 'often', and so on). For example the term 'frequent' was expressed on average as equivalent to nearly 70% in one study, but with a wide range around this figure (Woloshin *et al.* 1994). Wide variations in the interpretation of numerical data among physicians are also described (Bryant and Norman 1980).

There is conflicting evidence about whether verbal or numerical representations of probability are preferred by patients (Mazur and Merz 1994). Studies in the literature describe how most people usually prefer numerical presentation of information but approximately one third of patients prefer verbal descriptions to numerical data (Freeman and Bass 1992; Shaw and Dear 1990). How people understand numerical information is affected by several factors, including the severity of the illness or other outcome concerned, and characteristics such as age, educational level, health status, and recent experience of illness (Mazur and Merz 1994). Single figures presented in isolation (e.g. 1 in 10,000) may be interpreted differently compared to those presented in a list of sequential risks. Presenting single figures may lead to over-weighting of low probabilities and under-weighting of high probabilities (Shiloh and Sagi 1989).

Furthermore people differ not just in their interpretation of the language of risk (different evaluation of the same terms) but also the meaning or significance they attach to different outcomes (Edwards *et al.* 1996). The 'utilities' or values that people will place on different outcomes are likely to affect their use of the risk information in modifying or not modifying their own risks. For example, people's understanding of the term 'stroke', and the significance they attach to it, may affect the degree to which they are motivated to choose anticoagulation treatment for atrial fibrillation.

The components of risk communication

Taking this into account, there is a growing body of opinion that professionals engaged in risk communication need to go beyond simple probabilities and to explore the effects of risk information on individuals. Many authors have proposed that risk communication should address both the patient's perception of the actual *probability* of an event occurring ('subjective probability') and also the *severity* of the eventualities for that individual ('outcome utilities') (Shiloh 1996). Other terminology used for the concept of severity include *adversity* and *burden* (Frets and Niermeijer 1990; Palmer and Sainfort 1993). In practical terms, discussion of the benefits and risks of treatment options, for example, should be complemented by discussion of patients' opinions about prescribed medications and their commitment and abilities to follow through with the treatment plans (Makoul *et al.* 1995).

Definitions of risk communication

This features in some of the definitions of risk communication available in the literature. Ahl *et al.* (1993) viewed risk communication as: 'the open two-way exchange of information and opinion about risk, leading to better understanding and better risk management decisions'. This definition is consistent with developments towards 'patient-centred medicine' (McWhinney 1996) and 'promoting patient choice' (Richards 1998). This definition may, however, be too restrictive for health care in general. Much of health care communication, and also 'mass' risk communication, does not take place face-to-face between professional and patient. Other modes of communication may include written or audio-visual modes and are not therefore 'two-way exchanges'.

In response to this Edwards *et al.* (1998c) specified a more inclusive definition to allow for these other modes: 'communication with individuals (not necessarily face-to-face) which addresses knowledge, perceptions, attitudes or behaviour relating to risk. The communication should include an element of weighing up of risks and benefits of a treatment choice or behavioural risk-reducing change'.

The component of weighing up of risks and benefits represents a shift away from what might be viewed as traditional health education messages in which information was simply presented to patients. The evidence for such strategies achieving their goals is highly limited and the philosophy underlying such strategies also lags behind current progress towards greater partnerships between professionals and patients (Coulter 1999).

The risk communication literature

Much has been described in the literature about risk communication. The way information is presented can have important influences on the interpretations made by patients. Risk communication is a vital component of enabling people to make informed choices. But there are dangers as well as potential benefits in using risk information. In some situations professionals may want to use certain techniques to influence people to make particular decisions or even manipulate their decisions when they feel justified. Previously it has been difficult to distil a clear message from the literature about the application of such findings to clinical practice. In view of the importance, however, to establish how professionals can use risk information to aid discussions with patients, Edwards *et al.* undertook a systematic review of this literature. The review focused on one-to-one health care encounters, and some of the method and results of this review will now be described (Edwards *et al.* 1998c; Edwards *et al.* 2000).

A systematic review of risk communication

This review sought to identify the evidence of effective risk communication interventions, and then to identify the characteristics of risk communication interventions which appear to be most effective. Such *'effect modifiers'* included:

◆ 'content' aspects such as, for example, the nature of risk information used, the theoretical model underlying the intervention, and the mode of delivery; and

◆ 'context' aspects such as the clinical topic, types of risk and choices, and the setting in which the risk communication occurred.

The review undertook an exhaustive search process. This included electronic searching of Medline, EMBASE, CINAHL, PsycLit, SCI, SSCI, CancerLit, and ASSIA databases (1985–96) and follow-up hand searching of key journals, contacting key authors, and examination of reference lists and trial registers. Data were then extracted from the relevant papers regarding clinical topic; content, nature, and models of interventions; settings and personnel; level of evidence; methodological quality and bias; 'signal' or value of research to this review (Edwards *et al.* 1998a; Edwards *et al.* 1999a); and effect sizes of key outcomes: knowledge, perception of risk, anxiety, attitudes, and behavioural changes.

Because of the heterogeneity among the included papers exploratory 'meta-regression' analysis was more appropriate than meta-analysis. This tested for associations of effect size variations and was performed on the principal outcomes for each paper. A complementary analysis of papers of high 'signal' for the review (as rated by members of the review group) was also undertaken, providing a qualitative supplement to the quantitative analysis.

Ninety-seven studies were included in the review according to relevant clinical content. These covered coronary heart disease risk (19 papers), smoking (15), mammography uptake and breast cancer gene testing (15), HIV risk (9), accident prevention (6), cervical screening (5), and 28 others. Of these, 85 had calculable effect sizes (i.e. the statistical data required for this analysis) but 2 were eliminated from the analysis due to marked heterogeneity of effect sizes in comparison with the others. Thus 83 studies were used for the final regression analyses. Modest beneficial effects of the interventions were demonstrated across this range of clinical topics (mean effect size 0.3; funnel plot midline of effect sizes was approximately 0.15). This is equivalent, for example, to a study demonstrating that adherence to a screening programme increased from 70% to 83% with the introduction of the risk communication intervention.

The most effective risk communication

Regarding the characteristics of risk communication which influence effectiveness it is perhaps worth first of all commenting on several features which did not appear significant. In general the setting, the characteristics of patients, the deliverer, and the mode of risk communication interventions were not associated with greater or lesser effectiveness. Other 'negative' findings include the addition of 'counselling' to the provision of risk information, the theoretical model underlying the intervention, or including a substantial behavioural change programme. Thus the 'benefits' of risk communication were evident in general, and apparently regardless of other trappings that are often provided in addition. This indicates continuing scope for risk communication interventions to be implemented across a broad range of settings and conditions, and that they are not the domain of any one professional group. The range of health care professionals can be encouraged that there is evidence that current efforts which involve risk communication are effective in terms of process, behavioural and health outcomes for patients, and that this applies across the range of disciplines.

Regarding the characteristics of risk communication in which the interventions were most effective, two significant variables were identified in the analysis. These were *'treatment choice'* clinical topics, and the use of *individualized (calculated) risk estimates* in the risk communication process. Risk communication interventions were most effective in these situations and, for example again, interventions which used individually calculated risk estimates were found, on average, to produce an increase in adherence (or other risk-reducing behavioural change) from 70% to 87%. This compares with an average of 81% for other interventions based on general or population risk estimates (Edwards A *et al.*, 2000).

'Equipoise' – where the professional has no clear preference for which treatment is chosen

Thus the context of making treatment choices is one area where risk communication appears to have greater effects on key outcomes. The types of 'choices' studied included whether or not to take cholesterol lowering therapy, blood pressure therapy, HRT, anti-epileptic treatments, and so on. Risk communication has greater clinical effects in these circumstances than, for example, in prevention or screening programmes. This may reflect professionals being nearer to clinical *equipoise* regarding the actual decision made in many (but not all) of these studies of treatment choices. That is, they may have no clear preference about which treatment (or no treatment) to choose, such as in discussing options for treatment of menorrhagia or prostatic symptoms (Elwyn *et al.* 1999b). This is in contrast with other studies, which aim (rightly or wrongly) for behavioural changes, such as smoking cessation, reduced alcohol consumption, or increased participation in screening (mammography, cervical smears). It appears much more difficult to achieve similar effects in these latter situations.

Achieving such behavioural changes may clearly be hindered by significant social and contextual influences on individuals, but the other factors relating to the consultation, such as equipoise, may be important too. The lack of professional equipoise perhaps makes it much harder to achieve a genuine partnership with patients who clearly have their own motivations and values. In these situations the professional goals of risk communication may be at odds with the spirit of partnership and 'evidence-based patient choice'. This must be addressed in further work in this field, perhaps by re-orientating and redefining what the goals of the communication are. The goals of communication, and the framing of information to achieve them, can be an ethical dilemma (Sarfati *et al.* 1998). As will be discussed below, perhaps the objective should be to enable 'informed choices' by patients, rather than simply to modify behaviour, even if the conventional public health gains from these newer approaches may be smaller.

It was also clear from the systematic review of risk communication that many of the studies have taken place in 'hypothetical' clinical scenarios. There is a challenge to demonstrate the apparent effects of risk communication in real practice also. If such work is undertaken, more specific cognitive, affective, and behavioural outcomes for the risk communication process could then be addressed (Llewellyn-Thomas 1995). For example, the outcomes or goals of risk communication could go beyond just intentions to take treatments. They could also include satisfaction with the communication process, understanding of the risks and benefits of the different options, certainty that the best choice has been made, the treatments actually chosen, and adherence to those choices (Edwards and Elwyn 1999). Many of these outcomes are now the focus of attention for current work in this field (O'Connor *et al.* 1999).

This represents something of a shift away from the more 'traditional' outcomes addressed in research and which were perhaps of more interest to professionals. These included knowledge levels and accuracy of risk perception, anxiety, and behavioural outcomes (especially adherence to treatment) (Edwards and Elwyn 1999). Many of these aspects are relatively easily measured, but some are arguably of little immediate relevance to patients. The other areas, such as satisfaction, understanding of, and usefulness of information to decision making, and certainty and being able to make decisions according to individual values ('decisional conflict' (O'Connor 1995)) may be of greater importance to patients. They may be more relevant at an everyday level, in terms of whether an individual feels that the process of arriving at a decision was satisfactory or reassuring, and that the best decision was made in their particular situation. Adhering to the chosen treatment is likely to be a very different prospect for those who are satisfied and 'certain' compared to those who are not and still in a position of 'decisional conflict'. Other issues which are of value to patients include whether they perceive the information provided to have been honest, clear, and accurate, and these may also be worthy of greater attention in continuing work in this field.

Using individually calculated risk estimates

Returning to the systematic review of risk communication literature, another feature of the interventions which was associated with apparent effectiveness was the inclusion of individually calculated risk estimates in the process. Interventions which used individual risk estimates were associated with larger (and beneficial) effects. The evidence to support this approach appears generalizable as it derives from a range of primary and secondary care settings, and from a range of countries from USA to European and Australasian countries. However, the studies had frequently only addressed a narrow range of clinical topics. Examples of these interventions include calculating individual breast cancer risks from the Gail formula (Gail *et al.* 1989) or cardiovascular risks, usually from the Framingham study data (Wilson *et al.* 1998).

Making individually accurate and relevant information available to patients appears effective (at least at a simplistic level). It may also be a highly acceptable and valued method for patients as it entails using the most pertinent information of all to the individual. It would seem that efforts to facilitate the use of such risk calculations in clinical practice are likely to be well received and very much in keeping with the promotion of evidence-based patient choice. These methods will enable patients to make choices that are informed by the most relevant and individual data. What is needed now is to ensure that such approaches to communication are more widely available for a more diverse range of clinical topics and applicable in the health care consultation. This means, firstly, that data needs to be accumulated to enable calculation of individual risks and benefits. Secondly, attention must then be paid to the ways it is used and presented in health care practice. This might entail developing simple software packages that can interface with commonly used systems. Alternatively it might involve developing multiple graphical presentations which are varied according to the level of risk factors, such as recently used by the Joint British Societies Coronary Risk Prediction Chart (Wood *et al.* 1999).

'Framing' of information

There is a crucial issue about which risks are discussed, and ensuring an adequate match between patient expectations and needs, and the information provided by professionals. When discussing any of the specific risks though, different ways of 'framing' the information can also have varying effects (Sarfati *et al.* 1998; Skolbekken 1998). Framing itself is defined as presenting 'logically equivalent' information in different ways (Wilson *et al.* 1988). For example, the risk of major osteoporotic fractures is 12% in women who take HRT for over 5 years, and 15% in those who do not. This can be framed as a 3% reduction in (absolute) risk, or that fractures are 20% less common in women who take treatment (relative risk reduction). Other framing variations include expressing the figures as '3% more people remaining free of fractures with HRT' (positive framing) or '3% more people suffering fractures if not taking HRT' (negative framing). These different expressions may all have different motivational effects and influence whether individuals choose treatment options or adhere to chosen plans. Furthermore, people have different preferences for the way they wish information to be presented and discussed with them. For example again, some people may not be comfortable with the use of numerical terms and may prefer the same 'facts' to be conveyed descriptively, such as 'fractures are slightly less common in those who take HRT'. Even here though, there can be framing effects of language. The words used may not be value neutral, such as 'undergoing' or 'enduring' operations.

The way facts and figures are expressed will often need to vary according to the needs of the individual patient. As above, some may prefer more descriptive terms, others may prefer numerical data, and others still may prefer graphical formats. From the professional's perspective one such method alone is likely to be insufficient for clinical practice (Edwards *et al.* 1998b). They usually wish to be able to choose the method or presentation format for information being used in a consultation (Edwards *et al.* 1998d). The clear implication is that they will therefore wish to have the information available to be able to do this in a manner that is flexible to the needs of the individual patient.

Having identified substantial differences in treatment choices made by patients when presented with absolute or relative risk information, Hux and Naylor (1995) concluded that 'multiple complementary formats may be most appropriate' and this is supported by other workers (Liao *et al.* 1996). A *range* of complementary formats (e.g. descriptive, absolute and relative risk, 'numbers needed to treat', and graphical presentations) may be more valued by professionals and patients (Edwards *et al.* 1998b). Having such information available would then empower them to engage in a partnership between professional and patient in the discussions in a consultation, one in which both are able to make an informed contribution. We will discuss more below about exactly how this could be put into practice.

Ethical challenges

A further issue arising is a concern about the ethical implications of presenting information in different ways to achieve different effects. For example, presenting risk information in 'relative' format is generally more persuasive than the 'absolute' risk format (Hux and Naylor 1995; Malenka *et al.* 1993; Slaytor and Ward 1998). In a specific case, the WOSCOPS trial of lipid lowering therapy showed that the risk of death was reduced by pravastatin from 1.7% to 1.2% per year (Shepherd *et al.* 1995). The absolute risk reduction is therefore 0.5% and the relative risk reduction is 31%. Figures are often presented in isolation and if it is the relative risk reduction of 31% then this could have a major effect on the decisions people make regarding whether treatment is worthwhile.

Identifying the components of the most persuasive message may be of great interest to professionals and policy makers alike. However, it raises ethical concerns about what the goal of risk communication is. Is the goal to achieve a desired behaviour change (taking a 'paternalistic' approach (Elwyn *et al.* 1999a)) or is it to facilitate an informed choice with greater autonomy for the patient? Relative risk information is persuasive but may also be over-dramatic and thus potentially misleading when used on its own. It fails to maintain a sense of perspective on the data (Edwards *et al.* 1999b). Thus some have suggested that absolute risk should be the preferred format for presentation of data (Skolbekken 1998). This may be a more balanced perspective of results, but both relative and absolute risk information in isolation can be criticized as only giving part of the picture. Furthermore, although absolute risk information is perhaps closer to a 'true' perspective, people often make decisions on the basis of making comparisons and this requires relative risk data. So if data are to be provided to assist a decision making process this is likely to include the relative risk format as well.

'Relationality'

Combined data presentation approaches may enable patients to make an informed choice based on the 'whole truth' rather than the 'truth'. In terms of ethical principles this appears closer to the 'relationality' principle proposed by Bottorff *et al.* (1996). It complements the standard ethical principles of (patient) autonomy, beneficence (doing good), non-maleficence (doing no harm), and justice. Relationality promotes the provision of accurate honest information in the context of the individual situation. It examines the ethics of care in terms of such factors as response, interpretation, accountability, and social solidarity, often counterbalanced against other values such as truth and confidentiality. This ethical principle of relationality is highly consistent with current trends towards 'patient-centredness' and patient choice in health care (McWhinney 1996; Richards 1998). If the relevant information is made available in this context, then perhaps some strides are being made towards 'evidence-based patient choice'.

Risk communication in practice

So if the current state of risk communication can be summarized as above, what can be said about the future and ways of implementing the best strategies for clinical practice? From the discussion about 'framing effects', it seems that a range of complementary data formats should be available to professionals (Hux and Naylor 1995). They are likely to want to be able to choose from a number of options for presenting information, according to the needs of the individual patient consulting with them. This could be referred to as a 'shopping basket' of options, with enough flexibility to address the needs of a great range in requirements of patients. The information should be available in numerical and graphical formats, or be easily transferable (i.e. if the numerical information is relatively uncomplicated) to description in qualitative terms such as 'commonly', 'rarely', 'sometimes', or whatever term is appropriate. The information should also be balanced, both in terms of which benefits and harms to cover, and including absolute and relative risk formats. The aim should be to avoid presenting information in isolation and to minimize the risk of manipulating decisions.

Decision aids

Having the shopping basket available is, however, only the first part of the story. Professionals will need to be sufficiently familiar with the types of information available to use them to maximize benefit. This includes addressing both the 'traditional' goals such as behavioural risk reductions and also especially the more patient-centred goals such as patient satisfaction, certainty about decision making, and concerns. But there is evidence that professionals are frequently not confident about their own ability to deal with the numerical data available. Training in the use of such risk communication tools or 'decision aids' to ensure (professional) familiarity and confidence with the information will be critical to the success of such approaches. It is also likely to be important for any training to address the ethical issues raised by risk communication, particularly relating to the risk of manipulating patient decisions or behaviour. Raising awareness of these issues should be the first step at least towards reducing the risks of professionals manipulating individual patients with data.

Once the packages (and the skills to use them) are available, further attention can then be paid to the value of different modes of communication. Several media have been used for decision aids produced to date. These include booklets, tapes, videodiscs and interactive computer programmes, paper-based charts, and so on. In general the type of medium may not be particularly crucial in determining outcomes (Holmes-Rovner *et al.* 1999; Street *et al.* 1998). Each of these is likely to have its place according to the nature of the setting and the clinical problem being addressed. A further variation occurs in terms of whether the packages are thought most helpful if used as support before, during, or after a consultation. Decision aids are described and discussed fully in Chapter 14 (O'Connor and Edwards). There is still a need for the content of decision aids to be developed further, but they offer potentially useful ways in which informed patient choices can be facilitated. That is, choices are more likely to take account of available evidence and to be consistent with the individual's personal values ('evidence-based patient choice'). The practical difficulties of using technological innovations across a range of clinical settings are also likely to be significant and suggest that interventions must remain simple if they are to be broadly implemented.

Some interventions have developed and broadened their aims. For example, Lerman *et al.* (1997) evaluated an 'educational' intervention which sought to enhance informed decision making in relation to breast cancer gene testing. There were three key parts of the intervention. In the first, the aim was to convey probabilistic information that was accurate, clear, fair, and useful to decision making. In the second part, patients received information about their personal risk factors, the inheritance of susceptibility to cancer, the benefits and limitations of tests, the risks of testing, and the limitations of prevention or surveillance. The third part comprised counselling about patients' experience of disease, the possible impact of test results, the implication of not being tested, coping resources, and communication of test results. This offers an example of how risk communication can be put into practice, based on current evidence of effectiveness and principles of best practice. Specific decision aids may often be an integral part of such approaches.

Relationship to the competences of shared decision making

Decision aids may in general be 'effective' in influencing a variety of health and 'patient-based' outcomes (Fitzpatrick *et al.* 1998), but they are clearly only part of the effort towards achieving informed patient choices. Training in the use of the decision aids and the information is necessary. Professionals will also need to acquire skills to identify patients' preferences for information (amount and formats) and to discuss it to their satisfaction. The broader picture of the 'competences' (Elwyn *et al.* 1999b; Towle and Godolphin 1999) of shared decision making then becomes relevant (Chapter 8, Elwyn and Charles). Risk communication is just one of these competences. Successful involvement of patients in decisions requires awareness and implementation of the whole of this process. Sometimes information is provided in isolation. If it is truly shared, discussed, reactions explored, and so on, it is perhaps unlikely that the presentation of information can be separated from patient involvement in decisions about treatment or care. Both risk communication and the more general competences of shared decision making constitute essential parts of a package (and an approach to care), which seeks to achieve informed patient choice. Within this, however, patients have varying requirements to be addressed. Patients are quite consistent in their expressed desire for information. They appear more variable in their desire for involvement in the decision making process itself (Elwyn *et al.* 1999a). The package, and the approach of the professionals in using this package must remain flexible enough to meet the needs of individual consumers.

Summary

There is a substantial literature on risk communication. A wide variety of interventions have been shown to be effective in terms of influencing consumer knowledge, anxiety, satisfaction, certainty about making the best choices, and adherence to treatments or other behavioural changes. Whilst in general there are small beneficial effects of risk communication in a wide range of settings, and covering several clinical conditions, there is also some inconsistency about the effectiveness of risk communication interventions. They have, however, been shown to be most effective when using individually calculated risk estimates, and in the context of patients making choices about treatments rather than, for example, screening or behavioural risk modification programmes. Risk communication efforts are increasingly being implemented in the form of 'decision aids' – packages containing information and approaches to discuss reactions to the information and consumer values of different outcomes. These need to be flexible enough to meet the needs of individual patients, and professionals desire a 'shopping basket' of different strategies from which they can use an approach which meets those individual needs. Risk communication itself is just one of the competences of shared decision making. The series of competences is a broader context within which to visualize how risk communication contributes to evidence-based patient choice.

References

Ahl AS, Acree JA, Gipson PS, McDowell RM, Miller L and McElvaine MD (1993). Standardization of nomenclature for animal health risk analysis. *Rev.sci.tech.Off.int.Epiz.* **12**: 1045–53.

Beck U (1992). *Risk Society*, London: Sage.

Becker MH (1990). Theoretical models of adherence and strategies for improving adherence. In: *The handbook of health behaviour change* (ed. SA Shumaker, EB Schron, JK Ockene, CT Parker, JL Probstfield and JM Wolle). New York, NY, Springer Publishing Co.

Bottorff JD, Ratner PA, Johnson JL, Lovato CY and Joab SA (1996). Uncertainties and challenges. Communicating risk in the context of familial cancer. Report to the National Cancer Institute of Canada. Vancouver: School of Nursing, University of British Columbia.

Bryant GD and Norman GR (1980). Expressions of probability: words and numbers. *New England Journal of Medicine* **302**: 411.

Coulter A (1999). Paternalism or partnership? *British Medical Journal* **319**: 719–20.

Edwards A, Pill RM and Stott NCH (1996). Communicating risk: use of standard terms is unlikely to result in standard communication. *British Medical Journal* **313**, 1483.

Edwards A, Russell IT and Stott NCH (1998a). Signal and noise in the evidence-base for medicine – going beyond hierarchies of evidence? *Family Practice 15*: 319–22.

Edwards A, Matthews EJ, Pill RM and Bloor M (1998*b*). Communication about risk: the responses of primary care professionals to standardizing the language of risk and communication tools. *Family Practice* **15**: 301–7.

Edwards A, Barker J, Bloor M, Burnard P, Hood K, Matthews E, *et al.* (1998*c*). A systematic review of risk communication – improving effective clinical practice and research in primary care. Cardiff: University of Wales College of Medicine, Department of General Practice. Report to NHS Executive.

Edwards A, Matthews E, Pill RM and Bloor M (1998*d*). Communication about risk: diversity among primary care professionals. *Family Practice* **15**: 296–300.

Edwards A and Elwyn G (1999). How should 'effectiveness' of risk communication to aid patients' decisions be judged? A review of the literature. *Medical Decision Making* **19**: 428–34.

Edwards A, Elwyn G, Hood K and Rollnick, S (1999*a*). Judging the 'weight of evidence' in systematic reviews: introducing rigour into the qualitative overview stage by assessing Signal and Noise. *Journal of Evaluation in Clinical Practice* **6**: 177–84.

Edwards A, Elwyn G and Stott NCH (1999*b*). Researchers should present results with both relative and absolute risks. *British Medical Journal* **318**: 603.

Edwards A, Hood K, Matthews EJ, Russell D, Russell IT, Barker J *et al.* (2000). The effectiveness of one-to-one risk communication interventions in health care: a systematic review. *Medical Decision Making* **20**: 290–297.

Elwyn G, Edwards A and Kinnersley P (1999*a*). Shared decision making in primary care: the neglected second half of the consultation. *British Journal of General Practice* **49**: 477–82.

Elwyn G, Edwards A, Gwyn R and Grol R (1999*b*). Towards a feasible model for shared decision making: focus group study with general practice registrars. *British Medical Journal* **319**: 753–6.

Fitzpatrick R, Davey C, Buxton M and Jones DR (1998). Evaluating patient-based outcome measures for use in clinical trials. Report No.14, pp.1–72. Health Technology Assessment NHS R&D HTA programme.

Freeman TR and Bass MJ (1992). Risk language preferred by mothers in considering a hypothetical new vaccine for their children. *Canadian Medical Association Journal* **147**: 1013–17.

Frets PG and Niermeijer MF (1990). Reproductive planning after genetic counselling: a perspective from the last decade. *Clinical Genetics* **38**: 295–306.

Gail MH, Brinton LA, Byar DP *et al.* (1989). Projecting individualized probabilities of developing breast cancer for white females who are being examined annually. *Journal of National Cancer Institute* **81**: 1879–86.

Holmes-Rovner M, Kroll J, Rovner D, Schmitt N, Rothert ML, Padonu G et al. (1999). Patient decision support intervention: increased consistency with decision analytic models. *Medical Care* **37**: 270–84.

Hux JE and Naylor CD (1995). Communicating the benefits of chronic preventive therapy: does the format of efficacy data determine patients' acceptance of treatment? *Medical Decision Making* **15**: 152–7.

Jacoby A, Baker G, Chadwick D and Johnson A (1993). The impact of counselling with a practical statistical model on patients' decision making about treatment for epilepsy: findings from a pilot study. *Epilepsy Research* **16**: 207–14.

Lerman C, Biesecker B, Benkendorf JL, Kerner J, Gomez-Caminero A, Hughes C and Reed MM (1997). Controlled trial of pretest education approaches to enhance informed decision making for BRCA1 gene testing. *Journal of the National Cancer Institute* **89**: 148–57.

Liao L, Jollis JG, DeLong ER, Peterson ED, Morris KG and Mark DB (1996). Impact of an interactive video on decision making of patients with ischaemic heart disease. *Journal of General Internal Medicine* **11**: 373–6.

Llewellyn-Thomas HA (1995). Patients' health care decision making: a framework for descriptive and experimental investigations. *Medical Decision Making* **15**: 101–6.

McWhinney I (1996). *A textbook of family medicine*. Oxford, Oxford University Press.

Makoul G, Arntson P and Schofield T (1995). Health promotion in primary care: physician–patient communication and decision making about prescription medications. *Social Science and Medicine* **41**: 1241–54.

Malenka DJ, Baron JA, Johansen S, Wahrenberger JW and Ross JM (1993). The framing effect of relative and absolute risk. *Journal of General Internal Medicine* **8**: 543–8.

Mazur DJ (1990). Interpretation of graphic data by patients in a general medical clinic. *Journal of General Internal Medicine* **5**: 402–5.

Mazur DJ and Merz JF (1994). Patients interpretations of verbal expressions of probability – implications for securing informed consent to medical interventions. *Behavioral Sciences and The Law* **12**: 417–26.

O'Connor A, Fiset V, Rosto A, Tetroe J, Entwhistle V, Llewellyn-Thomas H et al. (1999). Decision aids for people facing health treatment or screening decisions [protocol for a Cochrane Review]. *Cochrane Library*. Oxford, Update Software.

O'Connor AM (1995). Validation of a decisional conflict scale. *Medical Decision Making* **15**: 25–30.

Palmer CG and Sainfort F (1993). Toward a new conceptualization and operationalization of risk perception within the genetic counseling domain. *Journal of Genetic Counseling* **2**: 275–94.

Prochaska JO and DiClemente CC (1992). Stages of change in the modification of problem behaviours. *Progress in Behaviour Modification* **28**: 183–218.

Richards T (1998). Partnership with patients. *British Medical Journal* **316**: 85–6.

Sarfati D, Howden-Chapman P, Woodward A and Salmond C (1998). Does the frame affect the picture? A study into how attitudes to screening for cancer are affected by the way benefits are expressed. *Journal of Medical Screening* **5**: 137–40.

Shaw NJ and Dear PRF (1990). How do parents of babies interpret qualitative expressions of probability? *Archives of Disease in Childhood* **65**: 520–3.

Shepherd J, Cobbe M, Ford I, Isles CG, Lorimer AR, MacFarlane PW *et al.*, (1995). Prevention of coronary heart disease in men with hypercholesterolaemia. *New England Journal of Medicine* **333**: 1301–7.

Shiloh, S (1996). Genetic counselling – a developing area of interest for psychologists. *Professional Psychology-Research and Practice* **27**: 475–86.

Shiloh S and Sagi M (1989). Effect of framing on the perception of genetic recurrence risks. *American Journal of Medical Genetics* **33**: 130–5.

Skolbekken JA (1995). The risk epidemic in medical journals. *Social Science and Medicine* **40**: 291–305.

Skolbekken JA (1998). Communicating the risk reduction achieved by cholesterol reducing drugs. *British Medical Journal* **316**: 1956–8.

Slaytor EK and Ward JE (1998). How risks of breast cancer and benefits of screening are communicated to women: analysis of 58 pamphlets. *British Medical Journal* **317**: 263–4.

Street RL, van Order A, Bramson R and Manning T (1998). Preconsultation education promoting breast cancer screening: does the choice of media make a difference? *Journal of Cancer Education* **13**: 152–61.

Towle A and Godolphin W (1999). Framework for teaching and learning informed shared decision making. *British Medical Journal* **319**: 766–71.

Wilson DK, Purdon SE and Wallston KA (1988). Compliance to health recommendations: a theoretical overview of message framing. *Health Education Research* **3**: 161–71.

Wilson PWF, D'Agostino RB, Levy D, Belanger AM, Silbershatz H and Kannel WB (1998). Prediction of coronary heart disease using risk factor categories. *Circulation* **97**: 1837–47.

Woloshin KK, Ruffin MTI and Gorenflo DW (1994). Patients' interpretation of qualitative probability statements. *Archives of Family Medicine* **3**: 961–6.

Wood D, Durrington P, Poulter N, McInnes G, Rees A, Wray R *et al.* (1999). Joint British recommendations on prevention of coronary heart disease in clinical practice. *Heart* **80**: S1–S29.

10 Decision analysis: utility for everyday use?

Glyn Elwyn, Adrian Edwards, Martin Eccles, and David Rovner

Introduction

The final chapter in this section examines some of the background and issues arising from the decision making approach known as 'decision analysis'. It is conceptually quite different from the other models or approaches just presented, although it includes the values of both professional and patient. Patient-centred medicine, shared decision making, and risk communication concern either the skills to engage the patient more directly in decisions about their treatment or care, or the nature of the information which may be most usefully provided or discussed with the patient. These approaches entail a transfer of responsibility from the professional more towards the patient.

Decision analysis is different because it prescribes the decision to be taken. It seeks to assess the patient's values regarding the outcomes of treatments or care options, which is then integrated with the professional's knowledge of the likelihood of these outcomes. Simple mathematical procedures result in a prescribed decision separate in some way from both members of the dyad. As we shall explore in more detail, this stage of combining values with outcome data may use software packages or more rough-and-ready calculations, but the emphasis is then on the analysis being able to provide a 'rational' decision.

The crux of this matter, and the differences between decision analysis and the other approaches, can be understood from a more formal perspective by examining the 'agency relationships' in health care. This has been highlighted by Gafni *et al.* (1998) who describe two key elements which are necessary for making the best decisions. These are:

- *information* about the different outcomes of treatment options (harms, benefits and their likelihood); and
- the patient's personal *values* about the significance and relative importance of these outcomes.

Gafni *et al.* identify a range of scenarios. At one end of the spectrum, the professional is seen as supporting patients to make their own decisions by providing information. In this circumstance, the patient then has both the necessary elements to arrive at the best decision: they have the information and they know their own values (and feelings, concerns, and so on). At the other end of the spectrum the professional may *act as the patient's agent –* making what is felt to be the best decision for them in their circumstances. In the traditional paternalistic approach the professional (who it is hoped has some of the knowledge required to make a decision) may feel they know what is best, based on their discussions or personal knowledge of the patient's values. Decision analysis comprises a formal and explicit assessment of the patient's values (or 'utilities') so that a decision can be made based on both information and values. In this approach however, as will be examined in more detail below, the responsibility remains with the professional, and the decision is *prescribed*. More recently however, some groups (Ranke and Dowie 1999; Tavakoli *et al.* 1999) are using the results of a clinical decision analysis simply as one more piece of information to aid decision making.

This chapter will provide an overview of this important topic area. It will summarize some of the background literature and the rationale for the approach, and will also identify the health care situations, particularly the types of treatment choices, to which it may be best suited. We will explore some of the problems that are encountered in decision analytic approaches. These include theoretical and ethical dilemmas and difficulties in application in practice. We recognize that other authors may portray decision analysis in a more positive light. A book such as this would be deficient without addressing this topic, but we find ourselves encountering greater weaknesses than strengths. We will introduce how other methods may overcome some of these problems, but seek to enable readers of this chapter to arrive at their own view about whether decision analysis can achieve its central aim – that of making 'better decisions'.

What is decision analysis?

Decision analysis examines potential outcomes under conditions of uncertainty. It is largely based upon the theory of expected utility (von Neumann and Morgenstern 1947). Expected utility is the product of the probability of an outcome (e.g. chance of avoiding a stroke by taking warfarin treatment for atrial fibrillation) and its utility or sense of worth, value, and importance. Decision analysis is based on the premise that a rational decision maker would normally carry out whichever plan of action results in the greatest expected utility. In this theory, the valuation of outcomes is measured in terms of strengths of preference (patient utilities), and the chances of uncertainties are presented as probabilities. The relevant information is usually portrayed in the form of a decision tree. An example taken from an analysis in gynaecological practice is shown in Fig. 10.1 (Thornton 1992).

Decision analysis is explicit, quantifying, and prescriptive (Weinstein, *et al.* 1980). The facts and the values that go into making decisions are (for the purposes of the decision) separated. In this way both the medical information (on the one hand) and the patient's preferences (on the other) are properly acknowledged. Both probabilities and patient utilities are quantified separately and then integrated (Dowie 1996a). The 'optimum' and prescribed choice is the decision outcome with the highest numerical score when the patient's utility for that event is multiplied by its probability. The decision produced is considered the 'rational' option. The process can have as its unit of analysis the individual patient, as is discussed here, or an entire population. When the whole population values are used the evaluation can be used for policy decisions.

The potential advantages for decision analysis are many. Ethically, it is considered to improve 'veracity' because it is explicit about the uncertainty within clinical practice and the complexity of decision making. Uncertainty and probability are an integral part of the process in everyday health care but are frequently not recognized. These uncertainties arise from various sources, including the variability within population or 'average' data, the interpretation of these data, and the relationship between clinical information and the presence of disease. Further complexity unfolds when one considers that treatment decision making usually unfolds over time and

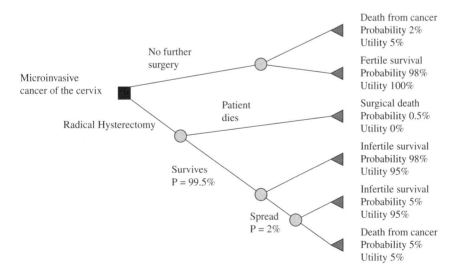

Fig. 10.1 Decision tree for microinvasive cancer of the cervix showing selected probabilities and possible utility calculations (adapted from Thornton J 1992).

circumstances and influences on the individual concerned inevitably vary. Usually there is more than one alternative action available to the professional or patient making the decision. Recognizing the choices and uncertainties ahead is one step towards improving the veracity of the decision making process.

Decision analysis also enhances patient autonomy because it allows a clear role for the patient's preferences (Dowie 1996b). It enables the patient to influence the decision making process, thereby influencing their health care in line with their own personal values (Dowie 1996b). Research evidence and patient preferences can be reconciled (Lilford and Royston 1998). Although clinical decision analysis does not usually consider costs, they can also be built in to a similar process and can inform the economic aspects of clinical management.

Another strength of decision analysis lies in the fact that it offers an approach to decision making which is both explicit and systematic. This is in contrast to the existing decision making approaches generally practised in health care, which are to say the least variable. The principles the professionals adopt or the methods of arriving at a decision by professional or patient are frequently vague. The rules of thumb or 'heuristic principles', which people use to make decisions, reduce complex tasks of assessing probability and predictive values to rather simpler operations. In general these heuristics are quite useful, but have been shown to perhaps over-simplify the process, and are liable to systematic errors. There are further factors such as the format of information presented, which can be highly manipulative. These 'framing' issues are examined in more depth in Chapter 9 (Edwards and Bastian). If not 'controlled' in the discourse between patients and professionals the decisions may not be fully informed or the best decision for the particular patient concerned. The issue of what exactly constitutes a good or 'the best' decision will be revisited later in this chapter. Decision analysis offers an explicit and systematic alternative, which may overcome some of the inherent problems in the heuristics of everyday unstructured decision making.

In offering a systematic approach to decision making, decision analysis firmly places itself in the paradigm of 'rational decision making'. This may offer certain advantages. It is difficult to balance the harms and benefits optimally in complex (multiple outcomes) situations with high levels of uncertainty. Decision analysis not only makes it possible to incorporate all the components into a decision, but also *ensures* that these are all incorporated. The decision may therefore be based on a fuller range of the relevant information than might be the case in an unstructured approach. Thoughtful health care professionals have always intended to carry out such tasks. However, with the increasing complexity of health care and medical knowledge, this is increasingly unrealistic. This applies both to diagnostic and therapeutic problems.

Techniques of decision analysis

Decision analysis was founded largely on the work of von Neumann and Morgenstern (1947). This work elicited an economic model for human decision making. It introduced the concept of utility as that attribute which motivates individuals to move in one direction or another. The model was developed to include the quantification of such utilities. From this template, the opportunity was taken to broaden its application to decisions in health care.

The four principal steps of clinical decision analysis are:

1. To identify and bound the question.
2. To structure the decision over time in a logical sequence.
3. To obtain the necessary data.
4. To make the decision with the highest expected utility (a term that takes into account both probability and utility).

The first step is the most important. It is vital that the exact question being addressed is identified, the decisions to be made, and the various outcomes from different choices that can arise for the patient. Crucially, this needs to be contextualized. The aspects of the patient's health that are of concern to the patient and the professional need to be specified, so that the probabilities of outcomes and utilities in relation to these issues are addressed. The choices in treatment or care must be identified and the clinical data which is relevant to these.

Secondly, the steps of the decision must be laid out in logical order. A decision tree is illustrated in Fig. 10.1. A decision to be made is depicted as a square node. Once a decision is taken, the outcome of that decision is a matter of chance. The chance of an outcome is depicted as a circle. A line connects nodes representing the passage of time. Thirdly, the data must be collected to 'populate' the tree. Two types of data are needed – the probabilities of events occurring (usually from standard evidence sources) and the utilities placed on them by the patient. These can be measured by a number of methods including 'time-trade-off', standard gambles, and so on. Finally, the product of utility and probability for each outcome at the end of the tree is calculated. This is the highest expected utility and identifies the 'best' decision.

To take an example, anticoagulation is frequently advised for atrial fibrillation of the heart. The patient's concern may be principally to reduce the risk of stroke from this condition, but they may also be concerned not to experience side-effects of treatment or to have as little inconvenience from treatment as possible. The incidence of side-effects of treatment and of stroke can be estimated for each of the three main management options: warfarin or aspirin treatment or no treatment. These will be derived from studies of populations of people with atrial fibrillation, and provide average data. They cannot, however, predict whether an individual will or will not experience such an event. The patient's utilities for the 'health states' of stroke or being stroke-free and for side-effects or being free of side-effects of treatment can be elicited (and will vary from one patient to another).

The probabilities and utilities can then be combined to identify the option with the highest expected utility. At one end of the spectrum, one can envisage a patient who places very high utility on remaining stroke-free, and is prepared to endure a high level of side-effects of treatment to achieve this (low utility attached to being free of side-effects). At the other end of the spectrum, another patient may not wish to risk side-effects of treatment at all (placing a high utility on remaining free of side-effects) and is less concerned with reducing the risk of stroke (low utility on being stroke-free). For the same probabilities of the events (stroke or side-effects of treatment), the expected utility of taking treatment such as warfarin will be highest for the first patient, but the 'no treatment option' will achieve the highest expected utility for the second. The decision analytic approach has formalized the process in which one patient was keen to do everything possible to reduce the risk of stroke, but the second one was reluctant to contemplate treatment for fear of side-effects. Arguably, this approach has also made the decision making more objective and rigorous. As will be discussed later though, the structure of the process should not be interpreted as indicating a more robust decision, which the patient is less likely to change. The process of assessing utilities is time-consuming and must be repeated each time the decision is revisited – as time goes by, the factors and influences which are important to the patient making the decision may change.

The decision analytic approach is most suited for situations of uncertainty, not for apparently clear-cut health care decisions. Thus it could be helpful to patients deciding on whether to have surgery for prostatic enlargement, but it would be superfluous in situations such as operating for appendicitis or treating pneumococcal pneumonia with penicillin. To be put into practice, the situations of uncertainty also need to be ones where data are available regarding the probabilities of events and utilities can be estimated. In this situation decision analysis is closely aligned with the evidence-based medicine paradigm because when there are a number of randomized clinical trials or meta-analyses available, these probabilities of outcomes are of the highest quality and will allow an accurate decision analysis.

Conceptual and practical problems with decision analysis

Despite the apparent advantages of decision analysis in systematicity, veracity, and objectivity, there are a number of fundamental concerns that arise if one examines the principles and practicalities in more depth. These need to be considered before deciding on whether the technique itself has great utility for everyday health care decision making.

Data about probabilities: availability and perception

The first issue concerns the availability and accuracy of relevant data. It is often extremely difficult to populate decision trees with probability data, even when apparently valid outcome information exists. Outcome data from systematic reviews are often derived from highly selected samples. They may not accurately reflect individual patient risk (Walsh PC 1993) or generalize to the whole population where decision making is required (Edwards and Pill 1996). In performing a decision analysis, a sensitivity analysis is part of the procedure. This analysis repeats the calculation for the entire range of data available. If the decision changes at the extremes, the analysis is said to be sensitive to the available data and is not very useful in decision making. It does however suggest further areas for study. This notion is difficult to convey to patients, quickly at least.

The availability of data should not obscure a further systematic influence on decision making. The quantification of probability (usually into a percentage risk) is inserted into a decision tree as if it were a mechanical factor. The patent's attitude to risk is not usually sought explicitly (Detsky *et al.* 1997), but if the determination of utility is done by the standard gamble technique, the patient is placed at some risk. In this manner, the patient's attitude towards risk of a definite outcome is incorporated. By removing probabilities from the patient's assessment of the outcomes (focusing only on utility) an assumption that all patients approach risk in the same way is made.

The assumption is not tenable because people value risk-taking in different ways. Some, but not all, are averse to risk-taking (Rothman and Salovey 1997). There are also important factors that affect an individual's response to a perceived risk. These include the potential lethality, its controllability through safety measures, the number of people simultaneously exposed, personal familiarity with the consequences and effects of the risks, and the degree of voluntariness of risk exposure (Vlek 1987). An even more fundamental concern is that people may not be able to assess utilities which are divorced from their probabilities. The two may be inextricably linked, such as can be seen from the utility attached to betting on horse-racing: the chances of success and the utilities attached to the process of both deciding and winning (or even losing) are intertwined. If people's decisions in other contexts are similar in terms of informally evaluating utilities and probabilities together, then the premise of decision analysis, which separates them, becomes shaky.

Problems of standardization: choosing outcomes

Patient values (utilities) in decision analysis are quantified in terms of strengths of preference for outcomes. Outcomes are the possible consequences of choices. But it can be argued that not all values can be elicited in terms of consequences. Kant (1964) suggests that no moral values could be elicited in this way. For example, individuals might wish to be involved in decision making even if it did not affect the outcome because they value the process of being involved *per se*. This puts a value on something that is excluded by decision analysis.

Designing a decision tree that is relevant to the decision at hand is difficult. It seems easy to do 'bad' decision analysis and not to ensure that preferences for all the relevant outcomes are sought. The more complex issues in a decision may not even figure in a decision about the use of drugs for a condition if the 'relevant outcomes' are defined too narrowly. It is usually the biomedical outcomes which are included and others such as the inconvenience of taking a tablet every day (or the implicit imposition of the 'patient' label on a previously fit individual) are not. Decision analysis will systematically influence decisions by taking account only of those aspects of outcomes most easily measured (Ubel and Loewenstein 1997), although frequently neither clinicians nor their patients make decisions in accord with formal decision analysis (Elstein *et al.* 1986; Holmes-Rovner *et al.* 1999). A ready-made decision tree may distort a patient's decision making by limiting the considerations available. For example, another decision tree shown in Fig. 10.2 portrays the choices of treatment for atrial fibrillation as either warfarin or no treatment. However, another reasonable treatment choice would be to take aspirin. If this is not presented then the decision making scope is restricted and the patient's decision is in effect not just limited but also *manipulated*. Clearly informal decision making is also at risk of manipulation, but the claims of decision analysis to improve the decision making in this regard are unfounded. This example is not alone in the literature. Frequently the options and outcomes portrayed in decision analysis trees fail to reflect the patient's personal concerns, the effect of context, or give them sufficient weight (Fitzpatrick *et al.* 1992; Redelmeier *et al.* 1995). The response to these problems of standardization is to allow patients to select outcomes of most concern to them (Tugwell *et al.* 1990) but this increases the complexity of tree construction, perhaps making them too unwieldy then to be useful.

Describing the outcomes

If the *relevant* outcomes have been identified, the next important step is the definition and description of these possible outcomes in order that patients

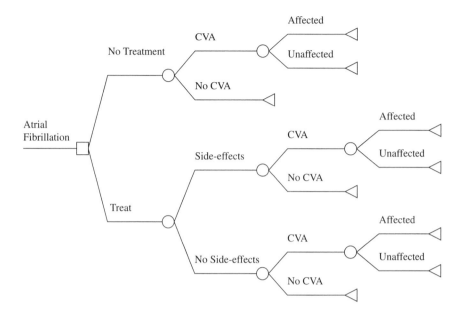

Fig. 10.2 Decision tree for atrial fibrillation. (Reproduced by permission of Dr T. Fahey).

can then attach their utilities to them. Standardization of outcome description is unavoidable in practical terms (and especially for research purposes).
When decision analysis is operationalized, these outcomes are portrayed
often by standardized vignettes, describing the future health states that the
patient could experience. Closer examination of this process shows that
this is not an easy task and is loaded with subjective bias. Choices have to
be made, such as who to interview in order to formulate the descriptions
(Wennberg *et al.* 1993; Stiggelbout *et al.* 1996) and then what language should
be used to portray them. The level of generality of the description is also
important (Torrance 1986) – should it be described in terms of general health,
quality of life, or specific health states? Judgements are required at each
stage of deciding what and how to portray the information. These notions
are widely discussed but there is little agreement (Mulley 1989). The variation of outcome descriptions (with words, images, or software formats) raises
issues about the consistency of presentation within consultations and the
different objectives and interests of professionals and patients involved
(Edwards *et al.*, 2001). This concern does not undermine the basis of decision analysis but it is an important problem that must be addressed.

Measurement of utilities by numbers

The quantification of patient utilities involves the assignment of cardinal numerical values. These are in terms of the natural numbers, one, three, seven, and so on. Ordinal values are expressible as 1st, 5th, last, and so on. Only the former can be used for measuring quantities. Patient utility is measured in terms of preference strengths. These preference strengths express an individual's evaluation of an outcome, in terms of her or his moral, aesthetic, hedonic, and personal values. These can naturally be *ranked* in terms of ordinal values. The methods of assessing utilities give cardinal values. A critical issue therefore is whether cardinal values capture the phenomenon of preference strengths.

To arrive at the utility for a future health state – a multidimensional and complex prospect – people have to 'weigh up' the different dimensions of an 'outcome' to arrive at 'a single index value' (EuroQOL Group 1990). This value is usually expressed as a value between 0 and 1.0, with 0 being death and 1.0 being perfect health. This is a cardinal measurement. However, we weigh things up without using cardinal measures, as when we consider options on a restaurant menu, where we end up with an order of preference, an ordinal measurement. Our ability using trade-off techniques such as the standard gamble to ascribe numerical units to 'preferences' are an attempt to 'rationalize' a more intuitive, heuristic approach to choice. Arguments for more pragmatic methods are appearing (Naylor and Llewellyn-Thomas 1998), although there are differing views on the feasibility of making such measurements in human affairs (Mulley 1989).

Another difficulty is that patients may attach different weights (perhaps at a social or emotional level) to the various outcomes even after ascribing a numerical utility. This is related, as before, to the patient's attitudes to the risk in question, familiarity, and so on (Vlek 1987). Although it can be argued that this is overcome by assessing individual utilities it assumes that the significance of outcome dimensions can still be expressed solely in numerical values. At the very least, it appears that the translation of utilities (an ordinal concept) into cardinal numerical values requires a leap of faith. If one is unable to make this leap, then a crucial part of the process of decision analysis is called into question and the process is potentially invalidated.

Heterogeneity of clinical conditions

Decision trees are brittle constructions and work best for conditions where probabilities are quantifiable (such as in economics where they originated). As above, the clinical scenarios in which decision analysis may be helpful are those in which there are legitimate treatment choices and data to bring to the different outcomes. However, clinical presentations are seldom 'typical'. This means that although a decision tree could be developed for a specific scenario, it is unlikely that the heterogeneity of the clinical presentation can be accommodated. For example, the attempt to improve diabetes control using diet, medication, or insulin raises a myriad of different decision making nodes. They will all be dependent on the severity of the disease, and the presence of co-morbidity such as obesity, hypertension, and ischaemic heart disease. These issues make it difficult to find accurate probabilities to construct decision trees which integrate the range of factors that must be considered when management choices are made.

Decision analysis may prove easier to use in settings with limited variability. Most attempts to use decision analysis have been in secondary care. Even by the time of arrival at a first outpatient appointment, much filtering of problems into specialized categories has already taken place (as also discussed in Chapter 12 by Rosenberg). There is therefore a degree of uniformity among the patients attending a certain clinic (such as those with cervical smear abnormalities or prostatic symptoms). It may be feasible to construct decision trees which accommodate the more limited variability in these patients. The undifferentiated nature of general practice presentations provides a particular challenge to the use of decision analysis.

Ethical considerations

Decision analysis values patient views. At first glance it achieves the goal of involving patients more in decision making. However, this increase in patient autonomy may not automatically lead to beneficence (de Haes and Molenaar 1997), and ethical principles may conflict. Clinical decision analysis is based upon population data and the principle of the greatest good for the greatest number or Utilitarian Ethics. Many ethicists have begun to question the usefulness of Utilitarian Ethics in that different individuals may come to harm or good than would otherwise have been true. The enhanced autonomy may also be an illusion, particularly if the decision analysis is not performed to the highest level of rigour. Autonomy may be undermined in fact, by influencing and restricting patient decisions by describing a narrow range of outcomes or by the way in which they are described.

Attitudes of clinicians

Examples of decision analysis being routinely incorporated into clinical practice are few and far between. An editorial (promoting the benefits of evidence-based practice) in 1996 commented: 'we note from the outset that potentially more powerful decision making models exist, but must report that these models currently lack practical application for most clinical decisions' (Haynes *et al.* 1996). It is important to explore whether this reluctance to apply decision analysis is simply a lack of 'practical application' or whether it reflects more fundamental concerns. Doctors appear wary of exploring the inherent uncertainty of decision making in medicine (Katz 1988) but this can perhaps be addressed in training. There may be other conceptual and ethical concerns about the claimed benefits of rational decision making, in keeping with those outlined above. Arguably, and though a number of specific applications have been developed in the research setting, decision analysis methods appear little closer to becoming reality in routine practice some 5 years after this key editorial (Haynes *et al.* 1996).

Patient responses to decision analysis

There is little published about the acceptability to patients of using decision trees in clinical practice (Wensing *et al.* 1998). Age, educational status, and social class are reported to have marked effects on preferences for participation in decision making. It is likely that these influences would be even more marked when decision analysis is introduced into the consultation (Guadagnoli and Ward 1998). Particularly when it comes to placing values on preferences and evaluating complex decisions, there also seems a real risk that decision analysis may be beyond the abilities of certain patients. Introducing it widely (if that were possible) might therefore accentuate inequalities in health care. Some patients would be able to participate and utilize the most up-to-date information and presentation packages, but others may not. These issues are revisited also in Chapter 17 with the developments in health informatics (Eysenbach and Jadad).

Shortage of time in consultations

There is evidence that a marginal increase in general practice consultation time has positive benefits, particularly in terms of 'patient enablement' or the ability to cope with an illness (Howie *et al.* 1998). Would this hold true for the extra time needed to use decision analysis? The current length of many primary care consultations in the UK is 6 minutes – which has been noted by others to be just the time it takes to boil two eggs, lightly of course. Professionals cite the lack of time as a reason for not exploring the reasons behind decision making in more depth (Edwards *et al.* 1998). But there is no work known to the authors which has measured the benefits of using decision analysis in routine consultations, in either secondary or primary care, outside the research setting. Using current decision analysis techniques in clinical practice requires either rescheduled appointments or invitations to extended consultations. This limits both research and implementation in routine practice.

Does decision analysis lead to the 'best' decisions?

Finally in this section of concerns about decision analysis, we must examine whether there is reason to believe that decision analysis is an improvement on current practice. Any technique for portraying options can be criticized for being selective, but is the attempt to be rational and explicit an improvement on the way clinicians may or may not involve patients in decisions? Does it achieve its aims of improving the decision making process? If so, greater efforts to overcome the difficulties described above would be justifiable.

If decision analysis does compromise aspects of patient autonomy by its choice of probabilities and outcome descriptors, it is morally necessary to identify which decisions are particularly sensitive to the calculation of utilities. Kassirer (1994) lists such circumstances, in which decision analysis may be especially helpful, as follows:

- when there are major differences in possible outcomes (for example, death versus disability);
- when there are major differences between treatments in the likelihood and impact of complications;
- when choices involve a trade-off between near-term and long-term outcomes;
- when one of the choices can result in a small chance of a grave outcome;
- when the apparent difference between options is marginal;
- when a patient is particularly averse to taking risks;
- when a patient attaches unusual importance to certain possible outcomes.

Ubel is more cautious, suggesting that many conditions are more suited to making decisions based on discussion rather than numbers (Ubel and Loewenstein 1997). Even Dowie (1996a), who is an enthusiastic advocate of decision analysis, suggests that patients should be asked whether the 'expected utility' calculation (the integration of probability and utility into a numerical conclusion), once completed, is acceptable to them.

Jungermann notes that little research compares the quality of patients' decisions arrived at via decision analysis with those arrived at by untutored choice (Jungermann and Schutz 1992). A decision tree presenting large amounts of information claims to enable the comparison of multiple options. It would seem therefore to guard against the over-simplification of complex decision making. But studies that attempt to define a 'gold standard' have found that a systematic approach to decision making does not always lead to better decisions. When decisions are analysed by their component parts, issues are identified that conflict with intuition. This may lead to lower satisfaction with the choices made (Wilson *et al.* 1993). But intuition can be rejected on the grounds that it is irrational, just as rational decision making can be rejected on the grounds it does not satisfy us intuitively.

Attempts to identify any gold standard 'best decision' presuppose opinions on such matters. Evaluations of interventions designed to improve decision making in clinical practice must grapple with the issue about which outcomes should be measured for evidence of making a good decision (Edwards and Elwyn 1999). Uptake of treatments or tests would certainly be an over-simplistic proxy measure of good decisions. For example, it is not necessarily a 'bad decision' for an individual to decline the offer of cholesterol lowering therapy on the grounds that the evidence of benefit does not justify the personal and family impact of being categorized as a life-long patient (Skolbekken 1998). O'Connor defines 'effective' decisions as informed, consistent with personal values, and acted upon (O'Connor 1995). This is an important guide to the evaluation of decision making approaches, which must address professional and patient valued outcomes (Edwards *et al.*, 2001). These issues are explored also in Chapter 9 (Edwards and Bastian).

Some responses to these issues

Enthusiasts argue that a substantial component of a decision making process can or even should take place outside the face-to-face consultation. This may overcome the issue of time constraints. There are other positive developments, either for groups of patients, or for individuals who may be asked to interact with audio-visual formats of information. This may indeed be a feasible avenue to pursue. It is possible that decision making techniques, such as decision analysis in more pragmatic guises, could liberate clinicians to consider using interactive media to complement the traditional interaction. Hybrid solutions, which combine a clinical guideline with a decision analysis tree, may provide the correct degree of pragmatism for day-to-day practice (Dowie 1998).

Decision *aids* which incorporate the use of 'weigh scales' to assess utilities may also be a relatively simple but effective and applicable way of integrating patient utilities into the decision making process (see also Chapter 14 by O'Connor and Edwards). They may also be a way of integrating patient utilities into a decision in which the patient is taking a significant amount of the responsibility onto themselves. This may overcome the very first issue raised in this chapter – that of whether decision analysis is open to criticism of remaining in (though developing) the paternalistic paradigm of decision making. Decision aids which use weigh scales allow the explicit contribution of patient utilities but in a paradigm of patient involvement and responsibility.

Other technological developments are also promising. Software packages (Helfand 1997) have simplified the task of decision tree construction and research is being conducted into utility assessment using automated interactive computer interviews. These techniques are reportedly well accepted and as reliable and valid as human assessors. The Stanford Centre provides this facility for a small number of clinical areas and is a resource for research work (Lenert 1997). Live desktop access to such tools may well facilitate the use of these methods.

Conclusion

Decision analysis is a structured and systematic development of decision making approaches. It may enhance the 'veracity' of decisions though this is unclear. The apparent promotion of patient autonomy may be an illusion when one considers the detailed process of decision analysis, and how outcome choices and portrayal may be restricted. If the approach is to permeate into routine practice these and other technical issues must be resolved. These would include the problem of estimating utilities at least partially with cardinal values, and the ability to address the heterogeneity of clinical conditions. Even if they can be resolved though, it seems that decision analysis remains fundamentally a *prescriptive* and in some ways paternalistic decision making approach. The professional provides the data she or he is best able to (probabilities) and patients those they are most cognisant with (utilities), and the analysis informs them both. This may be progress from the unstructured subjective decision making method used in conventional consulting styles. It may not, however, meet the aspirations of many who advocate greater involvement and responsibility of patients in decisions about their treatment or care. Other methods such as decision aids (which will be described in Chapter 14, O'Connor and Edwards) offer attractive and potentially very applicable solutions to these concerns. Decision making can be structured and perhaps examine patient utilities but without the paternalistic model. Time will tell which if any of these attempts to enable a better decision process produce better outcomes in the long run. For now, and in conclusion, we agree with Gafni *et al.* (1998) who suggest that it is better, and easier, to provide risk information to patients (who have the preferences) than for doctors (who have the information) to try and collect patient preferences, in other words to attempt decision analysis.

Acknowledgments: The authors gratefully acknowledge the contributions to earlier discussions of these issues from: Neil Pickering and Sue Sullivan. They also acknowledge contributions to earlier drafting of this text from: Nigel Stott; Samantha Speakman; Martyn Evans; and Richard Grol.

References

de Haes HC and Molenaar S (1997). Patient participation and decision control: are patient autonomy and well-being associated? *Medical Decision Making* **17**: 353–4.

Detsky AS, Naglie G, Krahn MD, Redelmeire DA and Naimark D (1997). Primer on medical decision analysis. *Medical Decision Making* **17**(2): 123–59.

Dowie J (1996a). 'Evidence-based', 'cost-effective' and 'preference driven' medicine: decision analysis-based medical decision making is a pre-requisite. *Journal of Health Services Research and Policy* **1**(2): 104–13.

Dowie J (1996b). The research practice gap and the role of decision analysis in closing it. *Health Care Analysis* **4**: 5–18.

Dowie J (1998). Decision analysis in guideline development and clinical practice: the 'Clinical Guidance Tree'. Guidelines in Health Care. WHO Conference Report (ed. H-K Selbmann). Baden Baden, Nomos.

Edwards A, Elwyn G, Smith C, Williams S, and Thornton H (2001). Consumers' views of quality: identifying the consultation outcomes of importance to consumers, and their relevance to 'shared decision making' approaches. *Health Expectations*, in press.

Edwards A and Elwyn GJ (1999). How should 'effectiveness' of risk communication to aid patients' decisions be judged? A review of the literature. *Medical Decision Making* **19**: 428–34.

Edwards A, Matthews E, Pill RM and Bloor M (1998). Communication about risk: diversity among primary care professionals. *Family Practice* **15**: 296–300.

Edwards A and Pill R (1996). Bridges from evidence to practice are fragile (letter). *British Medical Journal* **312**: 51.

Elstein AS, Holzman GB, Ravitch MM, Metheny WA, Holmes MM, Hoppe RB, *et al.* (1986). Comparison of physicians' decisions regarding oestrogen replacement therapy for menopausal women and decisions derived from a decision analytic model. *Am J Med* **80**: 246–58.

EuroQOL Group (1990). EuroQOL – A new facility for the measurement of health-related quality of life. *Health Policy* **16**: 199–208.

Fitzpatrick R, Fletcher A, Gore S, Jones D, Spiegelhalter D and Cox D (1992). Quality of life measures in health care. I: Applications and issues in assessment. *British Medical Journal* **305**: 1074–7.

Gafni A, Charles C and Whelan T (1998). The physician–patient encounter: the physician as a perfect agent for the patient *versus* the informed decision making model. *Social Science and Medicine* **47**: 347–54.

Guadagnoli E and Ward P (1998). Patient participation in decision making. *Social Science and Medicine* **47**(3): 329–39.

Haynes RB, Sackett DL, Gray JAM, Cook DJ and Guyatt GH (1996). Transferring evidence from research into practice: 1. The role of clinical care research evidence in clinical decisions. *Evidence-Based Medicine Journal* **1**(7): 196–8.

Helfand M (1997). TreeAge: book and software review. *Medical Decision Making* **17**(2): 237.

Holmes-Rovner M, Kroll J, Rovner D, Breer L, Schmitt N, Rothert ML, *et al.* (1999). Patient decision support intervention: increased consistency with decision analytic models. *Medical Care* **37**: 270–84.

Howie JRG, Heaney D, Maxwell M and Walker JJ (1998). A comparison of a Patient Enablement Instrument (PEI) against two established satisfaction scales as an outcome measure of primary care consultations. *Family Practice* **15**: 165–71.

Jungermann H and Schutz H (1992). 'Personal decision counselling: counsellors without clients?' *Applied Psychology* **41**: 185–200.

Kant I (1964). *Groundwork of the metaphysics of morals*. New York, Harper Torchbooks.

Kassirer JP (1994). Incorporating patients' preferences into medical decisions. *New Engl J Medicine* **330**: 1895–6.

Katz J (1988). Why doctors don't disclose uncertainty. In: *Professional judgement* (ed. J Dowie and A Elstein). Cambridge, Cambridge University Press.

Lenert LA (1997). The Stanford Centre for study of patient preferences: an Internet-based clinical trials resource (http://preferences.stanford.edu/definitions/background.html).

Lilford R and Royston G (1998). Decision analysis in the selection, design and application of clinical and health services research. *Journal of Health Services Research* **3**: 159–66.

Mulley AG (1989). Assessing patients' utilities: can ends justify the means? *Medical Care* **27**(3 (Supplement)): S269–81.

Naylor CD and Llewellyn-Thomas HA (1998). Utilities and preferences for health states: time for a pragmatic approach. *Journal of Health Service Research Policy* **3**: 129–31.

O'Connor AM (1995). Validation of a decisional conflict scale. *Medical Decision Making* **15**: 25–30.

Ranke MB and Dowie J (1999). KIGS and KIMS as tools for evidence-based medicine. *Horm Res* **51** Suppl 1: 83–6.

Redelmeier DA, Koehler DJ, Liberman V and Tversky A (1995). Probability judgement in medicine: discounting unspecified possibilities. *Medical Decision Making* **15**: 227–30.

Rothman AJ and Salovey P (1997). Shaping perceptions to motivate healthy behaviour: the role of message framing. *Psychological Bulletin* **121**: 3–19.

Skolbekken J (1998). Communicating the risk reduction achieved by cholesterol reducing drugs. *British Medical Journal* **316**: 1956–8.

Stiggelbout AM, de Haes JC, Kiebert GM, Kievit J and Leer JW (1996). Trade-offs between quality and quantity of life: development of the QQ Questionnaire for Cancer Patient Attitudes. *Medical Decision Making* **16**(2): 184–92.

Tavakoli M, Davies HT, Thomson R *et al.* (1999). Aiding clinical decisions with decision analysis. *Hosp Med* **60**: 444–7.

Thornton JG (1992). Decision analysis in medicine. *British Medical Journal* **304**: 1099–103.

Torrance GW (1986). Measurement of health state utilities for economic appraisal. A review. *Journal of Health Economics* **5**: 1–30.

Tugwell P, Bombardier C, Buchanan W, Goldsmith C, Grace E, Bennett KJH, *et al.* (1990). Methotrexate in rheumatoid arthritis: impact on quality of life assessed by traditional standard item and individualized patient preference health status questionnaires. *Archives of Internal Medicine* **150**: 59–62.

Ubel PA and Loewenstein G (1997). The role of decision analysis in informed consent: choosing between intuition and systematicity. *Soc Sci Med* **44**: 647–56.

Vlek C (1987). Risk assessment, risk perception and decision making about courses of action involving genetic risk: an overview of the concepts and methods. *Birth Defects: Original Article Series* **23**(2): 171–207.

von Neumann J and Morgenstern O (1947). *Theory of games and economic behaviour*. Princeton, NJ, Princeton University Press.

Walsh PC (1993). A decision analysis of alternative treatment strategies for clinically localized prostate cancer. *Journal of Urology* **150**: 1330–2.

Weinstein MC, Fineberg HV and Elstein AS (1980). *Clinical decision analysis*. Philadelphia, WB Saunders Company.

Wennberg JE, Barry MJ, Fowler FJ and Mulley A (1993). Outcomes research, ports and health care reforms. *Annals of the New York Academy of Sciences* **703**: 52–62.

Wensing M, van der Weijden T and Grol R (1998). Implementing guidelines and innovations in general practice: which interventions are effective? *The British Journal of General Practice* **48**: 991–7.

Wilson TD, Lisle DJ and Schooler JW (1993). Introspecting about reasons can reduce post-choice satisfaction. *Personality and Social Psychology Bulletin* **19**: 331–9.

Section 4
Evidence-based patient choice in practice

11 Evidence-based patient choice in primary health care

Theo Schofield

Many countries such as the UK have an established system of primary health care in which a large proportion of all illness episodes are managed. The elements of this system include personal doctoring, generalist whole person care, and the requirement that patients are usually only seen in secondary care after referral. This chapter examines how the structures and processes of primary care affects the opportunities that patients have to make evidence-based choices about their health care.

General medical practice

The definining characteristic of primary care is that patients may present with a very wide range of clinical problems and this poses particular difficulties for the practice of evidence-based medicine. The obvious one is the impossibility of any doctor being able to keep up to date in all areas of medical knowledge. One response of course would be to refer all patients with significant problems to specialists. Such a response however is neither feasible nor desirable. A second response is to attempt to remember information that is made available from a large number of sources including general journals, reviews, and postgraduate education. This is in fact the strategy that is adopted a large proportion of the time and is one of the reasons why there is such strong evidence of a gap between evidence and practice (Bero *et al.* 1998).

Two other approaches however are more promising. The first is to take the time to use new evidence and published guidelines to develop local or practice-based protocols for the management of particular problems (Feder *et al.* 1999). There is evidence that the process itself can influence clinical behaviour, and if the protocol is coupled with reminders that are available when the patient is seen, for example record cards or computer screens, that this change in clinical behaviour can be maintained (Buntinx *et al.* 1993). Many practices have protocols for the management of some chronic illnesses, for example diabetes and asthma, and the need for these has been increased with the development of team-based care where doctors, nurses, and others are working together to deliver consistent care for their patients. Similar work has been done to develop evidence-based guidelines and protocols for the referral and shared care of particular problems between primary and secondary care.

The other approach is to enable family doctors to be able to look up the necessary information at the time that it is required. This ranges from the provision of an up-to-date copy of the *British National Formulary* to all general practitioners in the UK, for example, to the development of computerized decision support systems, particularly for prescribing (Walton *et al.* 1999).

All these approaches presuppose that the information that is available is relevant to the decisions that have to be made. There is much more evidence and many more guidelines about treatment than about investigations and diagnosis. The majority of this information, however, is based on evidence obtained from controlled clinical trials on patients treated in secondary care. Many trials have criteria that exclude many patients with more complex problems or complicating factors which form the majority of those that are seen in primary care. Guidelines can be seen as providing the 'correct' evidence-based decision on management without acknowledging the scope for patient preference or choice.

Diagnosing the whole person

The second characteristic of primary health care is that patients present with symptoms of undifferentiated illness rather than with labelled diagnoses. It is possible to characterize the response of the doctor to these presentations in two ways. The first is the so-called medical model in which significance is attached to particular symptoms that may increase, or decrease, the probability of disease and there is some evidence to guide the doctor in this. For example, a 50-year-old man who has symptoms of heartburn and is also overweight, smokes, and has a stressful job is likely to have oesophageal reflux. However at that age there is also the possibility that he may have a malignancy. Therefore evidence-based guidelines would recommend that he be referred for an upper gastrointestinal endoscopy. A very large proportion of all these endoscopies do not reveal any serious pathology.

Under the second, holistic or patient-centred model, the doctor deals with the whole of the patient's illness experience and in the context of the patient's own life and community. This approach seeks to understand the interaction between the physical, psychological, and social factors that contribute to the patient's problem. Initially the case for this approach was made on the basis of experience in practice (Balint 1957). However there is growing evidence to support the effectiveness of this approach in relieving the patient's symptoms as well as increasing patient satisfaction (Stewart 1995).

Bensing (2000) argued that the term *patient-centred* consultations could be contrasted with the term *disease-centred*, and pointed out that patients also have a choice about which of these two approaches they wish to adopt. They may wish to confine the discussion to biomedical explanations for their health problems, for example some patients with chronic fatigue, or to pay attention to the non-medical aspects of their illness as well.

Both approaches may require the use of diagnostic tests or investigations. From the professional's point of view the decision to investigate may involve the likelihood of the condition, whether it would benefit from treatment, and the risks of failing to make the diagnosis. Tests vary in their sensitivity and in their specificity, and the predictive value of a positive result will vary with the prevalence of the condition in the population tested. Tests also have risks and costs, and many investigations, for example scans or endoscopies, have limited availability.

One reason for arranging investigations is to reduce uncertainty both for the professional and for the patient. There is therefore a natural tendency not to share the uncertainties about investigations with patients or to involve them in choices about them. Patients on the other hand will have their own views about risks, possible benefits, and their ability to tolerate uncertainty. Evidence-based patient choice in diagnosis has until now received far less attention, both in the consultation and in research, than choices about treatment.

The use of time

Primary care consultations have tended to be short. In the UK the average length is about eight minutes. It is frequently argued that this limits the range of issues that can be explored, the amount of information that can be given, and the amount that patients can be involved in choices in the consultation. The available evidence would support this view. Howie for example (1989) showed that short as against long consultations resulted in less attention being given to psychosocial issues. Howie *et al.* (1999) showed a strong correlation between the length of time in the consultation and the extent to which the patient felt 'enabled' by it. Doctors' ability to enable was also linked to the percentage of patients who said they knew them well.

These constraints have major implications for evidence-based patient choice in primary care. The first is that any evidence presented in the consultation must either be already known by the professional or very rapidly available. Patients still report that their professional is their main source of health information but this is changing rapidly, particularly through the Internet. Patients are also being helped to assess the quality of this information (Shepperd *et al.* 1999). Patients can obtain this either before they present with a problem or after an initial consultation as part of the process of choice and decision making.

This has implications for the professional–patient relationship. Patients may arrive in the consultation better informed than the professional and they may use this information to question decisions. There is no guarantee that this will be received warmly by the professional, and in one study of prescribed medication, doctors rated a patient asking another person about their prescription before they took it as a very undesirable behaviour (Makoul *et al.* 1995). On the other hand, if we embrace the concept of patient partnership, a more informed patient becomes a more equal participating partner. Professionals will need to come to recognize the value of this partnership.

Professionals can also participate in this partnership by giving or directing the patient towards further information and inviting the patient to return to discuss it and come to a decision at a later date. Consultations are not isolated events but are part of a cycle of care in which the patient's health understanding continues to develop in the light of the information they have been given in previous consultations and their experience of their outcomes (Pendleton 1983).

It has to be accepted that all the steps proposed to be taken by professionals to promote evidence-based patient choice – familiarizing themselves with the literature, developing policies and protocols, accessing information in the consultation, inviting patients to return for subsequent consultations before decisions are made, and the provision and use of appropriate time in each consultation – would all add to professional workload in the short-term. There may be potential gains in that more enabled patients make more appropriate use of health care services in the future. There is no evidence however that they would use them less.

Prevention and screening

Primary care is concerned not only with the care of the individual patient but also with promotion of the health of the population. For much of the time these aims are complementary but there are occasions in which they may conflict, particularly in the areas of immunizations and screening.

Immunizations against infectious diseases are effective not only because they protect the individual, but also because they create herd immunity. In this way each individual is not in fact exposed to the disease at all. An individual patient could refuse an immunization confident in the knowledge that they have been protected by the actions of others who have accepted. Thus they avoid any risk of side-effects or adverse reactions for themselves. This of course breaks down if a significant number of individuals take this choice and therefore all patients are advised to accept immunization. This is both for their own benefit and for the benefit of others. Population coverage rather than individual choice becomes a target for the health care system and in some countries payments are attached to the achievement of these targets. There is no conflict if all patients accept their responsibility to their community. However there are greater tensions when parents are being asked to make these decisions for their children in the face of public anxiety about the risks of immunizations.

There are similar difficulties with gaining informed consent for screening (Austoker 1999). The costs to the many patients who have false positive results and require further investigation need to be balanced against the possible benefit to those found to have a disease. This not only applies to programmes such as cervical cytology and mammography but also to the screening for risk factors for heart disease. Part of the rationale for screening programmes is that they benefit not only the individual patient but also reduce the burden of disease on the health care system. Again the health care system can provide rewards to professionals for achieving population coverage, but this may shift the focus of the encounter with the individual patient from informed choice to *persuasion*.

More subtle pressures are created by the process of standard setting and audit. A current example would be the proportion of patients with atrial fibrillation in a practice who are taking anticoagulants, with the clear implication that this is a marker of good quality care. However patients, balancing the evidence of benefit with the risks, and taking account of their own values, may well make an informed choice to decline the treatment (Howitt and Armstrong 1999). Informed choice in preventive care is much more difficult to measure than coverage or uptake. However from the perspective of the individual's right to choose it needs to be recognized as the most important outcome for preventive care and screening.

Referral

In many health care systems with established primary care, access to secondary care is achieved largely by referral. There are many reasons why patients may be referred (Coulter and Roland 1992), including to advance a likely diagnosis, to exclude unlikely but serious problems, to obtain treatment, or to reassure the patient. The decision to be referred has major implications for the patient. It should ideally be made on the basis of evidence and with the full involvement of the patient. However there are a number of issues that influence the extent to which this can be achieved.

Involving patients in the referral decision when the issue is an uncertain diagnosis or a potentially serious one involves the sharing of uncertainty. This may be uncomfortable for the professional and unsettling for the patient. On the other hand, acknowledging the fallibility of medicine may lead to a more mature professional–patient relationship in future and reduce the sense of grievance when things do not turn out as hoped.

The value of avoiding referral as a means of cost containment is increasingly being recognized even though other rationales, for example protecting patients from unnecessary investigations and treatment, have also been advocated (Franks *et al.* 1992). The health care system may place varying degrees of pressure on the doctor to take the issues of cost and the appropriate use of resources into account in the decision to refer. Again these difficulties can be shared with the patient in a mature relationship, but it cuts across the desire and expectation that the best will be done for each individual patient.

There is a complex sequence of events in the pathway between making the initial diagnosis and the start of specialist treatment. When a general practitioner identifies a problem, for example menorrhagia, for which there are a variety of treatment options, he or she may decide to share those options, and the evidence for them, with the patient. Only if the patient decides on specialist treatment, for example an operation, would she be referred. Alternatively, the doctor may take the view that this is a problem for which the patient requires specialist advice and offer to refer her for that advice.

The specialist may respond by explaining the options, or by assuming that as the patient has been referred for specialist treatment that is what the patient wants and requires. The patient may be offered time to consider the options or the specialist's advice. She may consult her family doctor again for his or her opinion. Exceptionally the specialist may have written to the family doctor detailing the options, and the evidence for them. In some settings, for example breast surgery, the patient will also be offered the opportunity to consult specialist nurses, or directed towards literature or other decision aids. And of course the patient can consult family, friends, or the Internet. On the whole, the communication that takes place during the referral process is under-researched. There is evidence however that decision aids do help patients make evidence-based choices (O'Connor *et al.* 1999), and that patients who are involved in decisions about their care are more satisfied and have better outcomes (Fallowfield 1994).

Patient's choice of doctor

The first choice that many patients have to make is which practice or doctor to register with for their primary care. Salisbury (1989) showed that patients in England displayed very little 'consumerist' behaviour and tended to choose the practice nearest to them. The evidence that would be available if patients sought it is limited to the information contained in the practice brochure. This lists the age and qualifications of the doctors in the practice and describes the services that they provide, including the range of services by other members of the primary health care team. Perhaps in the future information about performance may be made available, but this is unlikely to reflect the personal qualities of a doctor that are important to many patients. In other countries patients may have the opportunity to be more consumerist.

Unless the patient registers with a single-handed practice they usually have a degree of choice about which professional in the practice to consult and whether to seek to consult the same one on each occasion. Freeman and Hjortdahl (1997) contrasted two concepts of continuity of care, *longitudinal continuity*, care given by one professional over a defined time, and *personal continuity*, an ongoing therapeutic relationship between patient and professional in which the nature and quality of the contacts are more important than the number. They reviewed the evidence of benefit from continuity of care. This included more appropriate use of tests and resources and an increase in the professionals' knowledge about and sense of responsibility towards their patients.

The costs of greater continuity are the possibility of increased waiting times for patients and the need for personal commitment and availability from professionals. Changes in society, in particular the pattern of work, are increasing these costs both for patients and for professionals. Freeman and Hjortdahl argued that the first element in a policy to encourage personal continuity is to make it worthwhile for patients if they have waited to see a particular professional in primary care. In effect they were arguing that it is the experience of a patient when they actually consult that will influence the choices that they make in future.

When to consult

The decision to consult a doctor is one of the most difficult and complex decisions that a patient has to make in the process of their health care. When patients experience symptoms of ill health they have to make sense of these themselves, though often with the support of friends and family. A large proportion of symptoms are not presented to primary care and Hannay (1979) described this phenomenon as 'the symptom iceberg'. Campbell and Rowland (1996) reviewed the literature on the complex mix of social and psychological factors that influence this decision. These include not only the patient's ideas about the nature of their problem, but also their concerns about what their symptoms may signify and their expectations of what health care may have to offer. These expectations will be influenced by their previous experience of health care.

When patients present their symptoms to a health professional, one of the roles of the doctor or nurse is to help patients organize and make sense of those symptoms. Kai (1996) described the difficulties that parents of young children had coping and making sense of their illnesses. Central to the parents' difficulties were their experiences of inadequate information sharing by professionals. Parents expressed a need for a range of accessible and specific information to support them through their negotiation of children's illness.

The information that is available to help patients with the decision when to consult is limited and of variable quality (Coulter *et al.* 1999). It may also be because the evidence about the natural history and significance of symptoms in an unselected population is very poorly researched. NHS Direct, which is a telephone information service being launched throughout the UK, is an attempt to provide patients with appropriate information on how to manage their problems themselves and on when to consult a health professional. Early experience is that the service is used most by the parents of young children, particularly when surgeries are closed. The fact that a significant proportion of them are then advised to consult a doctor could be seen as a measure of its effectiveness at empowering patients to make a difficult choice, rather than evidence of failure to reduce demand.

Stott and Davis (1979) described 'modifying help seeking behaviour' as one of the potential tasks of each primary care consultation. More recently Howie *et al.* (1998) have argued that patient enablement is an appropriate outcome measure for effective consultations. If one of the major choices facing patients is whether or not to consult a doctor, then helping them make sense of their symptoms and how to respond to them appropriately is an essential part of promoting evidence-based patient choice.

Primary care and the community

Primary care takes place in the community, and one of its rationales is the ability to provide services that respond to and meet the community's needs. Methods of identifying these needs and of tapping into the views of consumers are well established if not universally used, but many of them offer the opportunity for a two-way dialogue. The content of this dialogue could be evidence-based and enable appropriate choices about the use of services by patients, as well as making the services responsive to patient needs.

This dialogue could also be about priorities for health care and the design of services, and the creation of partnerships between professionals and the public to address these difficult issues. The evidence that is valuable in these discussions is about the effectiveness in meeting patients' needs and this is not always available. Increasingly patients are being involved in the design of research so that this deficit can be corrected (Goodare and Lockwood 1999).

Conclusion

It is being increasingly recognized that improvements in the quality of health care require a critical examination of the system as well as the individuals who work within it. If we are to achieve evidence-based patient choice in primary care many parts of the system require modification. Many changes are being considered, but the fundamental part of any change must be to allow adequate time for patients and professionals to come to well-informed and shared decisions.

References

Austoker J (1999). Gaining informed consent for screening. *British Medical Journal* **319**: 722–3.

Balint M (1957). *The doctor, his patient and the illness.* London, Tavistock.

Bensing J (2000). Bridging the gap. The separate worlds of evidence-based medicine and patient-centred medicine. *Patient Education and Counseling* **39**: 17–25.

Bero L, Grilli R, Grimshaw JM, Harvey E, Oxman AD and Thomson MA (1998). Closing the gap between research and practice: an overview of systematic reviews of interventions to promote implementation of research findings by health professionals. *British Medical Journal* **317**: 465–8.

Buntinx F, Winkens R, Grol R, *et al.* (1993). Influencing diagnostic and preventative performance in ambulatory care by feedback and reminders. *Family Practice* **10**: 219–28.

Campbell S and Rowland M (1996). Why do patients consult the doctor? *Family Practice* **13**: 75–83.

Coulter A and Roland M (1992). *Referrals from general practice.* Oxford, Oxford University Press.

Coulter A, Entwistle V and Gilbert D (1999). Sharing decisions with patients: is the information good enough? *British Medical Journal* **318**: 318–22.

Fallowfield LJ, Hall A, Maguire P, Baum M and A'Hern RP (1994). Psychological effects of being offered choice of surgery for breast cancer. *British Medical Journal* **309**: 448.

Feder G, Eccles M, Grol R, Griffiths C and Grimshaw J (1999). Using clinical guidelines. *British Medical Journal* **318**: 728–30.

Franks P, Clancy CM and Nutting PA (1992). Gatekeeping revisited; protecting patients from over-treatment. *N Engl J Med* **327**: 424–9.

Freeman G and Hjortdahl P (1997). What future for community care in general practice? *British Medical Journal* **314**: 1870–3.

Goodare H and Lockwood S (1999). Involving patients in clinical research. *British Medical Journal* **319**: 724–5.

Hannay DR (1979). *The symptom iceberg: a study of community health.* London, Routledge and Kegan Paul.

Howie JGR, Porter AM and Forbes JF (1989). Quality and the use of time in general practice: widening the discussion. *British Medical Journal* **298**: 1008–10.

Howie JGR, Heaney DJ, Maxwell M and Walker JJ (1998). A comparison of a Patient Enablement Instrument against two established satisfaction scales as an outcome measure of primary care consultations. *Family Practice* **15**: 165–71.

Howie JGR, Heaney DJ, Maxwell M, Walker JJ, Freeman GK and Rai H (1999). Quality at general practice consultations: cross sectional survey. *British Medical Journal* **319**: 738–43.

Howitt A and Armstrong D (1999). Implementing evidence-based medicine in general practice: *British Medical Journal* **318**: 1324–7.

Kai J (1996). Parents' difficulties and information needs in coping with acute illness in preschool children: a qualitative study. *British Medical Journal* **313**: 987–90.

Makoul G, Arntson P, Schofield T (1995). Health promotion in primary care: physician–patient communication and decision making about prescribed medications. *Soc Sci Med* **41**:1241–54.

O'Connor AM, Rostrom A, Fiset V, Tetroe J, Entwistle V, Llewellyn-Thomas H, *et al.* (1999). Decision aids for patients facing health treatment or screening decisions: systematic review. *British Medical Journal* **319**: 731–4.

Pendleton D (1983). Doctor–patient communication: a review. In: *Doctor–patient communication* (ed. D Pendleton and JC Hasler). London, Academic Press.

Salisbury CJ (1989). How do people choose their doctor? *British Medical Journal* **299**: 608–10.

Shepperd S, Charnock D and Gann B (1999). Helping patients access high quality health information. *British Medical Journal* **319**: 764–6.

Stewart MA (1995). Effective physician–patient communication and health outcomes: a review. *Canadian Medical Association Journal* **152**: 1423–33.

Stott N and Davis RH (1979). The exceptional potential in each primary care consultation. *Journal of the Royal College of General Practitioners* **29**: 201–5.

Walton R, Dovey S, Harvey M and Freemantle N (1999). Computer support for determining drug dose; systematic review and meta-analysis. *British Medical Journal* **318**: 984–90.

12 Evidence-based patient choice in secondary care

William Rosenberg

Introduction: the characteristics of secondary care

The consumer's burden of expectation

The problems faced in secondary care differ in many ways from those seen in primary care. Patients first encounter secondary care in two settings, the outpatient clinic and the emergency room. In either situation the portents preceding that first hospital consultation carry a greater burden of expectation and anticipation than most primary care consultations. Often the primary care professional will have talked to the patient about their clinical problem, the likely content of the hospital consultation, and possibly even a description of the hospital setting and staff. The patient will arrive primed with ideas, concerns, and expectations, partially shaped by their previous experiences and a range of opinions coming from sources as diverse as their primary care team, their friends, and the daily media. Because of the magnitude of the step undertaken when entering the secondary care consultation, the patient entering outpatients arrives carrying a bundle of issues in addition to their clinical problem. All of these must be addressed if their experience of secondary care is to be beneficial.

More 'differentiated' conditions

By definition the vast majority of requests for a consultation in secondary care arrive with a 'label', suggesting a far more differentiated condition, than those encountered in primary care. With the passage of time from first presentation to hospital appointment the diagnosis may become clearer. Preliminary tests may also have shed some light on the nature of the patient's problem. The 'generally feeling unwell' may have been narrowed down by the primary care physician to 'abnormal liver function' or 'microcytic anaemia' by the time the referral letter reaches the hospital. Although this prior knowledge never removes the necessity to confirm the diagnosis (stories change and even the best primary care physicians make as many mistakes as hospital doctors!) the first attempt at diagnosis usually permits the primary care physician to select the appropriate secondary care specialist. It also alerts the secondary care clinician to consider a number of tests and treatment options prior to the consultation. In the most specialized areas prepared patient information can be identified and even distributed before the consultation.

More homogenous groups of patients in secondary care

Secondary care is not just characterized by the more limited range of clinical problems encountered. A further feature is that the patients often share common characteristics. Whilst respecting the unique individuality of each patient, all clinicians will recognize that the majority of patients attending an alcohol clinic will share at least something in common and probably more than the range of patients attending the average primary care morning surgery. This greater homogeneity amongst patients attending secondary care clinics allows adjustments to be made. Clinic times and locations can be tailored to a specific patient group. Information sheets addressing common problems can be provided (e.g. cardiac rehabilitation advice sheets), appropriate support service staff can be available in neighbouring clinics (e.g. joint surgery and medicine clinics for inflammatory bowel disease; chiropody next to the diabetic clinic), and appropriate facilities can be made available (visual aids in the hearing department, a ground floor neurology clinic with ramp access).

Breadth or depth of information available compared to primary care

The narrower and more specialized nature of the information required by professionals in secondary care is complemented by the greater volume of research that is conducted in secondary care. More research is conducted in secondary care settings than primary care for many different reasons. Assembling suitably large numbers of patients with similar problems is easier in a specialist referral clinic which draws from a wide population base than in primary care clinics seeing patients from a single area. Diagnostic and treatment facilities are usually concentrated either in, or close to hospitals and are thus more accessible for secondary care researchers. Secondary care also has a longer academic tradition of research. For these reasons most specialists in secondary care are able to draw from a greater body of evidence than their colleagues in primary care.

However in some specialist areas this may not be the case. So, for example, the primary care professional caring for elderly patients with hypertension can call upon systematic reviews of randomized controlled trials of treatment, but the general physician in secondary care trying to treat the second case of Castleman's disease she has ever seen will find difficulty in locating any useful trial evidence. Here patients may play an active role in expanding the body of evidence available to professionals involved in their care. While the case of Castleman's may be a 1 in 10,000 diagnosis for the professional, for the patient it is the only significant disease he will ever have and well worth attention. In a number of areas consumer organizations have lobbied for research in specific areas such as osteoporosis and have often raised funding to support research, such as has been the case in HIV/AIDS, cystic fibrosis, Huntington's Disease, and renal failure, to name but a few.

Obstacles to 'evidence-based patient choice' in secondary care

Many of the challenges posed by 'evidence-based patient choice' are common to the primary and secondary care sectors. Both sectors need to adopt a more collaborative approach to clinical management and the need to use information effectively in the consultation. Some of the obstacles to meeting these challenges differ between the care settings.

The patient–professional relationship

Traditional representations of secondary care professionals portray us as the caricatured and authoritarian 'Sir Lancelot Spratt' figure, barking orders and allowing no dissent from our cowering patients. While not denying that we might have encountered one or two such consultants during training, we doubt that they still exist and trust that 'clinical governance' will see them off for good. However this change is not yet recognized by all patients. Many arrive at a hospital consultation with feelings of inferiority to embark on what should be an equal relationship with a caring professional. It must be recognized that a consultant wielding a sigmoidoscope (to investigate the bowel) in the context of a ten-minute outpatient consultation is in a position of some power, no matter how caring her approach to the patient.

Continuity of relationships

The idealized view of primary care values the continuity of the relationship between patient and professional through health and disease. Although group practices and emergency out-of-hours services have eroded this relationship, the benefits of continuity still provide strong support for maintaining the traditional family doctor role. In many areas of secondary care patient–professional relationships are fragmented and lack continuity. The cardiologist managing a heart attack or the surgeon repairing a hernia is likely to meet the patient only on a very limited number of occasions.

The brevity and infrequency of patient–professional interactions, and team-working in secondary care all place burdens on professionals. They must rapidly assimilate an understanding of the patient's perspective, and communicate complex information in a limited number of meetings. Similarly burdens are placed on the patient: to assimilate information and to express and explain preferences to a 'stranger' in the same few meetings. However, this lack of continuity and pressure of time can be circumvented in outpatient clinics with careful planning.

The management of chronic disorders such as rheumatoid arthritis and inflammatory bowel disease provides more opportunity for the professional and patient to establish rapport and for treatment options to be explored more thoroughly in the course of repeated meetings. Many secondary care professionals begin to function as primary care deliverers for patients with chronic diseases, such as renal failure. They provide the first calling point for a variety of ailments unrelated to the original reason for referral. In this way continuity of care is restored for the patient but delivered by secondary care professionals. Here the benefits of an established professional–patient relationship can be realized. In the UK, however, increasing pressures on the NHS are now forcing the management of even complex chronic disease back into primary care to the detriment of the secondary care professional–patient relationship. This transfer does not necessarily benefit the patient. While continuity might be provided in primary care, much of the knowledge base remains in secondary care – to the dissatisfaction of the patient and both primary and secondary care professionals.

Continuity of care for in-patients in the secondary setting has also changed in recent years. This is perhaps largely attributable to the reduction in doctors' working hours, moves away from the old 'firm-based' division of labour (i.e. small teams under one consultant), and the introduction of more shift work in secondary care. The 'care package' may be delivered by up to four or five professionals servicing the same role. Lack of continuity between members of the secondary health care team often results in the patient having to offer the same information to five or six individuals sharing the same role on a rota. While professionals recognize the need to reduce working hours, many express regret at the loss of continuity of care which has an adverse effect on the professional–patient relationship. It also fragments experiential learning to the point of confusion.

Despite hospitals operating 'named nurse' and 'consultant-led' services, in reality while responsibility may stay with key professionals, care through night and day is passed from shift to shift. Emergencies and discharges cannot wait for shifts to change and professionals who have only just met the patient often take crucial decisions with little opportunity to establish their preferences and values. The changes in working practices place intense demands on the skills of professionals to communicate with one another and with patients. Insufficient attention has been given to developing effective methods for ensuring that communication occurs to the maximum benefit of both parties.

Time available for discussions

If the average consultation in primary care takes ten minutes and the average outpatient consultation in secondary care takes twenty minutes for a new patient, one might assume that secondary care professionals have more time to deliver 'patient-centred' care. This would ignore the complexity of the information exchanged, the time taken over examinations and tests, and the relative scarcity of 'simple' consultations in secondary care. In order to reduce the time pressure on communication many specialist teams have chosen to compartmentalize interactions with patients so that different members of the professional team can deliver differing components of the consultation. In our clinic for people with hepatitis C, patients are first seen by a hepatologist who confirms the diagnosis and assesses the severity of the disease. Preliminary information is given to the patient and their ideas, concerns, and expectations are explored. After a brief interval they are then seen by a nurse-specialist who has more time to repeat explanations, clarify uncertainties or misunderstandings, and establish care preferences.

In another setting a patient requiring an operation for colon cancer might be seen first by a surgeon who confirms the diagnosis and explains the plan of management. The patient will then see a stoma therapist who will discuss stoma care. Then the nutritionist will assess the individual concerned, discuss nutritional support issues, and establish intravenous feeding prior to the operation. By fragmenting the delivery of secondary care in this way a patient can spend a large total period of time in consultation, covering many aspects of their care with several different professionals, each of whom commits a brief period of their time to any one patient. The net effect is that each professional completes more consultation episodes than they would if they had to cover all aspects of the consultation.

The benefits of this highly specialized approach are that it allows individual professionals to develop expertise in a limited area. With communication skills to match they may then be in a position to practice 'evidence-based patient choice' in the secondary care setting. However the patient is confronted by a bewildering array of professionals, each of whom contributes a limited amount to their total care. The potential for the professionals to present contrary or confusing information is great, as is the opportunity for both parties to 'get along' or 'fall out.' It is unclear whether the benefits of this type of approach outweigh the disadvantages resulting from discontinuity in the patient–professional relationship.

Management drives to shorten the duration of in-patient admissions have increased the pressure to make diagnoses, share information, select treatment options, and initiate therapy as rapidly as possible. Some therapies, such as the use of thrombolysis for myocardial infarction, require early or immediate action. However confirming diagnostic criteria for infarction, excluding all contraindications to thrombolysis and obtaining informed consent take skill and time. It only requires a professional to witness one stroke during a thrombolytic treatment for them to become fully aware that 'haste' and 'speed' are different properties of time: quicker is not always better. Effective communication, even in emergency situations encountered in secondary care, takes time.

The setting for discussions

There should be no reason for the outpatient setting in secondary care to be any less comfortable or private than primary care consulting rooms. If it is less comfortable, this may reflect patients' expectations, the fact that hospitals are usually further away and thus represent a more 'foreign' territory for the health care encounter, or that more people may be involved in the running of the clinic. However, the in-patient setting most certainly differs markedly from primary care settings. Professionals often have to 'break bad news' to a bed-bound patient in an open ward with only thin curtains to create a pretence of privacy. It is difficult to engage in delicate but important discussions with patients in such situations, exploring concerns and identifying their preferences and values. Side-rooms and offices are useful for exploring issues with relatives or patients who can be moved. Such facilities though are often left empty for much of the day, and are then taken over for other uses. Their importance is only valued when they are lost.

When the research base is weaker or the choices less distinct

It is difficult to provide 'evidence-based patient choice' when the research base is weak, the evidence inconclusive, and professional approaches more idiosyncratic. While some patients will welcome a professional's honesty in communicating uncertainty, other patients will expect and desire a more authoritative approach. In some cases health care choices are indistinct. Is it better for a woman with severe menopausal symptoms and a weak family history of breast cancer to take HRT and tolerate an increased risk of cancer or put up with the symptoms? Such choices are best resolved through a face-to-face consultation where there is the flexibility for both sides to ask and answer many questions. The lack of information which is specifically relevant to the individual patient's situation will remain an obstacle, and discussions may inevitably be left with a sense of missing vital ingredients for the decision making process.

When the benefits and harms are more marginal and subject to variation in patient values

In many situations the objective benefit of an intervention is either uncertain or marginal. I am a middle-aged man. In some health care sectors middle-aged men are encouraged to undergo testing for levels of Prostate Specific Antigen (PSA) in the hope of detecting prostate cancer (a significant cause of morbidity and mortality) at an early stage. Offering this test might appear to go some way to redressing the sexual inequality in the screening tests offered by modern medicine. We men regard breast and cervical cancer screening programmes with envy and wonder why we are the neglected second sex. However, as a health care professional, I would find it very hard to discern what benefit I can derive from having the test. Furthermore I cannot imagine my anxiety if it came back with a false positive, or even worse a true positive result.

Now suppose I also read about the advantages of surveillance colonoscopy on reaching fifty to detect early bowel cancer. This is the tumour most likely to kill me, rather than the prostate cancer mentioned above. But the investigation carries a small but definite risk of bowel perforation and a fairly certain risk of discomfort. Explaining to me the balance of risk and benefit of this investigation would require more than a simple leaflet. In either prostate or bowel cancer screening, however, the eventual decision (in which the objective benefits are marginal) is likely to be heavily swayed by my personal values. My understanding of what bowel cancer or prostate cancer means, their seriousness, treatability, and impact on lifestyle and life expectancy are all important. Personal experience of others with these conditions will affect my perception of the disease and the outcomes being discussed by my health care professional. The situations in which personal values show particularly wide variation are ones where it is especially challenging to adopt 'evidence-based' approaches to decision making with patients.

Simple information sheets and decision aids are unlikely to provide the flexibility or depth of information required to help patients make informed choices. There appears to be no substitute for an informed, articulate, and sensitive professional spending time with the patient. In order to function effectively the professional will need to take time to understand the evidence (such as it is). They will need to develop strategies for communicating with patients from a range of educational backgrounds, using a variety of approaches tailored to the individual's needs.

Challenges for secondary care to answer the questions of patients

Patients' desire for information

The patient referred to secondary care generally comes armed with a battery of questions and a greater desire for information than that usually encountered in primary care. The complexity and detail of the information required will vary between settings. Within any setting, individual patients will differ widely in the beliefs, knowledge, and the desire for information that they bring to the consultation.

Frequency of being asked for detailed information in secondary care

The frequency with which professionals in secondary care are asked for detailed information reflects both the complexities of the specialist area and the consumer's desire for information. For example, there are many ways of managing breast cancer and navigation through the care pathways necessitates mastery of a considerable body of knowledge. Treatment choices vary depending on disease severity and the availability of treatments. Treatment availability itself may be dependent on the professional's knowledge, the physical availability of the treatment, and the funds to pay for those treatments. Each of these factors increases the need for detailed information and contributes to the complexity of decision making.

Variations in desire for information

For any given clinical condition individual patients differ in their desire for detailed information. Some patients wish to know about the minutiae of each decision, requiring the professional to be able to communicate sufficient relevant information. In this scenario, professionals need to have access to and be familiar with the relevant information. Decision aids are becoming increasingly popular as a way of conveying and discussing information about treatment options and these are discussed fully in Chapter 14 (O'Connor and Edwards). In contrast there are still patients who do not wish to know in such detail and prefer the professional to take more responsibility. It is still common, in the UK at least, to hear the phrase 'whatever you think is best, doctor' even if this attitude is now on the wane.

The profusion of information will not fully meet patients' desires. A distressed or anxious patient may not easily assimilate information that has taken professionals years to comprehend, even when the information is presented clearly. By the nature of the issues confronted in secondary care the information is often complex and the decisions of great significance. Many patients express their preference to be guided through management choices by a professional, perhaps using an information leaflet, but not being handed the leaflet and left to make a decision.

Variations in consumer preferences for involvement in their health care decisions

There is some variation in patients' desire for information though in general this desire is high. There is a much greater variation, however, in patients' desires for involvement in decisions about their treatment or care. Such differences in patient preferences show recognizable patterns of variation. These patterns represent gross generalizations but they may help to inform clinical management. As above, it may vary according to the significance of the decision to the individual. Also, younger and better-educated patients tend to request more detailed information and desire to be involved in the decision making more than older or less-educated patients. Similarly North American patients have tended to expect greater involvement than UK residents, and some professionals report a gradient of expectation from rural to urban areas within the UK.

The same patient may express different preferences for information in different situations. The patient who wishes to be fully informed and take an active part in decision making about the management of his asthma may prefer to allow the professionals in the emergency room to take the decision to ventilate him during a sudden attack. Similarly the patient actively involved in making treatment choices about her breast cancer is unlikely to discuss with the emergency physician which is the best route to drain fluid from the lung in the event of such a complication.

Challenges to involve consumers according to their preferences

The principal challenge to professionals is how to accommodate this range of patient preferences – both for information about the condition and for involvement in decision making about treatment. Increased awareness of the need to better inform patients has led to a profusion of information monographs, leaflets, communication aids, and videos. Almost inevitably each information source can usually take only one stance. While this may be beneficial in providing a single view of a subject it lacks the flexibility that an interview might provide, including greater opportunity for interaction and an individualized 'patient-centred' approach (Chapter 7, Stewart and Brown). They are also unable to take account of how different patients will react to the information provided.

So, for example, while one patient may be reassured to learn that only 25% of people with chronic hepatitis C will develop liver cirrhosis, and then only after 15 to 20 years of infection (Poynard *et al.* 1997), another patient may be terrified at the chance of this outcome. Similarly providing the information that alcohol consumption will worsen disease progression is of limited use to the 'teetotaller' but vitally important to the 'social drinker' of four pints (eight units of alcohol) per day. Whilst many professionals are eager and willing to help produce materials to which patients can refer, some are less willing to discuss with patients the implications of the information and how to use it. It is almost as if the dispensing of a leaflet allows the professional to tick the 'good communication box' in the notes. Within organizations the development of patient information sources has been used to reduce consultation times and personal input from professionals in clinic. This may be a false economy and certainly not to the benefit of the patient.

The potential for 'evidence-based patient choice' in secondary care

Clearly a balance must be sought between making optimal use of the professional's time and ensuring that patients have the opportunity and resources to take a full and active part in their own care. Although there will be an optimum number of consultations that provides this balance, that number will vary between conditions, between patients, and between professionals. Broad guidelines might be possible in time but any recommendations will have to accommodate wide intervals. A variety of more specific strategies are already employed in an attempt to enhance consumer participation in secondary care consultations.

Information and decision aids

In a number of secondary care specialist areas professionals have developed packages containing a range of material from background information to complex decision aids that can be used by patients prior to meeting professionals. Patients can consider treatment for hysterectomy, the management of prostatism, HRT, and non-valvular atrial fibrillation prior to or between their outpatient consultations. These materials can provide an invaluable adjunct to the consultation, allowing patients to develop, at their own pace, an understanding of the information and choices that confront them. They can help both patients and professionals make optimal use of time in the consultation, by approximating the knowledge base of both parties. By disseminating information prior to the consultation decision aids may also help to share power and place the patient–professional relationship on a more equal footing. Their successful use assumes that the professionals using the aids are familiar with their content and in agreement with the perspective represented in the document. For the patient it is essential that the aid is accessible and comprehensible. The preparation and presentation of these materials requires careful consideration and they should be tailored for their audience. These issues are discussed more fully in Chapter 14 (O'Connor and Edwards). Even if information and decision aids are produced according to current 'best practice' it is worth noting as well, though, that the availability of a decision aid or information sheet does not imply that it is informative, accurate, or useful. Critical evaluation of these materials is as important as critical evaluation of primary research literature. Effective implementation strategies are also vital and these are discussed in Chapter 16 (Holmes-Rovner *et al.*).

While a few examples have been cited above there are only a very limited number of conditions for which published decision aids exist. Whether their scarcity reflects a lack of awareness of their utility or the limited number of conditions for which they can be prepared with any degree of consensus is unclear. For common conditions such as cardiovascular disease and diabetes, numerous information sheets have been produced by national and local bodies and the quality of many of these is high.

Further examples

Other examples are being pursued. Within the field of liver disease the British Liver Trust has co-ordinated the development of a whole range of patient information leaflets covering all the common and some rare liver diseases. These are also available over the Internet at *www.britishlivertrust.org*. We make use of locally developed written materials explaining the use and meaning of diagnostic tests in liver disease. Decision aids for treatment of hepatitis C are being piloted using visual, verbal, and numerical representations of treatment outcomes. Patients can choose the formats that are most readily accessible. Similar materials are being developed to help patients with haemochromatosis. These explain disease risks and the benefits of biochemical and gene testing for their relatives – this is currently managed in a pilot project to cascade information through affected families but without involving large numbers of professionals in separate consultations.

It is also important that these efforts, which are being made in situations where research evidence is reasonably strong and the choices distinct, are then applied to the situations where the research is less strong and the choices less distinct or the 'benefits' even more subject to the wide variation in patient values attached to the outcomes. As discussed above such situations might include the benefits of HRT in menopausal women with a weak family history of breast cancer, or the possible benefits of surveillance for bowel cancer.

Scope for EBPC to be directed towards groups as well as individuals

As secondary care becomes ever more specialized so patient groups become more tightly defined. The general physician of the 1970s would see patients with a variety of very different problems in one clinic, encompassing everything from gallstones to asthma. His successor in 2000 is likely to work in a single speciality area such as gastroenterology and see only patients with gastrointestinal disorders. Indeed he or she often specializes further than this nowadays. Most patients attending a consultant's clinic might only have one of two or three chronic conditions which she is expert in managing.

This super-specialization can work to the benefit of individual patient groups. Through specialization the professional is better able to maintain her awareness of all available evidence. Through repetition she is more likely to develop optimal means of sharing that evidence with patients.

Having patients with shared problems in one outpatient clinic or hospital ward opens up possibilities for patients to share their experience with one another. Although this self-help may occur spontaneously it can be facilitated by professionals to good effect. Health care teams working in the fields of breast cancer, stoma therapy, and cardiac rehabilitation have all helped facilitate patient–patient support. Specialist clinics and wards provide an ideal forum for the provision of information in a range of formats. For example, patients may view a video on arrival in outpatients, have access to leaflets, and leave the consultation with an audio or video tape.

Consumer perspectives on health care delivery in groups

As above, there may be potential benefits from sharing experiences. A trouble shared can be a trouble halved. Merely learning that others share the same difficulties and anxieties can restore confidence and strengthen resolve. However, not all individuals are equally assertive or articulate and functioning in a group is not a universal skill. Many patients also report difficulties in expressing their personal views in a group setting and some describe feeling influenced by group opinions with which they do not feel comfortable. If groups are the only forum in which patients can express their views some problems will undoubtedly fail to be aired or addressed.

Professional perspectives on health care delivery in groups

Working with patient groups offers the professional the advantage of maximizing the number of patients who hear each fact and explanation. It thus appears to be a highly efficient use of the professional's time. In addition the professional has the opportunity to experience a spectrum of patients' views and opinions in one session. The disadvantage to the professional (as well as the patient) of working in this way is that it is impossible to maintain confidentiality and it is often difficult to explore individual patient's views or problems. Sometimes it can be hard to gauge the breadth and depth of understanding among individuals within a group or even of the whole group.

Implications for effectiveness and efficiency

The professionals working with patient groups are often nurses. This probably reflects the nursing profession's readiness to adopt this role rather than a carefully considered strategy designed by the whole health service. In some fields doctors are beginning to take an active role in working with patient groups and multidisciplinary group working is also developing. Working with groups appears to be an efficient use of professional time, increasing the number of patients contacted by one professional in a single 'consultation'. As yet though there is little or no evidence to show how effective such groups are, and whether they are most effective if they include nurses, doctors, Professions Allied to Medicine (PAMs), or a mix of professionals. Undoubtedly providers of health care will be eager to identify which professionals can deliver effective care for the lowest cost. Before such cost-effectiveness can be determined it is vital to identify appropriate measures of effectiveness. These should include disease-specific measures of health as well as measures of the efficiency of clinical care and patient satisfaction.

The roles of consumer groups

Many of the most successful consumer groups have been formed by patients and for patients without input from the health care professions. In the field of genetic disorders patients have formed numerous societies for the support of sufferers and their relatives. One highly successful example is the Haemochromatosis Society. The Internet has fostered the globalization of such organizations. There is a rapid cascade of information and sharing of experiences. It is now a common experience for specialists in secondary care to meet patients carrying pages of computer print-out that have generated dozens of questions. This living network can benefit patients and professionals alike. A popular chocolate bar was well known amongst patients with coeliac disease (gluten sensitive enteropathy) to be a good and tasty source of gluten-free nourishment. When the manufacturers brought out a mini-sized bar a number of patients reported unpleasant reactions to the Coeliac Society. The manufacturers were questioned and explained that gluten was added to the mini-bars only. The first gastroenterologists heard of this was when patients and the Coeliac Society made them aware of the change in manufacture.

In diseases ranging from AIDS through hepatitis C to haemochromatosis, well organized patient groups have played a major role in changing health policy, societal attitudes, and even research strategies. Professionals working in harmony with these consumer groups can do much to improve 'evidence-based patient choice' for groups and individuals in these and similar areas. The roles of patients and consumer groups in influencing health care services are discussed more fully in Chapter 3 (Entwistle and O'Donnell).

Conclusions

Secondary care is only beginning to embrace evidence-based patient choice. There is a sound evidence-base underpinning many of the treatments used in secondary care (Ellis J *et al.* 1995) and there are well developed mechanisms for involving consumer groups in a number of areas of clinical care. However we have much to learn about the most effective ways of communicating complex information to patients, of how patients and professionals might reach consensus over treatment or care options, and how to make best use of the secondary care consultation.

The two major challenges for evidence-based medicine are how to incorporate patient choices in clinical care and how best to include evidence from qualitative research. Much of this is concerned with patients' experiences of clinical care and thus of direct relevance to patient choice. These two challenges are as important for professionals in secondary care as for workers in any other health care sector.

For 'evidence-based medicine' (EBM) to develop towards 'evidence-based patient choice' it must incorporate patient choices and their ideas, concerns, and expectations about their condition and possible treatments. These must be addressed at all stages in the practice of EBM: when determining the questions that need to be answered; when considering which sources of evidence to search; when appraising the evidence; and when using it in clinical care. If patients are to play a full and active part in this process they may require education and this will need to be part of any strategies that seek to promote evidence-based patient choice.

There are some obstacles to the implementation of evidence-based patient choice, particularly in the secondary care setting. There are however several examples already of good practice, and there should be no reason why some of these examples of best practice should not be generalized throughout secondary care. This should begin with the areas where there is sufficient evidence to inform patient choices. Where the evidence is currently lacking there are opportunities for research and development of services and these should be exploited. There is little reason to believe that evidence-based patient choice is not achievable. The steps of evidence-based medicine provide a sound enough framework (Rosenberg W and Donald 1995; Sackett

DL *et al.* 1997). The key stages can be followed in the future, from identifying the clinical questions, searching for the evidence, critical appraisal, and then applying the evidence in patient care. Ascertainment of patients' desire for information, their preferred formats for receiving or discussing this information, and their preferred level of involvement in their health care decisions are the crucial elements which complement this process.

References

Ellis J, Mulligan I, Rowe J and Sackett DL (1995). In-patient general medicine is evidence-based. A-Team, Nuffield Department of Clinical Medicine. *Lancet* **346**: 407–10.

Oxman AD, Sackett DL and Guyatt GH (1993). Users' guides to the medical literature. I. How to get started. The Evidence-Based Medicine Working Group. *Journal of the American Medical Association* **270**: 2093–5.

Poynard T, Bedossa P and Opolon P (1997). Natural history of liver fibrosis progression in patients with chronic hepatitis C. The OBSVIRC, METAVIR, CLINIVIR, and DOSVIRC groups. *Lancet* **349**: 825–32.

Rosenberg W and Donald A (1995). Evidence-based medicine: an approach to clinical problem-solving. *British Medical Journal* **310**: 1122–6.

Rosenberg W, Lusher A, Dooley G, Snowball R and Sackett D (1998). Improving searching skills and evidence retrieval. *Journal of the Royal College of Physicians, London* **32**(6), 557–63.

Sackett DL, Richardson WS, Rosenberg W and Haynes RB (1997). *Evidence-based medicine: how to teach and practice EBM*. London, Churchill Livingstone.

13 Narrative and patient choice

Trisha Greenhalgh

What is narrative?

This chapter is about the patient's unique story and how it fits in with 'evidence-based decision making' and 'shared decision making' about health interventions. As Brian Hurwitz and I have argued in more detail elsewhere (Greenhalgh and Hurwitz 1998), five features of narrative distinguish it from other linguistic forms:

- It has a finite and longitudinal time sequence – that is, it has a beginning, a series of unfolding events, and (we anticipate) an ending.

- It presupposes both a narrator and a listener, whose different viewpoints are brought to bear on how the story is told.

- It is concerned not only with the events that happen, but also with the feelings and motives of the individuals they happen to.

- It provides items of information that do not pertain simply or directly to the unfolding of events. The choice of what to tell, and what to omit, lies entirely with the narrator.

- It engages the listener and invites an interpretation.

Narratives of clinical interest tend to take the form of a *plot* – that is the story is constructed with the general aim of establishing meaning and with the specific aim of answering the question 'why?' (what best explains this patient's experiences?) (Greenhalgh and Hurwitz 1998). Thus, as Forster says, the statement 'The king died then the queen died' is a story; but 'The king died then the queen died of grief' is plot, because it reveals a deeper meaning within the sequence of events, and helps us to understand why the events happened as they did (Forster 1970).

Leder (1990) has argued (in an article I have summarized elsewhere (Greenhalgh 1998)) that the doctor–patient encounter takes place in a highly structured transactional space, in which the behaviour of both parties is determined by socialized expectations. In Leder's view, the 'text' that constitutes the diagnostic encounter, and which distinguishes it from other human narratives or modes of communication, is a story about the *person-as-ill*. This, in turn, integrates four separate secondary texts:

◆ the *experiential* text – the meaning the sufferer assigns to the various symptoms, deliberations, and lay consultations in the run-up to the clinical encounter;

◆ the *narrative* text – what the doctor interprets to be 'the problem' from the story the patient tells – the traditional medical history;

◆ the *physical* or perceptual text – what the doctor gleans from a physical examination of the patient; and

◆ the *instrumental* text (what the blood tests and X-rays 'say').

Far from 'evidence' and 'narrative' being mutually exclusive dimensions of clinical practice, a genuine evidence-based approach to decision making actually *presupposes* an interpretive paradigm within which the patient experiences illness and the professional–patient encounter is enacted (Greenhalgh 1998).

Let us begin, then, with a unique personal illness story. The case of Sally P is fictitious but is based on four different true stories in my own practice. Details have been changed to protect confidentiality.

Framing the questions – and seeking evidence

Part 1 of Sally's story reflects the type of information and the approximate level of detail that a family doctor might glean during an initial 10-minute consultation. What I knew by the end of Part 1 was that this was a healthy and health-conscious woman with a few months' history of galactorrhoea. I also knew from Sally's behaviour that she found the symptom surprising but not apparently distressing, and that she knew – and seemed to accept – that a sinister cause was a fairly unlikely possibility.

My encounter with Sally was a very typical primary care case. Even with only cursory details of her story, I was able to provide important expertise on the medical aspects of her problem. The nature of the 'white stuff' was, for example, a mystery to Sally but a perfectly straightforward diagnosis to me. Whereas the textbook chapter had focused (not unreasonably) on the management of symptomatic prolactinomas, and discussed surgical interventions in considerable detail, this patient had almost nothing in the way of symptoms and was undoubtedly at the benign end of the spectrum of disease. Even my own limited and out-of-date knowledge of pituitary neoplasms allowed me to place her concerns about a brain tumour in perspective.

Looking back, my decision to send her for another blood test was probably a subconscious stalling move while I collected more information from the research literature on the diagnostic possibilities, natural history of the

Box 13.1   **Sally's story – Part 1**

Sally P was a new patient on my list. She was an attractive professional woman in her early thirties and attended the last booked appointment of the day. From the preliminary interview that my nurse had already completed, I could see that she exercised daily, did not smoke or drink alcohol, and followed a 'mostly vegetarian' diet. Her boyfriend, David, who had accompanied her to the surgery, waited outside, offering to come in if she chose to summon him (she didn't).

Sitting opposite me in the consulting room, she was clearly somewhat uncomfortable being a 'patient'. 'I must say I don't generally have much to do with doctors', she confided, laughing. Her problem was the loss of 'white stuff' from both nipples. She showed me, and I confirmed that the 'stuff' was almost certainly milk. 'Humph!', she said, looking incredulously at her leaking breasts, and laughing again.

I examined Sally briefly, and noted that her breasts were otherwise normal, she had no features of androgen excess, and no visual field defect. Sally's previous doctor had ordered a blood test, which had shown a serum prolactin level of 840 mu/L – approximately double the upper limit of normal. He had written her a letter reassuring her that high prolactin levels are very common in young women, and that she should commence the drug bromocriptine, which would soon alleviate her symptoms. He had enclosed a prescription for the drug, and advised her to have another blood test in three months' time.

Sally asked me what might have caused her bizarre symptom. I told her that the causes of galactorrhoea (leaking milk when not breast-feeding) included physical stimulation of the nipple (she said she didn't do this), and certain drugs – both medicinal and recreational (she wasn't taking any). She said that her boyfriend had discovered on the Internet that these symptoms might indicate a brain tumour and he felt that she should get her head scanned. I said that given her fairly low prolactin levels and lack of other symptoms, a tumour was highly unlikely. I pulled down a large medical textbook from my shelf, and we read the relevant section together, with me explaining some of the technical terms. The text reminded me that psychological stress is a cause of galactorrhoea, and she admitted to a 'quite stressful' job. She was visibly relieved to find an explanation for her symptoms that felt plausible.

Sally agreed that a referral to a consultant was not needed at this stage. But my own knowledge of this problem was limited, and I felt that the textbook had given insufficient detail on key management choices. I wanted to go and look things up in the journals. In the meantime, I asked Sally to get the prolactin test repeated along with a test of thyroid function.

End of part 1

condition, and management options. In particular, I wished to find answers to four key questions with a view to informing a shared decision about investigation and monitoring:

- What is the chance that Sally's problem is serious – and how hard should I try to exclude rare but sinister diagnoses?
- If it isn't serious, will it get better on its own?
- Should she be taking the bromocriptine given by her previous doctor?
- What if she wants to get pregnant?

For evidence-based decision making, these questions must be expressed in a more focused and standardized way as described below:

1. What is the likelihood that a healthy 32-year-old woman with a short history of galactorrhoea and mildly raised prolactin levels has a pituitary tumour?

This is an example of a question about *diagnosis*. Ideally such a question should be answered using an investigation (or set of investigations) that have been independently validated against an established gold standard, and administered to a representative population sample – that is to a sample of young women with mild symptoms, no sinister features, and only mildly raised prolactin levels. Using the free public access Medline service 'PubMed Clinical Queries' (http://www.ncbi.nlm.nih.gov/PubMed/) and a somewhat rough and ready search string – 'hyperprolactinaemia OR hyperprolactinemia' and selecting the 'diagnosis' filter – I found around half a dozen studies conducted in the past five years but none that exactly matched my criteria. The abstracts of several review articles stated that in such cases pituitary microadenoma is 'rare', and macroadenoma 'very rare' (Fossati *et al.* 1985), but without sending for the full text articles I could find no reliable figures for how rare.

It appeared from this brief (and far from exhaustive) search that mildly raised prolactin levels commonly occur in otherwise healthy women with no ill effects except galactorrhoea. There was no explicit advice as to whether investigations to exclude prolactinoma were indicated in all cases or only selected ones, and there appeared to be some controversy about the investigation of choice. In particular, there was apparently little to choose between a specialized (dynamic serial) CT scan and an MRI scan in the only published study comparing the two, which showed that both techniques had a sensitivity of around 90% and a specificity of 82% (Stadnik *et al.* 1994).

2. Assuming that no prolactinoma is found, what is the prognosis of galactorrhoea with mild hyperprolactinaemia in a healthy 32-year-old woman?

This is a question about *prognosis*. The ideal clinical research study to address this question is a prospective cohort study of a representative population sample as described above. I repeated my search, this time using the 'prognosis' filter on PubMed. I found one small prospective study of so-called 'idiopathic' hyperprolactinaemia (i.e. in patients with no evidence of pituitary enlargement), which suggested that this condition rarely if ever progresses to adenoma and often resolves spontaneously (Sluijmer and Lappohn 1992).

3. What are the benefits, and what are the risks, of bromocriptine therapy – and is there any other medication available with a better risk-benefit profile?

This time, I searched using the 'therapy' filter – and again, there wasn't a great deal in the literature directly relevant to my question. There were, however, countless articles describing trials in which bromocriptine success-fully reduced prolactin levels and alleviated a range of symptoms from which Sally did not suffer (including hirsutism, menstrual irregularity, and subfer-tility). The number of trials in which medication was *not* offered to some groups of patients was much fewer!

In the prospective study of idiopathic hyperprolactinaema described above (Sluijmer and Lappohn 1992), medication (usually bromocriptine) was not routinely offered to patients for simple galactorrhoea. Rather, it was used for specific indications (anovulatory infertility or hypogonadism). The authors concluded that 'there is a high tendency to spontaneous cure' and that 'dopaminergic medication had no appreciable impact on the course of the disease' (but it should be noted that this was not a randomized trial). The abstract of one major review article (Fossati *et al.* 1985) suggested that other studies had found similar outcomes, and promised a more detailed description of different medications. But by this time I was already fairly sure I had enough information to continue my discussions with the patient.

4. What are the chances of achieving pregnancy in idiopathic hyperprolactinaemia, and if pregnancy is achieved, what are the risks to the foetus if any?

Sally had not volunteered any plans for a pregnancy, but it was clearly impor-tant to establish any potential risk to a foetus of both the underlying condition and the medication she had already been advised to take. My searches described above had turned up two small prospective studies of pregnancy outcome in hyperprolactinaemia, both of which suggested that, if pregnancy is achieved (either on or off bromocriptine), its outcome is no different from that in normal women (Ampudia *et al.* 1992; Randall *et al.* 1982). But when I did a further search using 'pregnancy' as a qualifier, I found an additional retrospective hospital-based study suggesting an increased risk of ectopic pregnancy in women with raised prolactin levels (Rossi *et al.* 1995). I repeated my search, this time going for recall rather than precision, and including 'tubal' and 'ectopic' as search terms – but I failed to corroborate this finding, so I concluded that its generalizability was in doubt.

Using 'infertility' as a qualifier for my general search on hyperprolacti-naemia, I found several studies suggesting that high prolactin levels are found in 20–40% of infertile women (Prathibha *et al.* 1994; Choudhury and Goswami 1995), but none describing what proportion of women with high prolactin levels are infertile! The studies suggested that bromocriptine therapy led to successful pregnancy in about half the cases. In any case, Sally hadn't yet complained of infertility so I did not need to pursue this aspect of the problem at this stage.

On the basis of all the above evidence, I felt far more confident to help Sally make her choices. My own interpretation of the literature can be summarized as follows:

◆ Isolated galactorrhoea with mildly raised serum prolactin levels is common in women of Sally's age and very unlikely to indicate serious pathology;

◆ There is no firm guidance on whether to investigate to exclude a prolactinoma in women with mild symptoms, but if this option is taken, specialized investigations include CT scan and MRI scan;

◆ In the absence of a prolactinoma, Sally's symptoms are very likely to resolve spontaneously (but this outcome cannot be guaranteed);

◆ She may achieve a pregnancy without any treatment (and hence must use contraception if she does not seek this yet), and the evidence, though conflicting, suggests that pregnancy outcome would probably not be adversely affected by her condition; and

◆ If she does wish to become pregnant in the future but has trouble con-ceiving, bromocriptine therapy may help – but success is not guaranteed.

The patient's narrative

The story so far has incorporated very little of the patient's narrative – that is, of Sally's personal story, told in her words, and of the meaning she assigns to her experiences. How can I access this information, and how will it impact upon the evidence-based shared decision making process we are both aiming for? Let us now consider Part 2 of her story.

In Part 2 of the story, I have given you more information about Sally than is generally presented in a medical case history, and considerably more than I myself had at my fingertips during the first consultation. I have elaborated on Sally's background to show you that even though *I* did not know much about aspects of her personal life that were likely to influence her management choices, she herself was, of course, an expert in these very details.

Box 13.2 **Sally's story – Part 2**

The result of the repeat prolactin test was 888 mu/L, and thyroid function was normal. Sally had been due to see me to discuss this but cancelled her appointment at the last minute because of pressure of work. I decided not to write to remind her to rebook, and she eventually came again seven weeks later.

Over the next few consultations, I learned more about Sally's background. She worked as a senior buyer in a leading fashion company and had moved into the area recently when her company relocated. She worked long hours but she loved her job, especially the opportunities for travel and the exciting social life. She was a member of the local private gym and did weight training several times a week. She had been a moderately successful ballet dancer in her teens, and had met David on a contemporary dance course four years ago. She described him as 'devoted to me', and I noted that he always accompanied her to her appointments and waited, somewhat anxiously, outside the door.

They were renting a smart flat in the more upmarket part of my practice area. Neither of them was interested in cooking, but both earned a comfortable salary, so they ate out most evenings. David bought vitamin and mineral supplements from the local health food shop, and also took garlic capsules 'to stay healthy', but Sally thought this 'a bit daft' and didn't take any herself. They both had private health insurance.

Sally had been taking the combined oral contraceptive pill until nine months ago, but had discontinued it because it made her moody. Her galactorrhoea had begun soon afterwards. They were now using condoms. Many years ago, in a previous relationship, Sally had become pregnant and had had an uncomplicated termination of pregnancy. She and David planned to have children in about three years' time, but they had a number of more pressing plans. Sally was trying for promotion, and they wanted to spend time choosing a house and decorating it. They were currently on the list of every estate agent in town.

End of Part 2

Unlike many of the patients who regularly fill my waiting room, Sally was not plagued by anxiety about her symptoms. In fact, having cancelled her first appointment she then forgot to rebook, and only did so on repeated prompting from her anxious boyfriend (whom I have to admit I was beginning to think of as 'Drippy David'). It did become clear, however, that Sally's self-image was strongly tied up with her strikingly attractive physique and sporty, health-conscious lifestyle. Going to the doctor wasn't part of this – and neither was having an illness or taking medication.

Combining research evidence with the patient's unique narrative

I hope you feel that Part 2 of the story would help you enormously if you were the clinician in my shoes. Whereas the 'raw' evidence about galactorrhoea and hyperprolactinaemia as presented earlier is very informative, it is dry and does not in itself lead us to a decision. Likewise, Sally's story paints a useful picture of what she is like, how she wants to live, her priorities and hopes for the future, and the other important individuals in her life, but taken in the absence of the research evidence, this doesn't help us much either. The key to effective shared decision making is to *place the research evidence in the context of the patient's unique narrative* – an interpretive task that is remarkably straightforward in practice once all the information is assembled.

Table 13.1 shows, in a somewhat artificial deconstruction, the information needed to make decisions about Sally's management – in particular, decisions about how far to investigate her problem and how (if at all) to treat it. I have represented this information in terms of the state of play at the end of the initial consultation, and the first thing to note is that *most* of the information needed lies *outside* the top left-hand box. After just a single consultation, either I know something important but Sally doesn't, or Sally knows it but I don't, or neither of us knows it!

Table 13.2 offers a general taxonomy of where the 'narrative' and the 'evidence' tend to lie early on in the clinical encounter. Note that as both Tables 13.1 and 13.2 demonstrate, the information known to Sally but not to me mostly comprises her personal narrative. The information known to me but not to Sally is generally the stuff of clinical experience and some rather unreliable technical data (neither good evidence nor relevant narrative – but useful nonetheless). The information known (initially) to neither of us mostly comprises the 'evidence' – in this case, the results of my Medline search described above.

There is one additional item of information that neither of us knows at the outset, and which we will not get from the research literature either, and that is how Sally's individual and unique clinical problem will pan out over the next few months. From my literature search, we can say with a fair degree

Table 13.1 Information available in the first consultation – Sally's example

	Known to me	Unknown to me
Known to Sally	Good general health On no medication or recreational drugs White fluid is coming from her nipples This symptom *could* indicate a 'brain tumour' The prolactin level is double the upper limit of normal The drug bromocriptine is a possible treatment	Symptoms began after stopping the pill Previous termination of pregnancy; plans a definitive pregnancy in about 3 years Self-image strongly associated with slimness, fitness, and ability to cope with highly stressful and demanding job Supportive partner who is anxious and rather overprotective Privately insured Finds my surgery times highly inconvenient Hates the idea of taking tablets, especially when 'not ill'
Unknown to Sally	The white stuff is almost certainly milk The normal female breast can produce milk in response to a range of stimuli Causes of galactorrhoea include physical stimulation, and a range of drugs A prolactin level of 840 mu/L is very unlikely to indicate a pituitary tumour Uncertainty in primary care is often appropriately managed by using a 'wait and see' strategy Research evidence is available which will help answer our questions	The likelihood that a healthy 32-year-old woman with a short history of galactorrhoea and mildly raised prolactin levels has a pituitary tumour is extremely low Both dynamic serial CT scan and MRI scan would exclude a pituitary tumour with a sensitivity of about 90% and specificity of 82% Idiopathic hyperprolactinaemia resolves spontaneously in most cases Hyperprolactinaemia is commonly found in infertile women, and bromocriptine therapy achieves pregnancy in about 50% of these Pregnancy outcome in hyperprolactinaemia is probably the same as in normal women but one study suggests an increased rate of ectopic pregnancy

of confidence that it is *likely* to resolve spontaneously (thus, *on average*, it will resolve spontaneously). But we cannot say with complete certainty whether it will *actually* resolve – nor indeed whether Sally's own condition will progress or recede more or less rapidly than average. Gould (1998) expands on this argument in his excellent chapter 'The median isn't the

Table 13.2 Information available in the first consultation – general taxonomy

	Known to health professional	Unknown to health professional
Known to patient	Declared aspects of the illness history and symptoms (volunteered spontaneously or accessed via a conventional medical history) Clinical knowledge and beliefs – unconfirmed, incomplete, and imprecise, from sources of unknown validity. Patient's and health professional's knowledge and beliefs may conflict Preliminary physical examination test results	Undeclared aspects of the illness history and symptoms (accessible via a more detailed conventional medical history) Totality of personal history – ill and not ill – including role of relatives and significant others (accessible via the patient's unique narrative) Priorities and preferences (accessible via the patient's narrative and via formal shared decision making techniques – see Chapter 8, (Elwyn and Charles)
Unknown to patient	Additional clinical knowledge – likely to be inaccurate, incomplete, or outdated (from clinical experience and general reading) Knowledge of where to access best evidence and how to use it (from prior training in searching and critical appraisal) Techniques for managing uncertainty (from clinical experience and, perhaps, academic training)	Best research evidence about diagnosis, prognosis, and benefits and harms of treatment (based on probabilities derived from population samples) Future behaviour of Sally's particular lesion – i.e. what point does her unique illness occupy on the population 'scatter plot' (from observation over time and judicious repeating of investigations)

message'. He argues that an *average* value has meaning and reliability when we are talking about a population (or a sample drawn from that population), but it becomes increasingly meaningless and unreliable when we try to apply it to a single individual. In clinical consultations, we tend to see patients one at a time, and all practising clinicians know the frustration of trying to portray an uncertain future in unique encounters. Gould himself was once diagnosed as having a 'median' of eight months to live with a rare cancer. He quickly made his way to a library in search of more detailed information about the differential survival of particular subgroups that allowed him to predict (rightly, as it turned out) that his personal prognosis was considerably better than the textbook average.

Let us return to the four key questions we posed earlier:

1. What is the chance that Sally's problem is serious – and how hard should I try to exclude rare but sinister diagnoses?

2. If it isn't serious, will it get better on its own?

3. Should Sally be taking the bromocriptine given by her previous doctor?

4. What if she wants to get pregnant?

We now know from the research evidence that Sally's problem is most unlikely to be serious. We know from her personal narrative that she herself has a laid back approach to the problem and might well be happy to take a 'wait and see' approach. But we also know that her partner is extremely anxious and is focused on the possibility of a tumour. Sally's private health insurance will cover her for a scan, so there is no material barrier to this option in her particular case (but note that a scan may not be on offer if she were uninsured).

Sally's desire to avoid doctors and not take medication is a powerful theme in her personal narrative, and the evidence fortunately supports an expectant approach to her current condition. The problem of what to do about a pregnancy is not an issue right now, except that I need to explain to both of them that the risk of successful pregnancy falls with increasing maternal age, and that Sally is, statistically, more likely than most women to require assisted conception.

As we leave this couple, we see that over the course of this chapter, much has changed both within and beyond the illness narrative. The clinical case history (what Leder (1990) calls the narrative text) is fairly unremarkable – someone is suspected of having benign idiopathic hyperprolactinaemia and this turns out to be the case. Similarly, there are no surprises from the physical examination or the investigations, and the progression of the 'disease' (it gets no better and no worse over the course of eight months) is pretty typical.

But consider the experiential text (Sally's interpretation of her symptoms and her assignment of medical or other meaning to them). Her 'illness' has changed from a bizarre and unexpected symptom with a possibly sinister explanation to a benign, predictable, but unwanted reminder of the prospect of motherhood. Placed within the broader narrative of Sally's life as a young, attractive, and successful professional whose immediate ambitions are no longer concordant with those of her long-term partner, the illness story moves on into its next phase – the contemplation (or not) of pregnancy and the wider future.

Summary – how has narrative helped decision making in this case?

I have tried to use Sally's story to illustrate six principles of the benefits of narrative in evidence-based shared decision making:

Box 13.3 **Sally's story – Part 3**

Eight months after our first meeting, following two more cancelled appointments, Sally's symptoms are unchanged and she has not taken any bromocriptine. In this consultation, she is a little tearful and confides that 'It's not very athletic, all this milk production, is it? I mean, I don't really see myself as an earth mother!' She explains to me that she accepts the scientific explanation – that milk production is a normal response of a healthy breast to the slightly high levels of prolactin in her blood, but she also realizes that she is having to come to terms with a significant alteration in her body image. For Sally, the significance of the unwanted milk is *not* that it raises the spectre of serious pathology – but that it raises the possibility of motherhood and the associated perceived loss of sexuality and freedom!

Since our first encounter, Sally and David have found a house to buy and are negotiating the final contract. David remains highly anxious about Sally's 'illness', and has suggested that she should reduce her work commitments and stop the energetic dancing. He has also started cooking macrobiotic food, which he believes will help. In Sally's words, 'He's beginning to wrap me in cotton wool'.

I can see that David's behaviour is now placing a palpable strain on their relationship. Sally and I discuss the evidence, and the options for investigation. Sally quickly decides that if a head scan will reassure him she should have one as soon as possible. I order an MRI scan of the pituitary fossa, which is reported as normal. We both agree that drug therapy is not indicated. We see no indication to repeat the serum prolactin level test at this stage but agree to do so in about a year's time if her symptoms remain unchanged.

With David present, we discuss the implications for future fertility. David is keen to start trying for a family immediately, in case it takes longer than anticipated, but Sally is more reluctant. She wonders if it matters whether they have children at all, and states that 'I can tell you now, I'm not doing any of that test tube baby nonsense'. The couple agree that they need to discuss this further outside the consultation, and I offer the services of my practice counsellor. They thank me for my input and say they will drop me a note if they decide they want a referral.

End of Part 3

1. Illness narratives are part of patients' wider life narratives; they therefore tend to promote a holistic and patient-centred approach to management.

2. Constructing a narrative allows the patient to make sense of his or her symptoms and explore the meaning (or potential meanings) of the illness experience.

3. The narrative enables the health professional to gain a deeper understanding of 'what the patient is going through'. Mismatches between the

meaning ascribed to aspects of the illness experience by the patient, the relatives, and the health professional can be identified and explored.

4. The interpretation of narrative by a health professional is based on linguistic and communication skills, and is thus part of the traditional art of medicine.

5. Contrary to popular belief, the incorporation of research-based evidence into the clinical encounter is usually a straightforward task, which extends rather than replaces the health professional's traditional skills.

6. The patient's unique narrative may assist the health professional in deciding on the relevance to this particular problem of research evidence expressed as an 'average' effect on a distant population sample.

Postscript

It is interesting to reflect on how Sally reached her decisions at the various key points in this story. As the professional whom Sally chose to consult (albeit reluctantly and infrequently), did I really produce the goods for genuine shared decision making? Or have I imposed a *post hoc* interpretation that gives the story a clear linear thread, accords the patient a high degree of empowerment, and overestimates my competence in the relevant areas of shared decision making as described in Chapter 8 (Elwyn and Charles)?

Certainly, at the time the sequence of events did not unfold in quite such a linear fashion as I have depicted here, and the gaps between the encounters were more prominent in my consciousness than the consultations themselves. My motive for looking up the evidence in Sally's case was my own clinical curiosity rather than a desire to provide the raw materials for her own evidence-based choices. I was not consciously aware of attempting to influence or guide her.

But perhaps this particular series of encounters was unusual in that there was relatively little social distance between Sally and me, and we both had a 'gut feeling' that her symptoms were probably not serious. There was thus a high degree of shared understanding, a natural concordance in perspective, and little or no conflict between us. As I have hinted in the narrative, the same cannot be said of my limited encounters with David – and I suspect that if and when I come to assist him with any decision making, I will need to pay more conscious attention to the tasks of developing a partnership, establishing his preferences and values, responding to his concerns and expectations, and so on. In Chapter 8, Elwyn and Charles suggest a formal framework for such an approach. In this individual situation this will always be easier or harder according to the interpersonal dynamics between patient and professional.

References

Ampudia X, Puig-Domingo M, Schwarzstein D, Corcoy R, Espinos JJ, Calaf-Alsina J, *et al.* (1992). Outcome and long-term effects of pregnancy in women with hyperprolactinaemia. *Eur J Obstet Gynecol Reprod Biol* **46**: 101–7.

Choudhury SD and Goswami A (1995). Hyperprolactinemia and reproductive disorders – a profile from North East India. *J Assoc Physicians India* **43**: 617–18.

Forster EM (1970). *Aspects of the novel.* Harmondsworth, Middlesex: Penguin Books.

Fossati P, Dewailly D, Thomas-Desrousseaux P, Buvat J, Fermon C, Lemaire A, *et al.* (1985). Medical treatment of hyperprolactinemia. *Horm Res* **22**: 228–38.

Gould SJ (1998). The median isn't the message. In: *Narrative-based medicine – dialogue and discourse in clinical practice* (eds T Greenhalgh and B Hurwitz). London: BMJ Publications.

Greenhalgh T (1998). Narrative-based medicine in an evidence-based world. In: *Narrative-based medicine – dialogue and discourse in clinical practice* (ed. T Greenhalgh and B Hurwitz). London: BMJ Publications.

Greenhalgh T and Hurwitz B (1998). Why study narrative? In: *Narrative-based medicine – dialogue and discourse in clinical practice* (eds T Greenhalgh and B Hurwitz). London: BMJ Publications.

Leder D (1990). Clinical interpretation: the hermeneutics of medicine. *Theoretical Medicine* **11**: 9–24.

Prathibha D, Govardhani M and Krishna PT (1994). Prolactin levels in infertility and bromocriptine therapy in hyperprolactinaemia. *J Indian Med Assoc* **92**: 397–9.

Randall S, Laing I, Chapman AJ, Shalet SM, Beardwell CG, Kelly WF, *et al.* (1982). Pregnancies in women with hyperprolactinaemia: obstetric and endocrinological management of 50 pregnancies in 37 women. *Br J Obstet Gynaecol* **89**: 20–3.

Rossi AM, Vilska S and Heinonen PK (1995). Outcome of pregnancies in women with treated or untreated hyperprolactinemia. *Eur J Obstet Gynecol Reprod Biol* **63**: 143–6.

Sluijmer AV and Lappohn RE (1992). Clinical history and outcome of 59 patients with idiopathic hyperprolactinemia. *Fertil Steril* **58**: 72–7.

Stadnik T, Spruyt D, van Binst A, Luypaert R, d'Haens J and Osteaux M (1994). Pituitary microadenomas: diagnosis with dynamic serial CT, conventional CT and T1-weighted MR imaging before and after injection of gadolinium. *Eur J Radiol* **18**: 191–8.

14 The role of decision aids in promoting evidence-based patient choice

Annette O'Connor and Adrian Edwards

Introduction

Health care decisions are often difficult to make. This may be because the outcomes are uncertain or because the options available to patients have different benefit and harm profiles which they value differently. Several 'decision aids' are being developed to supplement existing communication between professionals and patients. In general their aim is for patients to:

- understand the range of options available;
- understand the probable consequences of options;
- consider the value they place on the consequences; and
- participate actively with their professionals in deciding about options.

This chapter provides a brief overview of patient decision aids and their role in promoting 'evidence-based patient choice'. We begin by defining decision aids, describe their methods and efficacy, and then discuss further issues in their development, evaluation, and dissemination.

What is a patient decision aid?

Decision aids prepare patients to participate with their health care professionals in making deliberated, personalized, choices about health care options. They supplement counselling by providing information on options. The aim is that patients are better able to judge the value of the benefits versus the harms. The Cochrane Collaboration has defined what decision aids include and do not include:

> Inclusion criteria: Interventions designed to help people make specific and deliberative choices among options by providing (at the minimum) information on the options and outcomes relevant to the person's health status.

Additional strategies may include providing: information on the disease/ condition; the probabilities of outcomes tailored to a person's health risk factors; an explicit values clarification exercise; information on others' opinions; and guidance or coaching in the steps of decision making and communicating with others. Decision aids are delivered using media such as decision boards, interactive videodiscs, personal computers, audio-tapes, audio-guided workbooks, pamphlets, and group presentations.

Exclusion criteria: Passive informed consent materials, educational interventions that are not geared to a specific decision, or interventions designed to promote compliance with a recommended option rather than a choice based on personal values.

(O'Connor et al. 1999a)

Decision aids have been developed for a range of situations (O'Connor *et al.* 1999b; O'Connor *et al.* 1999c) such as:

(a) medical therapies for: atrial fibrillation; benign prostatic hypertrophy; low back pain; cancers of the breast and lung, leukaemia, lymphoma; circumcision; and ischaemic heart disease;

(b) diagnostic tests such as: amniocentesis; and screening for colon and prostate cancers;

(c) preventive therapies such as: hepatitis B vaccine; and hormone therapy at menopause;

(d) clinical trial entry decisions; and

(e) end-of-life decisions such as resuscitation in seniors.

The media used to present decision aids are varied, and it is important to note that each of these is likely to have its place according to the nature of the setting and the clinical problem being addressed. A further variation occurs in terms of whether the packages are thought most helpful if used as support before, during, or after a consultation. Some decision aids are provided for patients to work through on their own (outside the consultation or at home) as a platform for discussions in a further consultation (Liao *et al.* 1996; Barry *et al.* 1997; Sawka *et al.* 1998; O'Connor *et al.* 1998; Davison and Degner 1997; Man-Son-Hing *et al.* 1999; Holmes-Rovner *et al.* 1999; Street *et al.* 1995; Bernstein *et al.* 1998;). These aids vary in their use of explicit links to the clinical encounter, such as guiding patients to communicate values, preferences for participation, and questions with their professional. Others are delivered within consultations (Whelan *et al.* 1995; Holmes-Rovner *et al.* 1999). Each is likely to have its place according to the situation, but where decision aids are discussed *outside* consultations, it is important to ensure that both patient and professional contribute to the process of making a decision about treatment (see also Chapter 8, Elwyn and Charles). Possible additional components of decision aids include structured counselling approaches for the professional (Lerman *et al.* 1997), the use of specific approaches to clarify or quantify patient values (e.g. 'weigh scales' (O'Connor *et al.* 2000)), and exploration of the patient's preferred level of involvement in the decision making itself (Man-Son-Hing *et al.* 1999). Decision aids do not need to be complicated. In some situations they can be simple graphical depictions of risks and benefits relating to a treatment choice to provide information for discussion between professional and patient (Elwyn 2000). As more literature accumulates it will become clearer whether these interventions may be the ones most likely to achieve the key goals of informed choices, satisfaction with decisions, and adherence to the chosen treatments as often currently promoted. All of the packages, however, seek to enhance patient involvement, on the basis of evidence, and thus facilitate 'evidence-based patient choice'.

Providing decision support involves preparing professionals for counselling with information on the scientific evidence regarding the options, and on how to counsel with the decision aid, preparing patients prior to counselling with a self-administered or group-administered decision aid, and structuring follow-up counselling. To examine one such decision aid as an example, we shall describe one of the Ottawa decision aids developed for patients with atrial fibrillation considering anticoagulant therapy (Man-Son-Hing *et al.* 1999). Patients with atrial fibrillation use an audio-tape, booklet, and worksheet to prepare for consultation. The audio-tape guides them to review key points in the booklet about: atrial fibrillation; complications of stroke including effects on functioning; and the benefits and risks of aspirin and warfarin. The probabilities of stroke are tailored to the patient's risk factors. As shown in Fig. 14.1, probabilities are presented numerically (e.g. 10 out of 100) accompanied by figures of 100 faces, which are shaded to illustrate the proportion of patients affected and not affected.

Next, the audio-tape guides patients to complete a *personal worksheet* (see Fig. 14.2). This seeks to: a) identify medical factors that may affect the choice of outcomes; b) clarify their values using a 'weigh scale' to indicate the benefits and risks that are most important to them; c) list their questions; d) identify their preferences for participation in decision making; and e) indicate their predisposition or 'leaning' toward taking treatments. Examples of how other patients complete their worksheets are provided to help them learn the steps in decision making and to illustrate the variable and individualized nature of deliberation.

Follow-up counselling between patient and professional begins with a review of the patient's completed personal worksheet. Professionals can then work through a number of aspects. These cover the patient's medical risks, their values as revealed by the patient's 'weigh scale', and the patient's questions. They can then facilitate decision making considering the patient's preference for decision participation and predisposition towards the options. Knowing a patient's preference for participation and predisposition can assist

Option #1 Taking No Medication to prevent stroke

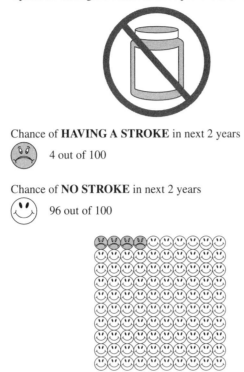

Chance of **HAVING A STROKE** in next 2 years

4 out of 100

Chance of **NO STROKE** in next 2 years

96 out of 100

Fig. 14.1 Example of presenting probabilities of outcomes for patients with atrial fibrillation.

the professional to judge how quickly they can move from facilitating decision making to follow-up planning.

In terms of the effects or outcomes of this package (Man-Son-Hing *et al.*
1999), more patients appeared to be ready to make a choice about treatment after receiving the decision aid than in the control group, and they
were more knowledgeable about the issues and had more realistic (evidence-
based) expectations of outcomes. The decision aid increased patients'
preferences for conservative therapy using aspirin rather than warfarin. As
would be expected, those with a greater risk of stroke were more likely
to choose warfarin. However, both control and decision aid groups had
similarly high levels of satisfaction and certainty about their choices, and
perhaps because of this did not show improvements in actual adherence to
the chosen treatments.

Step 1 My Medical Situation
Do I have these factors . . .

❐ Previous stomach ulcer or bleeding
❐ Stomach pain or heartburn on aspirin
❐ Allergy to aspirin
❐ Take more than 1–2 drinks of alcohol per day

❐ Take medications for arthritis
❐ Previous falls
❐ Usual activities make me prone to injury
❐ Specify:...

Step 2 My Opinions in Weighing the Pros and Cons of Therapy

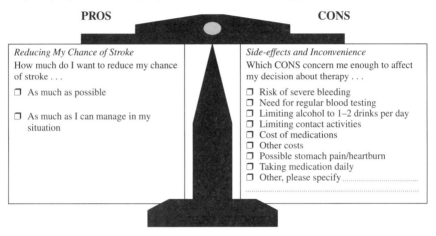

PROS

Reducing My Chance of Stroke
How much do I want to reduce my chance of stroke . . .

❐ As much as possible

❐ As much as I can manage in my situation

CONS

Side-effects and Inconvenience
Which CONS concern me enough to affect my decision about therapy . . .

❐ Risk of severe bleeding
❐ Need for regular blood testing
❐ Limiting alcohol to 1–2 drinks per day
❐ Limiting contact activities
❐ Cost of medications
❐ Other costs
❐ Possible stomach pain/heartburn
❐ Taking medication daily
❐ Other, please specify.............................

Step 3 My Questions answered

_____
_____
_____
_____

Step 4 Who Should Decide

❐ I should, after considering the opinions of my doctor, family or others
❐ My doctor and I together
❐ My doctor
❐ Unsure

Step 5 My Overall Leaning

❐ ❐ ❐ ❐ ❐ ❐ ❐ ❐ ❐ ❐ ❐

Warfarin   Coated   No treatment to
                  Asprin   prevent stroke

Fig. 14.2 Example of personal worksheet guiding people to consider the steps in decision making.

When do you need a decision aid?

The development of decision aids across North America and Europe is motivated by several trends:

- the rise of consumerism with an emphasis on informed choice rather than informed consent;

- the evidence-based practice movement disseminating evidence to patients as well as to professionals;

- the use of patient-focused strategies to reduce regional practice variations;

- the identification of treatment decisions that are 'utility', or 'value' sensitive from decision analyses;

- related clinical practice guidelines which indicate that certain choices are sensitive to patient preferences and that patients should be involved in decision making;

- the proliferation of overviews and outcome studies which provide estimates of outcomes for use in decision aids;

- the evolution of patient preference-orientated health policy that reserves interventions for those individuals who consider the treatment benefits to outweigh the harms (e.g. reserving palliative surgery for those who consider symptom relief worth the surgical risks, rather than basing a surgical policy on the average patient's utilities);

- the expansion of evaluation criteria by quality improvement groups to include the quality of counselling regarding options, such as at the time of menopause.

Kassirer (1994) lists some of the situations when it is most valuable to elicit patients' preferences in clinical practice. Firstly, when options have major differences in outcomes or complications; secondly, when decisions require trade-offs between near-term and long-term outcomes; thirdly, when one choice can result in a small chance of a grave outcome; and finally, when there are marginal differences in outcomes between options. In these situations a decision aid may be particularly helpful. Patient characteristics may also determine the need for a decision aid, for example, if patients are very risk-averse, or attach unusual importance to certain possible outcomes.

Another useful strategy for determining the need for a decision aid is to classify treatment policies as standards, guidelines, or options using Eddy's definitions (1992). For standards of care where outcomes are known and patients' preferences are generally consistent in favouring an intervention, decision aids may be less useful and conventional informed consent procedures more appropriate. Examples would include insulin treatment for Type

I diabetes or antibiotics for an infection. In contrast, decision aids may be indicated for the scenario in which there are genuine treatment options. These arise when outcomes may be more uncertain, or the values for the benefits relative to the harms are more variable or unknown. For example, there is good evidence that amniocentesis for pregnant women over thirty-five is effective in detecting abnormalities, but not all women choose the procedure because their values differ. Another example would be the treatment of benign prostatic hypertrophy with its multiple options (watchful waiting, drugs, surgery) and potential outcomes (amount of symptom relief versus drug side-effects or surgical risks of incontinence and impotence).

Do decision aids work?

Evaluation studies from a Cochrane systematic overview of trials (O'Connor *et al.* 1999a) and two general reviews (O'Connor *et al.* 1999b; Molenaar *et al.* 2000) have shown that decision aids generally improve decision making by:

- reducing the number of patients who are uncertain about what to do;
- increasing patients' knowledge of the problem, options, and outcomes;
- creating realistic personal expectations of outcomes;
- improving the match between choices and patients' values;
- reducing decisional conflict (uncertainty) and the factors contributing to decisional conflict such as feeling ill informed, unclear about values, and unsupported in decision making; and
- increasing participation in decision making without adversely affecting anxiety.

The evidence about the effects on altering choices is less clear. Trials have generally been under-powered, options may have been under-used or over-used at baseline, and the research has not taken into account that patients respond differently to different types of decisions. However, it is noteworthy that when provided with information and opportunity for greater involvement in *major surgical* decisions, patients generally became more wary of the treatments offered and made more conservative choices. In their reviews of this specific area of the literature O'Connor *et al.* (O'Connor *et al.* 1999a; O'Connor *et al.* 1999b) found that, on average patients were 26% less likely to choose treatment in studies where information was provided and choices offered (relative risk of choosing treatment 0.74; 95% CI 0.6–0.9). Such findings are likely to be of great interest not just to consumer-representative groups but also to purchasers of care – decision aids may be highly cost-effective interventions in regions where surgical procedures are over-used.

The direct patient benefits demonstrated for changes in 'affective' outcomes such as satisfaction with decision making and decisions made, and confidence about making the best choice appear less consistent (O'Connor *et al.* 1999b). There is still a need for further development of the content and use of decision aids in practice if these outcomes are to be influenced. More research is also needed on which decision aids work best with which decisions and which types of patients. In addition, we need to evaluate the acceptability of decision aids to professionals and diverse groups and cultures, their impact on patient–professional communication, and their effects on adherence to choices, health-related quality of life, practice variation, and use of resources.

There also remain questions about the essential elements in decision aids. Although decision aids have been quite beneficial relative to usual care, the differences between simpler and more detailed aids often have been quite marginal. The simpler methods produce similar effects on patients' knowledge and satisfaction. However, more intensive methods are generally superior in terms of user acceptability and the extent to which choices are based on realistic expectations and personal values. The clinical importance of these differences and the cost-effectiveness of decision aids remain to be established.

In particular, as it is the individually calculated risk information which has greatest influence on outcomes (compared to average or population data), attention is required as to how this can be implemented in practice (Edwards *et al.* 2000a). To date most decision aids have used population data, integrated, for example, into an individualized counselling package (Lerman *et al.* 1997). Interactive media may be required to enable individually calculated risks to be used in consultations. The practical difficulties of using technological innovations across a range of clinical settings are also likely to be significant and suggest that interventions must remain simple if they are to be broadly implemented.

How do you develop and evaluate a decision aid?

There are several issues that need to be considered during the process of development and evaluation (O'Connor *et al.* 1999b). These issues are listed below and summarized in more detail in Fig. 14.3.

Steps in developing, evaluating, and disseminating a decision aid

- Assess *need*.
- Assess *feasibility*.
- Define the *objectives* of the aid.

- Identify the *framework* of decision support.
- Select the *methods of decision support* to be used in the aid.
- Select the *designs* and *measures* to evaluate the aid.
- Plan *dissemination*.

1. Is there a need for a decision aid?

As summarized in Fig. 14.3, developers need to ascertain the decision making needs of patients facing the decision and the professionals who counsel them. Developers also need to appreciate the factors that make the decision inherently difficult, for example, options with different benefit and harm profiles. Methods for needs assessment are varied and data are obtained from primary or secondary sources. It is important that needs are defined from the perspective of potential users of decision aids (both patients and professionals) as well as potential third party payers.

2. Is it feasible to develop a decision aid?

Feasibility concerns whether the aid can be developed with the available evidence and resources. The aid would then need to be delivered and updated in a timely, accessible, and acceptable manner. Evidence is needed regarding the numbers affected and their burden of illness, practice, and preference variation, and availability of aids elsewhere. Important resources include access to evidence databases, experts with external credibility, and dissemination networks. Another crucial factor is ongoing commitment to updates. Therefore, developers need to forge strong linkages with organizations such as the Cochrane Collaboration whose mandate is to summarize and update evidence.

3. What are the objectives of the decision aid?

The objectives are key to making decisions about the remaining steps of development and evaluation. They should be clear, specific, and measurable, and stated from the perspective of the user. Entwistle *et al.* (1998) illustrate the variability in opinions about which goals are desirable. Some see 'evidence-informed consumer choice' as the desired goal. This means that patients or consumers make a choice that is informed by the scientific evidence about the potential benefits and harms of the available options. It is based on the belief that we have a basic moral obligation to provide individuals with sound information as well as choice about their health care. Therefore if a person makes a choice based on adequate knowledge of options and realistic expectations of potential benefits and harms, then the desired goal has been achieved.

1. Is there a need for a decision aid?

What are the decision making needs of patients and professionals? Conduct key informant interviews, focus groups, or surveys (O'Connor AM *et al.* 2000; O'Connor AM *et al.* 1997) to elicit patients' and professionals' perceptions of: decisions perceived as important & difficult; usual roles and decision making practices; barriers & facilitators in providing/accessing decision support, potential strategies for overcoming barriers. Conduct marketing surveys regarding demand for an aid and preferred method of delivery.

What makes the decision difficult? Review systematic overviews, decision analyses, and preference studies to determine whether: benefits marginal or uncertain; risks material/uncertain; value trade-offs between benefits and risks; variation in preferences for outcomes

Are sufficient numbers affected and how are they affected? Review databases, demographic, morbidity statistics; population surveys

Is there sufficient variation in utilisation? Review practice atlases, utilisation data, practice variation studies

Are there decision aids available to meet these needs? Review published overviews, reports. Contact centres that produce aids.

2. Is it feasible to develop a decision aid?

Are there adequate resources?
Assess finances, availability of experts with credibility, networks, and commitment to ongoing update. Link to established overview & dissemination networks.

Is there enough evidence of benefits and risks to incorporate into a decision aid?
Review systematic overviews with appraisals of the quality of evidence.

How quickly is the evidence expected to change? Review ongoing trials.

Can delivery be accessible/acceptable to users? Conduct focus groups, market surveys.

3. What are the objectives of the decision aid?

Improve decision making of patients and professionals.
Improve knowledge of the clinical problem, options, outcomes, variation in patient opinions and practices.
Create realistic expectations of outcomes, consistent with available evidence.
Clarify personal values for outcomes and promote congruence between patients' values and choice.
Reduce patients' and professionals' decisional conflict (uncertainty) (O'Connor A, 1995) about the course of action to take.
Promote implementation of choices. Improve patients'/ professionals' satisfaction with decision making.
Improve outcomes of decisions.
Promote patients' continuance of preferred option. Reduce patients' distress from consequences of decision.
Improve patients' health-related quality of life. Promote informed use of resources by patients/practitioners.

4. Which framework will drive its development?

Charles *et al.* distinguish shared decision making from other decision making approaches (Charles C *et al.* 1997)
Entwistle *et al.* define evidence-informed choice; outlines different criteria for evaluation's depending on objective (Entwistle VA *et al.* 1998)
Hersey & Lohr Framework for AHCPR with a health services and informatics perspective (Hersey J *et al.* 2000)
Llewellyn-Thomas Framework has a special focus on types of preferences; placement in socio-political context (Llewellyn-Thomas, 1995)
Mulley places shared decision making in the context of outcomes research. (Mulley A, 2000)
O'Connor's Ottawa Decision Support Framework prepares professional and patient with clinical and behavioural focus (Hersey J *et al.* 2000)
Rothert *et al.* describe mutual roles of patients and professionals in decision making;focus on information and values (Rothert M and Talarczyk G, 1987)

5. Which methods will be included in the decision aid?

Patient Decision Support

1. Information about Options and Outcomes (a) content: clinical problem, options, outcomes; (b) detail in describing outcomes: define outcomes; describe physical, emotional, social impact; use narrative/scenario styles; (c) probabilities: none; numerical frequencies/ percentages (Barry *et al.* 1997; Man-Son-Hing M *et al.* 1999); graphic pie charts (Whelan TJ *et al.* 1995); 100 people qualitative (low, moderate, high); (d) tailored probabilities: not tailored; stratified by personal risk factors; (e) evidence for statements: references included/not

2. Values clarification: (a) Implicit (Barry *et al.* 1997; Whelan TJ *et al.* 1995); (b) explicit methods such as weigh scale exercise (O'Connor A *et al.* 2000); treatment trade-off task; relevance chart; decisional balance sheets ; formal utility assessments(Pauker and Pauker, 1987)

3. Information on others: none; cases of different choices (Barry *et al.* 1997; O'Connor A *et al.* 2000; Rothert ML *et al.* 1997); statistics on variation in patients' decisions or professionals' opinions

4. Coaching or guidance in deliberation, communication, and implementation: not included; steps in weighing the benefits, risks (O'Connor A *et al.* 2000; Rothert ML *et al.* 1997); steps in discussing decision with a professional; tips on managing consequences of choices.

5. Delivery: personal counselling supplemented by: generic tools; decision board; take home audio-guided workbook (O'Connor A *et al.* 2000); interactive videodisc or linear video (Barry *et al.* 1997); computer based tool; group lecture, workshop (Rothert ML *et al.* 1997)

Professional Decision Support

1. Content: scientific evidence about decision; rationale for decision aid; efficacy of decision aid; timing and use in practice; scientific references (Edwards A *et al.* 1999).

2. Delivery: manual; video; lecture; workshop; hot-line; academic detailing

Fig. 14.3 Developing and evaluating decision aids: questions and methods.

6. Which designs and measures will be used to develop and evaluate decision aid?	
Development Panel	Participants: researchers, clinicians, educators, patients, opinion leaders
	Methods: iterations of drafts, feedback, revisions, feedback etc.
Review Panels	Participants: potential users (professionals, patients who have already made decisions)
	Methods: focus groups, personal interviews, questionnaires to elicit acceptability, etc.
Pilot Studies	Participants: patients at the point of decision making
	Before/after study - baseline questionnaire, decision aid, post-test questionnaire
	Post-test only, with pre-established criteria for success (e.g. 70% knowledge test)
Trials	Participants: patients at point of decision making; professionals
	Designs: Quasi experimental, or randomized controlled trial

Criteria For Evaluation	Measurement Tools
Knowledge	Knowledge/Comprehension test
Expectations of outcomes	Probability scales (likelihood scales)
Clarity of values	Values sub-scale of Decisional Conflict Scale (O'Connor A, 1995)
Agreement between choice & values	Statistical relationship between values and choices (O'Connor A *et al.* 2000)
Realistic perceptions of others	Perceptions of % of professionals/patients choosing options; subjective norms
Decision (O'Connor A *et al.* 2000)	Choice Question (option x, option y, unsure); choice predisposition
Decisional conflict	Decisional conflict scales for patients and providers (O'Connor A, 1995)
Skill in decision making	Self-efficacy scale (Lerman *et al.* 1997), Implementation data
Satisfaction with decision making	Decision Satisfaction Inventory (Barry *et al.* 1997); Satisfaction with Decision (Holmes-Rovner M *et al.* 1996; Michie S *et al.* 1997) Satisfaction with Preparation for Decision Making (Rothert ML et al. 1997)
Acceptability	Acceptability Questionnaires (Liao L *et al.* 1996)
Use of decision aid	Utilisation data
Participation according to needs	Congruence between preferred and actual role in decision making (Elwyn GJ *et al.* 1999)
Persistence with decisions	Survey of decision over time; implementation data
Reduced distress from outcomes (Lerman *et al.* 1996)	Condition-specific symptom and side-effects distress scales; distress from risk
Health related quality of life	Generic, condition-specific, preference-based
Use of resources	Analysis of utilisation data
Costs	Cost-effectiveness model

7. How should the decision aid be disseminated?
What are potential 'adopters': attitudes toward innovation/change; knowledge, attitudes and skills to use aid; preference for shared decision making?:
Conduct focus groups, key informant interviews, environmental scans, surveys of potential users.
What are the environmental barriers & supporters? Conduct focus groups, surveys to identify the following factors:
Social: likely supporters & opposers; presence of opinion leaders as supporters; predominant belief system regarding shared decision making.
Structural: operational tools & processes, regulations, quality assurance criteria, to encourage/hinder use of aid; resources to support dissemination of aid.
Other incentives and disincentives
Will the evidence-based innovation meet expectations of target audience?
Conduct focus groups, surveys.
Which transfer strategies should be used?
Tailor strategies according to needs.
Diffusion strategies: advertisements, publications, Internet
Dissemination strategies: targeted mailings
Implementation strategies: education programmes, feedback, administrative changes
Is the aid being adopted and is it having the expected effect on outcomes?
Analyse databases, conduct quality assurance studies, surveys and implementation studies to determine whether the aid is being used by the expected audience in the expected manner and whether it is having the expected effect on health and economic outcomes and evidence-based decision making among patients/clinicians.

Fig. 14.3 continued

In contrast, others argue that evidence-informed choice is not sufficient unless it leads to other beneficial outcomes such as greater clinical effectiveness, health gain, individually appropriate resource utilization, reduced expenditures on inappropriate interventions, reduced litigation, and so on. The short-term objective of making an informed choice is therefore viewed as a means to another desirable end. Fig. 14.3 provides specific examples of potential objectives.

4. Which decision support framework will drive its development?

Depending on the objectives, several frameworks are available to guide decision aid development. Firstly, there are *prescriptive* frameworks that use decision trees and expected utility maximization principles to guide decision making (Keeney and Raiffa 1976). Developers using this framework maintain that many decisions are too complex for unaided human processing. A more 'rational,' theoretically valid approach is to:

(a) create a decision tree describing options, outcomes, and their associated probabilities;

(b) elicit the patient's utilities or values for each outcome in the tree using techniques such as the standard gamble, time trade-off, or category rating; and

(c) calculate the expected utility of each option.

The prescribed or recommended option is the one with the highest expected utility. This recommendation is often the starting point for discussion with patients about which option they prefer (Pauker and Pauker 1987; Sox 1999). These approaches are explored more fully in Chapter 10 (Elwyn *et al.*).

Secondly, there are *descriptive* frameworks that use decision trees only to structure the presentation of options (O'Connor *et al.* 2000; Llewellyn-Thomas 1995; Hersey *et al.* 2000; Sox 1999). Developers use the underlying structure of the trees to describe options, outcomes, and probabilities so that patients are better able to judge the value of the benefits versus the harms. Their presentation of information conforms more closely to usual patient education approaches in clinical practice. 'Values clarification' is simpler than utility assessment, and placed in the context of the options being considered; this will be described later in this chapter. Expected utilities are not calculated nor are options prescribed because expected utility maximization does not conform to the way people make choices. Formal utility assessments are not used because they are complex, elicited outside the context of the choice, impractical in most practice settings, and fraught with their own measurement errors that often shift recommendations. Many of the descriptive frameworks also take into account determinants of decisions beyond perceived probabilities and values, for example, stage of decision making, the influence of others, personal and external resources, characteristics of participants, and socio-political influences.

The third group of frameworks (Rothert and Talarczyk 1987; Charles *et al.* 1997) are those that describe patient and professional *transactional roles* in a clinical encounter. They classify roles between professionals and patients based on their level of mutuality and direction of exchange of information about options, outcomes, values, and control over choices. These frameworks offer some insights into how decision aids can facilitate patient participation in decision making. Many decision aids based on these frameworks also stress the need to take into account patients' preferences for participation in decision making so that counselling can be tailored according to the preferred role (Elwyn *et al.* 1999).

5. Which methods should be included in the decision aid?

The methods and sequencing of information in the aid depend on the frameworks driving its development. Those using a descriptive framework usually start by presenting the clinical condition, the options, the outcomes, and the probabilities of outcomes. Values for outcomes are elicited implicitly or explicitly. Decision aids may also include information on others' decision making and guidance or coaching in deliberation, communication, and implementation. Those using a prescriptive framework need to decide how much of the tree to show to the patients at the start and in what sequence. Thus according to the objectives and framework, it may be desirable to show the whole tree or just the outcomes. Similarly, the sequence might be to elicit preferences for outcomes first, then calculate expected utility, show the rest of the tree, and discuss patient views, though this could vary.

Other important issues are the method of delivering decision support and the amount of preparation provided to the patient and the professional. The specific decision support methods, content, and delivery methods depend not only on the framework but also on the nature of the decision, the needs of the users, feasibility constraints, and the objectives of the decision aid. The 'essential content' in decision aids is still a matter of debate. Each of the content issues is discussed below.

Information about clinical condition, options, and outcomes Most decision aids include a description of the clinical situation that has stimulated the need to consider certain options and outcomes. Patients need to know about the conditions or diseases they face, common manifestations, and complications. Health care options are laid out and then usually described in detail, for example, what the treatment option is, how it is delivered, and how the patient is involved in its use.

An important hallmark of decision aids, no matter what the framework, is a detailed description of the outcomes of each option so that users can understand what it is like to experience such an outcome. This is important because people will often underestimate the likelihood of an option that they cannot imagine or identify with. Moreover, people cannot judge the value of an outcome that is unfamiliar. In many decision aids, the functional impact of the outcome is described (such as how the person can expect to respond physically, emotionally, and socially). The evidence to support the description of outcomes can be found in quality of life studies. In the absence of quality of life data, a panel of experienced patients consumer-representatives and professionals can be helpful in describing outcomes. Some decision aids that are delivered by video include interviews of patients describing what it is like to experience the 'outcomes'. The presentation of experiences and outcomes to patients is a matter of intense research interest in the UK. (DIPEX project http://www.dphpc.ox.ac.uk/primarycare/research/medical_communications/dipex/) and the US Agency for Health care Research and Quality (the 'People Like Me' project).

Presenting probabilities of outcomes One of the consistent benefits of decision aids is to create realistic expectations of outcomes. This is achieved by presenting probabilistic information about the likelihood of benefits and harms. Patients who have unrealistic expectations (for example, overestimating the benefits and underestimating the risks) can be helped with this information. The many issues in presenting risk information are summarized in Chapter 9 (Edwards and Bastian) and a recent monograph of the National Cancer Institute, USA (Journal of the National Cancer Institute Monograph-Risk Communication in Cancer, Number 25 1999).

Values clarification exercises Patients clarify their values in two possible ways. First the descriptions of outcomes provide vicarious experience from which to judge their value. Second, and more specifically, some decision aids ask patients to consider explicitly the personal importance of each potential benefit and harm.

In those that use explicit valuing approaches, some handle probabilities and values for outcomes separately, asking patients to value each outcome via formal utility assessments. These are then combined with the associated probabilities using expected utility decision analysis (Dowie 1996*a* & 1996*b*). Others ask patients to value treatments, by considering both probabilities and values together, using probability trade-off tasks, relevance charts, and 'weigh scale' exercises. The purposes of these valuing exercises are to structure and provide insight into how values affect personal decision making about options and to communicate their values to others.

For example, the Ottawa decision aids use 'weigh scales' in which patients are presented with the potential benefits and harms of the options. They are then asked to add any other positive or negative factors that are important to them, check or shade each item in the weigh scale to indicate how important they are to them in the decision, and finally to indicate their predisposition or leaning toward the options (see Figs 14.2 and 14.4). At a

A) list 'other benefits' and 'other concerns' in the boxes below

B) shade the benefits and risks that are most important to you

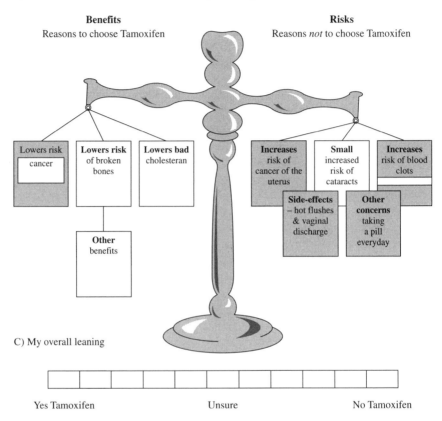

Fig. 14.4 Example of values clarification exercise using 'weigh scale' depicting importance a woman high risk for breast cancer places on tamoxifen outcomes.

glance, professionals and family members involved in the decision are able to appreciate and acknowledge what is relevant to the patient in deliberating about the options.

Information about others' opinions Whether decision aids should include information about others is still open for debate. Some developers of decision aids include no examples in order to remain neutral. Others provide balanced information on different points of view. Their rationale is that some patients like to learn from the examples of others. Often, it is easier to recognize opinions that correspond to your own (and those that do not) than to try formulating them from scratch. One survey of the public's decision making needs (O'Connor 2000) indicated that 50% of respondents obtained information about how others make choices but only 21% thought it was essential for decision making.

Guidance and coaching in decision making and communication Guidance and coaching has been found to be helpful in promoting better coping strategies, health practices, and outcomes (O'Connor *et al.* 1999a). Whether it is a helpful element in decision aids is still under investigation. Some decision aids include them whereas others do not.

Methods of delivering decision aids Decision aids can be delivered in various forms: decision boards, interactive videodiscs, personal computers, audiotapes, audio-guided workbooks, pamphlets, and group presentations. The method used depends on the preferences of the users and the resources and expertise of the developers. The efficacy of different methods is under active investigation, though it is perhaps likely that each will have its place in different situations. Most developers now use more than one delivery method, and many are moving toward Web-based delivery strategies. Having a choice of methods available to the professional or patient may make the decision aid more flexible and helpful for an individual's needs (Edwards *et al.* 1998). Consequently the application of the decision aid in practice may be greater (Edwards and Elwyn 2001; Street *et al.* 1998).

Preparing the professional There are several methods of preparing the professional including with manuals, videos, educational workshops, and so on. The content of these materials usually include scientific information on the decision and information on how to use the decision aid in practice (Edwards *et al.* 1999). This is an underdeveloped area of research, however, and there is increasing attention now among developers of decision aids as to how professionals can be encouraged to use and apply the aids in practice.

6. Which designs and measures should be used to develop and evaluate the aid?

Development and evaluation depend on the objectives of the decision aid in question. Developers need to decide on the sampling and design architecture, the criteria for evaluation, and the measurement tools. There is still considerable debate on the criteria for evaluation of decision aids. The range of scales which have been used to evaluate decision aids are summarized in Fig. 14.3. The issues about what constitutes 'effectiveness' and the types of outcomes which should be assessed have been discussed in Chapter 9 (Edwards and Bastian). There are doubts about whether the outcomes addressed in the existing literature are fully consistent with the outcomes of greatest importance to patients (Edwards *et al.* 2000*b*; Edwards and Elwyn 1999). However, some evidence of consensus in opinions is emerging among decision scientists, professionals, and patients and consumer-representatives (O'Connor *et al.* 1999*b*; O'Connor *et al.* 2000). There is most agreement that the goal is to achieve informed decisions that are compatible with personal values.

Evaluating whether this has been achieved should therefore be the focus of outcome assessment in these cases. There is also some consensus that further important goals are for patients to be satisfied with the decision making process and able to implement their choices. These should also form part of the evaluation of decision aids. If decision aids are to be used widely in health care, outcomes of interest to third party payers will need to be addressed. In our experience, improved decision making is not sufficient to convince third party payers that these aids should be adopted. Funders want to see their impact on choices, adherence to choices, appropriate use of resources, and costs.

Methodological problems   Most randomized clinical trials of decision aids are fraught with methodological difficulties. They cannot be double-blind. Those that randomize patients rather than professionals have contamination problems that narrow the differences that will be detected. Estimates of effects are therefore likely to be conservative. Those that randomize professionals need to be very large, because of cluster sampling. Moreover, they may have selection biases because clinicians, knowing their assignment, can be more or less enthusiastic about recruiting patients or they recruit different types of patients to the study. Despite the researchers' best efforts, it is very difficult in a real world setting to present the decision aid at the appropriate time to those patients who are eligible to consider all of the options in the aid. Furthermore, efficacious interventions may have no impact if either patients or professionals, or both, are extremely polarized towards one of the options at baseline. When post-intervention measures are administered after the consequences of the choice are known, it is very difficult to avoid having the outcome colour their evaluation of satisfaction with the decision making process and the decision.

Future clinical trials should:

◆ examine the impact of decision aids on a broader range of decisions with a more comprehensive range of patient and professional outcomes;

◆ select patients who are at the point of decision making for whom the choices in the aid are relevant (though in practice this is difficult to capture);

◆ measure patients' and professionals' baseline predispositions towards the choices;

- have sample sizes large enough to detect clinically meaningful differences in decisions among the undecided subgroup of patients;

- measure patients' perceptions of professionals' opinions;

- have a usual care arm and describe clearly what usual care comprises; and

- describe clearly what was in the decision aid and how it was used in the diagnostic/treatment trajectory.

There are also several methodological challenges associated with evaluating the incremental efficacy of various elements in decision aids in controlled situations or pragmatic trials. Most studies are under-powered to detect clinically important differences between aids with and without the elements. Many studies have healthy participants whose responses may not be generalizable to patients actually faced with the options. Actual patients have more to gain or lose, and they use more than the information in the aid to arrive at decisions. Despite the wide variation in the complexity and cost of decision aids, little attention has been paid to this issue. Therefore, evaluation of decision aids should address the elements with most potential to influence decisions, and those in which baseline variation is greatest. It is also important to evaluate those elements which contribute significantly to the cost, complexity, and time required to administer decision aids. Moreover, clinically important differences should be defined a priority and studies should be adequately powered. Finally, efforts should be made to include patients actually faced with the decisions and cost-effectiveness should be examined.

If such requirements are met in future evaluations of decision aids, this will improve the quality of the evidence available. It will then be possible to judge the benefits or otherwise of these innovations and to encourage professionals and patients alike to use them more widely.

7. How should the decision aid be disseminated?

Dissemination involves the targeted distribution and promotion of the use of the decision aid. Although there may be a growing body of evidence indicating the benefits of decision aids, there is likewise a realization developing that these aids are not being taken up readily in practice, particularly by professionals. The reasons for this are likely to be multiple. Some will be shared with any innovation and the delay in transferring research findings into routine clinical practice (Haines and Jones 1994). As shown in Fig. 14.3, five key elements of research transfer and use are recognized and can be addressed: potential adopters; practice environment; the evidence-based innovation (e.g. the decision aid); strategies for transferring the evidence into practice; evidence adoption, and outcomes. These elements should be systematically monitored prior to, during, and following any research transfer efforts in order to address potential obstacles and provide direction for continuing transfer strategies. Although dissemination is identified as a final step, it should be addressed early in the development process so that the aid is acceptable to potential users and has a greater potential for adoption. Therefore, dissemination questions can be posed during the needs and feasibility assessment phases. Development and review panels can include potential users (professionals and patients) and partners who may assist with dissemination (consumer groups, health professional organizations, disease foundations, and public education agencies).

But some difficulties, which restrict wider implementation of decision aids, are specific to the content and context of using them. The innovations may be highly efficacious, but not found to be effective in routine practice. Reasons for this include the complexity and time required to work through some decision aids. A further reason is that the clinical decisions and choices of real life often may not fit exactly into the choices and information provided by decision aids. Thus although a professional may be aware of the decision aid as a resource, they may remain reluctant to use it (or make it available to the patient) if it is not thought to fit the individual clinical situation. Complexity of decision aids can be addressed with a view to producing simpler (and quicker) aids (Elwyn 2000). Whether these are then implemented more widely requires evaluation. There remains also a challenge for the developers of decision aids to address the need for flexibility to the individual patient's situation (Edwards *et al.* 1998; Hux and Naylor 1995; Liao *et al.* 1996). Dissemination may be less problematic if the aids more closely meet the needs of professionals in routine clinical practice.

Conclusion

In this chapter we have defined patient decision aids, their rationale, their efficacy, and issues in their development, evaluation, and dissemination. We have illustrated how the process has been applied, particularly by reference to some of the Ottawa aids. From the wider literature on decision aids it is clear that initial progress has been made and there is a large body of evidence about their benefits in the research setting. Study populations may be highly selected though. The indications are that implementation of decision aids in routine practice (away from the realms of the enthusiasts) is perhaps limited. Whilst some of the reasons for this are generic to the transfer of any research into practice, some more specific issues are also relevant. Developers of decision aids must continue to refine their methods and content. Meeting the needs of the individual patient with a package developed for many remains a challenge. However, if these needs continue to be addressed in developing future aids then there is great potential for the benefits currently shown in research to be available to patients across a wide range of settings and for a variety of health care choices. Decision aids build on the conceptual frameworks of shared decision making and seek to implement effective risk communication and values clarification. As such they offer a very practical way in which evidence-based patient choice can be facilitated.

References

Barry MJ, Cherkin DC, Chang Y, Fowler F and Skates S (1997). A randomized trial of a multimedia shared decision making programme for men facing a treatment decision for benign prostatic hypertrophy. *Disease Management and Clinical Outcomes* **1**: 5–14.

Bernstein SJ, Skarupski KA, Grayson CE, Starling M, Bates ER and Eagle KA (1998). A randomized controlled trial of information-giving to patients referred for coronary angiography: effects on outcomes of care. *Health Expectations* **1**: 50–61.

Charles C, Gafni A and Whelan T (1997). Shared decision making in the medical encounter: what does it mean? (Or it takes at least two to tango). *Social Science and Medicine* **44**: 681–92.

Davison BJ and Degner LF (1997). Empowerment of men newly diagnosed with prostate cancer. *Cancer Nursing* **20**: 187–96.

Dowie J (1996*a*). Evidence-based, cost-effective and prefernce driven medicine: decision analysis-based medical decision making is a pre-requisite. *Journal of Health Services Research and Policy* **1**: 104–13.

Dowie J (1996*b*). The research practice gap and the role of decision analysis in closing it. *Health Care Analysis* **4**: 5–18.

Eddy D (1992). *A manual for assessing health practices and designing practice policies: the explicit approach.* Philadelphia, American College of Physicians.

Edwards A, Matthews EJ, Pill RM and Bloor M (1998). Communication about risk: the responses of primary care professionals to standardizing the language of risk and communication tools. *Family Practice* **15**: 301–7.

Edwards A and Elwyn GJ (1999). How should 'effectiveness' of risk communication to aid patients' decisions be judged? A review of the literature. *Medical Decision Making* **19**: 428–34.

Edwards A and Elwyn G (2001). How well do patients understand the concept of risk? Lessons for clinical risk communication. Medical Research Council Health Services Research Collaboration Workshop Proceedings No 1. Medical Research Council, Bristol. In press.

Edwards A, Elwyn GJ and Gwyn R (1999). General practice registrar responses to the use of different risk communication tools in simulated consultations: a focus group study. *British Medical Journal* **319**: 749–52.

Edwards A, Hood K, Matthews EJ, Russell D, Russell IT, Barker J, *et al.* (2000*a*). The effectiveness of one-to-one risk communication interventions in health care: a systematic review. *Medical Decision Making* **20**: 290–297.

Edwards A, Elwyn GJ, Smith C, Williams S and Thornton H (2001). Consumers' views of quality in the consultation and their relevance to 'shared decision making' approaches. *Health Expectations*. In press.

Elwyn GJ (2000). Explaining risks to patients. *British Journal of General Practice* **50**: 342–3.

Elwyn GJ, Edwards A and Kinnersley P (1999). Shared decision making in primary care: the neglected second half of the consultation. *British Journal of General Practice* **49**: 477–82.

Entwistle VA, Sheldon T, Sowden A and Watts IS (1998). Evidence-informed Patient Choice. *International Journal of Assessment in Health Care* **14**: 2.

Haines A and Jones R (1994). Implementing findings of research. *British Medical Journal* **308**: 1488–92.

Hersey J, Matheson J and Lohr K (2000). Consumer health informatics and patient decision making. 98-N001, Research Triangle Institute, Agency for Health Care Policy and Research.

Holmes-Rovner M, Kroll J, Rovner D, Schmitt N, Rothert ML, Padonu G, *et al.* (1999). Patient decision support intervention: increased consistency with decision analytic models. *Medical Care* **37**: 270–84.

Holmes-Rovner M, Kroll J, Schmitt N, Rovner D, Breer L, Rothert ML, *et al.* (1996). Patient satisfaction with health care decisions: the satisfaction with decision scale. *Medical Decision Making* **16**: 58–64.

Hux JE and Naylor CD (1995). Communicating the benefits of chronic preventive therapy: does the format of efficacy data determine patients' acceptance of treatment? *Medical Decision Making* **15**: 152–7.

Kassirer JP (1994). Incorporating patients' preferences into medical decisions. *New England Journal of Medicine* **330**: 1895–6.

Keeney R and Raiffa H (1976). *Decisions with multiple objectives: preferences and value trade-offs*. New York, John Wiley and Sons.

Lerman C, Biesecker B, Benkendorf JL, Kerner J, Gomez-Caminero A, Hughes C and Reed MM (1997). Controlled trial of pretest education approaches to enhance informed decision making for BRCA1 gene testing. *Journal of the National Cancer Institute* **89**: 148–57.

Liao L, Jollis JG, DeLong ER, Peterson ED, Morris KG and Mark DB (1996). Impact of an interactive video on decision making of patients with ischaemic heart disease. *Journal of General Internal Medicine* **11**: 373–6.

Llewellyn-Thomas, HA (1995). Patients' health care decision making: a framework for descriptive and experimental investigations. *Medical Decision Making* **15**: 101–6.

Man-Son-Hing M, Laupacis A, O'Connor AM, Biggs J, Drake E, Yetisir E, *et al.* (1999). A randomized controlled trial of a decision aid for patients with atrial fibrillation. *Journal of the American Medical Association* **282**: 737–43.

Michie S, Smith D, McClennan A and Marteau TM (1997). Patient decision making: an evaluation of two different methods of presenting information about a screening test. *British Journal of Health Psychology* **2**: 317–26.

Molenaar S, Sprangers MAG, Postma-Shuit FCE, Rutgers EJT, Noorlander and DeHaes H (2000). Feasibility and effects of decision aids. *Medical Decision Making* **20**: 112–27.

Mulley A (2000). Outcomes research: implications for policy and practice. In: *Outcomes in clinical practice* (ed. R Smith and T Delamothe). London, BMJ Publishing Group.

O'Connor AM (1995). Validation of a decisional conflict scale. *Medical Decision Making* **15**: 25–30.

O'Connor AM, Llewellyn-Thomas HA, Sawka C, Pinfold S, To T and Harrison D (1997). Physicians' opinions about decision aids for patients considering systemic adjuvant therapy for axillary-node negative breast cancer. *Patient Education and Counseling* **30**: 143–53.

O'Connor AM, Tugwell P, Wells GA, Elmslie T, Jolly E, Hollingsworth G, *et al.* (1998). Randomized trial of a portable, self-administered decision aid for postmenopausal women considering long-term hormone therapy. *Medical Decision Making* **18**: 295–303.

O'Connor AM, Fiset V, Rosto A, Tetroe J, Entwhistle V, Llewellyn-Thomas H, *et al.* (1999*a*). Decision aids for people facing health treatment or screening decisions [protocol for a Cochrane Review]. *Cochrane Library*. Oxford, Update Software.

O'Connor AM, Rosto A, Fiset V, Tetroe J, Entwhistle VA, Llewellyn-Thomas HA, *et al.* (1999*b*). Decision aids for patients facing health treatment or screening decisions: systematic review. *British Medical Journal* **319**: 731–4.

O'Connor AM, Fiset V, DeGrasse C, Graham I, Evans W, Stacey D, *et al.* (1999*c*). Decision aids for patients considering health care options: evidence of efficacy and policy implications. *Journal of the National Cancer Institute* Monograph No 25, 67–80.

O'Connor AM, Tugwell P, Wells GA, Elmslie T, Jolly E, Hollingworth G, *et al.* (2000). A decision aid for women considering hormone replacement therapy after menopause: decision support framework and evaluation. *Patient Education and Counseling* **33**: 267–79.

O'Connor AM (2000). National survey of Canadians' health care decision making needs. ISHTAC Conference 2000.

Pauker SP and Pauker SG (1987). The amniocentesis decision: ten years of decision analytic experience. *Birth Defects: Original Article Series* **23**: 151–69.

Rothert M and Talarczyk G (1987). Patient compliance and the decision making process of clinicians and patients. *Journal of Compliance in Health Care* **2**: 55–71.

Rothert ML, Holmes-Rovner M, Rovner D, Kroll J, Breer L, Talarczyk G, *et al.* (1997). An educational intervention as decision support for menopausal women. *Research in Nursing and Health* **20**: 377–87.

Sawka CA, Goel V, Mahut CA, Taylor GA, Thiel EC, O'Connor AM, *et al.* (1998). Development of a patient decision aid for choice of surgical treatment for breast cancer. *Health Expectations* **1**: 23–36.

Sox H (1999). What is a good decision? *Effective Clinical Practice* **2**: 185–200.

Street RL, van Order A, Bramson R and Manning T (1998). Preconsultation education promoting breast cancer screening: does the choice of media make a difference? *Journal of Cancer Education* **13**: 152–61.

Street RL, Voigt B, Geyer C, Manning T and Swanson GP (1995). Increasing patient involvement in choosing treatment for early breast cancer. *Cancer* **76**: 2275–85.

Whelan TJ, Levine M, Gafni A, Lukka H, Mohide EA, Patel M, *et al.* (1995). Breast irradiation post-lumpectomy: development and evaluation of a decision instrument. *Journal of Clinical Oncology* **13**: 847–53.

Section 5
The next and possible future developments

15 Education and training of health care professionals

Angela Towle and William Godolphin

Hope (1996) defines the focus of evidence-based patient choice (EBPC) as the use of evidence-based information to help people make choices when they, or those close to them, are in need of health care. Neither he, nor other writers, have identified the knowledge, skills, and attitudes which health professionals require in order to practice EBPC nor described the ways in which EBPC can be implemented within the doctor–patient encounter. Our work has been based on the concept of informed shared decision making. We believe there are many similarities in terms of the knowledge, skills, and attitudes needed for both. We will therefore use our work on shared decision making as a model for exploring the teaching and learning of EBPC, the problems likely to be encountered, and possible solutions. In this chapter we focus particularly on the education and training of physicians. However, our preliminary work with dentists, pharmacists, physiotherapists, and occupational therapists suggests that the competences required for physicians are generalizable to other health care professionals.

This chapter looks first at the knowledge, skills, and attitudes required for EBPC and the gap between this 'ideal' and current practice. We will discuss the types of training and education that are needed to bridge this gap, and how these might be implemented. Certain barriers to this implementation are already recognized and we will describe these as well as the strategies which are likely to overcome them.

Defining the knowledge, skills, and attitudes of professionals for evidence-based patient choice models of care

The practice of EBPC is not just a matter of having positive attitudes towards patient choice and involvement in decision making. It requires good knowledge of treatment options, critical appraisal skills, and sophisticated communication skills, such as an ability to elicit patients' preferences, present evidence-based choices, and negotiate conflict. These knowledge, skills, and attitudes need to be explicitly taught throughout the continuum of medical education, beginning in medical school and continuing through postgraduate training and into continuing medical education (CME).

The first step in planning educational programmes is to define the competences (knowledge, skills, and attitudes) necessary to practice EBPC. That is, what is it that professionals need to be able to do? Based on the literature, interviews, and focus groups, we have defined a set of competences for informed shared decision making (ISDM) (Towle and Godolphin, 1999) shown in Table 15.1. An alternative framework is described in Chapter 8 (Elwyn and Charles).

In order to develop specific educational programmes, the competences need to be broken down further to define the specific knowledge, skill, and attitudinal components. For example, competency 4, which is not specific to EBPC but is necessary for any successful consultation, is at the heart of patient-centred care (finding common ground). An extensive set of educational objectives have been defined to achieve this component (Stewart 1995).

Table 15.1 'Informed shared decision making' competences for physicians

1. Develop a partnership with the patient.
2. Establish or review the patient's preferences for information (e.g. amount, format).
3. Establish or review the patient's preferences for role in decision making (e.g. risk taking; degree of involvement of self and others), and the existence/nature/degree of decisional conflict. (Decisional conflict is a state of uncertainty about the course of action to take.)
4. Ascertain and respond to patient's ideas, concerns and expectations (e.g. about disease management options).
5. Identify choices (including ideas and information patient may have) and evaluate the research evidence in relation to the individual patient.
6. Present (or direct to) evidence taking into account 2 and 3 above, framing effects, etc. and help patient to reflect upon and assess the impact of alternative decisions vis-à-vis his/her values and lifestyles. (Framing effects are said to occur when the presentation of the same information in different formats changes the decisions that people make.)
7. Make or negotiate a decision in partnership and resolve conflict.
8. Agree upon an action plan and complete arrangements for follow-up.

Informed shared decision making may also:
   Involve a team of health professionals;
   Involve significant others (partners, family);
   Differ across cultural, social, and age groups.

As another example, Sackett *et al.* (1997) identified the 5-stage process of evidence-based medicine (EBM) which is relevant to competency 5:

♦   Formulate for each chosen clinical problem an answerable question;

♦   Search, with maximum efficiency, the medical literature and other sources of information pertaining to that question;

♦   Assess the validity (closeness to the truth) and usefulness (relevance to the problem) of the evidence identified;

♦   Manage the patient accordingly;

♦   Evaluate one's own performance.

So a number of goals for health care practice and EBPC in particular are beginning to come together. A range of tasks and skills are required for EBPC to become a reality. We will now look at how far off these are from current practice.

The gap between 'ideal' and current practice of EBPC

Real needs: the evidence

There is a wealth of evidence that doctors and patients do not communicate well. In relation to EBPC, where good communication is fundamental, problems of information sharing are of special importance. It is well documented that physicians do not provide sufficient information: they overestimate what they give; they give less than patients want; they are not good judges of patients' needs. The scale of the problem can be illustrated by three well conducted studies.

Waitzkin (1985) analysed 336 encounters (34 physicians) in diverse practices in the USA. In encounters that averaged 16.5 minutes, doctors spent an average of 1.3 minutes (9% of total interaction time; range 0 to 11.6 minutes) in information giving; patients spent an average of 8 seconds (1%; range 0 to 97 seconds) in questioning behaviour. Doctors overestimated the amount of time giving information by a mean of 7.6 minutes. In 65% of encounters physicians underestimated the patient's desire for information.

Makoul *et al.* (1995) studied communication and decision making about prescribing medications in 271 consultations between 36 family doctors and their patients in Oxford, UK. Physicians overestimated the extent to which they accomplished specific consultation tasks: eliciting the patient's opinion about the prescribed medication; discussing the patient's ability to follow the treatment plan; discussing risks of the medication. Doctors estimated that they accomplished these three tasks in 49, 49, and 42% of the consultations respectively. Video tape analysis showed actual accomplishment occurred in

34, 8, and 3%. Of particular relevance to EBPC is the fact that side-effects, precautions, and risks were not mentioned by either physician or patient in 68% of interactions. Moreover, 23% of patients left the consultation with an 'illusion of competence' – that the physician had fully explained the risks of the prescribed medication when the video analysis had shown no mention of side-effects, precautions, or risks.

Braddock *et al.* (1999) analysed audio tapes of 1057 consultations (with primary care physicians and surgeons) in the USA. Only 9% met the criteria of informed decision making as defined by the authors. Among the elements of informed decision making, discussion of the nature of the intervention occurred most frequently (71%) and assessment of patient understanding least frequently (1.5%). There was seldom elicitation of the patients' preferences (21%), or discussion of alternatives (11%), pros and cons (8%), the patients' role in decision making (6%), or uncertainties associated with the decision (2%). Basic decisions (e.g. laboratory tests) were most often 'completely informed' (17%), while no intermediate (e.g. new medication) decisions and only one (0.5%) complex decision (e.g. procedure) was completely informed.

A competence gap can also be identified when EBPC skills other than communication skills are examined. For example, a survey of 311 family doctors in Australia by Young and Ward (1999) found that 22% were aware of the Cochrane Library, although only 6% had access to it and 4% had ever used it. A survey by McColl *et al.* (1998) of British family doctors found that 40% knew of the Cochrane Databases, but only 5% made use of them; the most popular sources of evidence-based information (Effective Health Care Bulletins) were only used by 28%. McAlister *et al.* (1999) found that 11% of 294 Canadian general internists reported always using EBM in their clinical practice and 59% used it often. However, only a minority used EBM-related information sources such as primary research studies (45%), clinical practice guidelines (27%), or Cochrane Collaboration Reviews (5%) on a regular basis. Fewer than half of respondents were confident in the basic skills of EBM such as conducting a literature search (46%) or evaluating the methodology of published studies (34%).

Perceived needs: educational priorities

Are these performance gaps recognized as important by practising physicians? A survey of 1248 family physicians in British Columbia by Lirenman (1996) showed the top five educational topics were: gynaecological problems, chronic back pain, hypertension, ischaemic heart disease, and headaches. The only problem topic on the list which was not a specific disease or condition was 'Dealing with difficult patients' which was ranked 13th on the list. However this item only appeared on the city practice lists (ranked 7th) and was not mentioned by family doctors in regional or rural practice. None of the items of relevance to EBPC, such as critical appraisal, assessment of therapeutic interventions, understanding, and avoiding sources of bias appeared on any of the lists of top 12 or 15 topics. In the study by McAlister *et al.* (1999) quoted above, respondents demonstrated a 'high level of interest in further education' about EBM skills.

Hulsman *et al.* (1999), in a review of communication skills training programmes for experienced physicians, noted that recruitment was generally of the order of 16–20% although recruitment of residents for such programmes approached 100%. From our own experience we agree with their conclusion that practising professionals are reluctant to partici- pate in communication skills training and are resistant to the suggestion that they have deficiencies. In order to get around this problem we devised a different kind of needs assessment to try to identify challenges in doctor–patient communication related to involvement of patients in decision making.

In 1999, we surveyed 285 family practice preceptors of medical students in British Columbia, all of whom have a vested interest in teaching good communication skills by example to medical students. Physicians were asked to rate on a scale of 1 to 5 the frequency and degree of challenge of each of nine problem scenarios requiring practice of shared decision making competences. The most challenging problem (mean score of 3.0) and frequent (3.5) problem identified was 'Dealing with a patient who wants something (e.g. test, prescription, or referral) you do not think is appropriate or necessary.' The second most challenging (3.0) was 'Handling a situation in which the patient is accompanied by a significant other (e.g. spouse, parent) and they interfere with your ability to identify the problem or discuss treatment.' Other difficult situations of relevance to EBPC were: 'Responding to a patient who wants to try an alternative or complementary therapy about which you have major concerns' and 'Responding to a patient who has lots of information' (e.g. from books, the Internet, friends) but is unable to assess its quality. The problems that the preceptors found most challenging were those that involved negotiating a decision and resolving conflict.

The needs identified here could often be addressed by communication approaches which are based on the shared decision making (and by extrap- olation also EBPC) competences. Although professionals may not often volunteer for such training they are identifying the difficulties for which such training is developed. It may almost be simply a marketing exercise of ensuring that professionals are aware that such help is available. There may also be an issue of how to reassure potential participants in such training about the process. We will now look at the nature and requirements of training in this area.

The education and training needed to support EBPC

An approach to educational design: the PRECEDE framework

Educational interventions are designed to bring about a change in the behaviour of the learner. A useful framework which has been used to guide the development and implementation of educational programmes, particularly for postgraduates, is the PRECEDE model (Green *et al.* 1980). The model describes three categories of factors which affect an individual's ability to change behaviour in response to education:

- *Predisposing factors* are those which predispose an individual to act in a certain way. These are generally personal factors and include such areas as knowledge, attitudes, perceptions, beliefs, etc.

- *Enabling factors* are those which enable a behaviour to occur. Even in the presence of appropriate knowledge and attitudes, behaviour may not change in the absence of certain skills or of access to and availability of resources.

- *Reinforcing factors* are those which determine whether a behaviour will continue and include things like the patient's or client's response and the attitudes of other health professionals.

It is through the interaction of these factors that the ability to effect and maintain change is determined.

Applying this model to education and training to support EBPC, it is possible to identify a set of predisposing, enabling, and reinforcing factors at each of the three levels of medical education (undergraduate, postgraduate, and continuing education). Some of these factors guide the development of educational interventions appropriate for each stage of professional development; others are important for implementation and putting learning into practice. These are laid out in Table 15.2 and we will now explore each of these three levels, with particular reference to the medical curriculum.

Undergraduate medical education

Medical students are not in a position to make independent management decisions or put EBPC into practice. At this stage they need to be predisposed to EBPC and to acquire the building blocks for later practice.

In terms of predisposing knowledge, the building blocks would include a knowledge of ethics and law relating to informed consent; a knowledge of the research on doctor–patient communication and the rationale for good communication skills; and importance of evidence-based treatment choices for common conditions. Skills would include basic communication skills, as for example listed in the Cambridge-Calgary checklist (Kurtz and Silverman

Table 15.2 Evidence-based patient choice: education and training of physicians

	Predisposing	Enabling	Reinforcing
Undergraduate (UG)	Development of attitudes (patient-centred care; shared decision making) Evidence about professional–patient communication (e.g. effect on outcomes)	Formal teaching – Evidence-based Medicine – Use of decision aids – Ethics (basis of informed choice) – Basic communication skills	Evaluation of relevant knowledge, skills and attitudes Consistent and cumulative messages Observation of influential role models Primary care experiences in clinical years
Postgraduate (PG)	Predisposed attitudes from undergraduate training Supportive culture of PG training Requirement for PG examinations	Formal teaching/skills development Self-assessment, e.g. through video review Availability of patient information or decision aids	Feedback from preceptors Evaluation of practice in postgraduate exams
Continuing Medical Education (CME)	Perceived need Anticipated preceptorship Recertification or accreditation CME credits Peer pressure Challenging self-perceptions (e.g. video review) Evidence on professional–patient communication Individual feedback Media profile for EBPC Influential opinion leaders	Formal CME workshops/activities Peer discussion Self-learning packages Working environment that supports EBPC Availability of good quality patient infor-mation or decision aids	Actual evaluation of performance Preceptorship Feedback from patients Personal satisfaction

1996), and skills of evidence-based medicine such as literature searching and critical appraisal (Sackett *et al.* 1997). With respect to attitudes, although medical students generally come into medical school predisposed towards involving patients in decision making (since for many students this is what they would want for themselves), care needs to be taken to ensure that these attitudes are promoted and maintained as students become professionalized into medicine (see below).

Postgraduate education

This is the stage at which EBPC can reasonably be put into practice. At the present time it is unlikely that trainees will have sufficiently acquired the prerequisites during their undergraduate course. For example, Elwyn *et al.* (1999a) found that registrars in general practice in Wales reported not having been trained in the skills required to involve patients in clinical decisions (although all had previously received 'training in communication skills').

For those postgraduates not already predisposed, it will require a new way of thinking about their relationships with patients. It will also involve some advanced communication skills such as explaining risk, negotiation, and conflict resolution. Educational programmes will probably need to include:

- ◆ a rationale for EBPC (based on ethics and law, evidence for improved outcomes, and so on);
- ◆ a conceptual framework for approaching EBPC (such as the list of competences) and an opportunity to discuss the ideas;
- ◆ a demonstration of what it looks like in practice; and
- ◆ an opportunity to try it and get feedback from patients.

Continuing medical education (CME)

CME is the last and perhaps most complex phase of the medical education continuum. It is distinct from undergraduate and postgraduate education in many ways, perhaps the most important of which is the necessity to determine learning needs. From a review of 50 randomized controlled trials of CME interventions, Davis *et al.* (1992) concluded that CME is more effective when it incorporates practice-based enabling and reinforcing strategies. Adequate assessment of physicians' needs leads to increased potential for change in physician behaviour. A variety of methods have been described for assessing these needs (Laxdal 1982). The commonest method of planning CME courses is subjective estimates by physicians. However, as indicated earlier, physicians' self-perceived needs may not coincide with real needs and are often better characterized as 'wants'. Response rates to questionnaire surveys are often below 50% which raises questions of how representative the results are and whether those who need CME the most in fact respond at all. Other methods, for example the use of standardized patients as described by Davis *et al.* (1997), offer a more promising approach for a needs assessment for EBPC, but are expensive and not practical other than in a research context.

Only physicians who have recently graduated or completed specialist training will have had any exposure to the kinds of predisposing and enabling factors for EBPC, so most practising physicians could benefit from all of the 'curriculum items' listed above. For those who have already mastered the basics, the focus of CME might be dealing with the more challenging situations in practice, such as those identified in our needs assessment survey earlier. The challenge is to convince physicians that learning skills for EBPC is relevant and useful in helping them to solve important problems in their practice.

Ideas for the teaching and assessment of competences for EBPC

Medical ethics

Fox *et al.* (1995) described the goals, methods, and trends in undergraduate medical ethics education in the USA during its 25-year history, with examples of courses and curricula, including a selected resource list. Johnson *et al.* (1992) described a unit on informed consent consisting of a pre-test, post-test, a lecture, readings, small group discussions, a model video-taped interview, and the students' video-taped interviews with one or two simulated patients. In the interviews students were most successful in establishing rapport and engaging the patients in discussion of treatment alternatives, and were less successful in perceiving the patients as unique individuals and in dealing with situations that involved conflict or confrontation. Hope *et al.* (1996) described a course which provides integrated training in ethics, medical law, and communication skills successfully implemented throughout the three years of the clinical course at Oxford, UK.

Communication skills

A useful resource book for curriculum development, teaching, and evaluation of communication skills in medicine is by Kurtz *et al.* (1998); the companion volume by Silverman *et al.* (1998) is a good summary of the evidence underpinning these communication skills. For quick reference the paper by McManus *et al.* (1993) is useful. The paper by Kurtz *et al.* (1999) contains a useful compilation of resources available for communication skills training. For a comprehensive review and comparison of the assessment instruments used to evaluate professional–patient interaction over the past decade, the paper by Boon and Stewart (1998) is recommended.

Hulsman *et al.* (1999) review the evaluation studies of communication skills training programmes for clinically experienced physicians (postgraduate and CME). Two interesting models of effective communication skills courses for physicians are those described by Roter *et al.* (1995) and Clark *et al.* (1998).

Risk communication is a specialized area of communication with particular relevance to EBPC. It rarely appears in discussions of doctor–patient communication skills. It has been discussed more widely in Chapter 9 (Edwards and Bastian), but in relation to education we mention Morris' (1990) overview of this complex and under-researched topic. Bottorff *et al.* (1998) in their review of communication of cancer risk information also summarize the current status of risk communication strategies. Edwards *et al.* (1999) piloted the use of a range of complementary risk communication tools in simulated primary care consultations (practice with a standardized patient followed by focus group) which has potential as an educational intervention for teaching about risk communication.

Evidence-based medicine

There is debate about whether all the steps of EBM need to be taught to all professionals. It is frequently noted that professionals do not have the time to undertake literature searches. One strategy which seeks to circumvent this issue is to provide professionals with a service which identifies the most relevant evidence to answer a clinical question. An example of this is the ATTRACT service in Wales, UK [http://www.tripdatabase.com]. This is one of the most frequently visited health evidence sites. If such services are available, the focus of educational strategies to promote EBM can be on question formulation and implementation of evidence. If they are not then attention must be given to the skills of ordinary professionals to undertake all the steps of EBM.

Norman and Shannon (1998) reviewed 10 studies of the effectiveness of instruction in critical appraisal, six involving undergraduates and four involving residents. Undergraduates showed consistent improvements in knowledge whereas the gains at residency level were small. Interventions for undergraduates were typically lecture or seminar courses of several weeks' duration; interventions in the residency studies were generally of the journal club format, with a meeting once a week, but attendance was typically sporadic. Alguire (1998) reviewed the goals, organization, and teaching methods of journal clubs in postgraduate medical education and found that a major goal of most is to teach critical appraisal skills. Clubs with high attendance were characterized by mandatory attendance, availability of food, and perceived importance by the programme director.

Sackett and Parker (1998) optimistically reported that as more curriculum planning committees become convinced of the need to teach the methods of EBM, literature searching and critical appraisal are being taught at multiple stages in pre-clinical and clinical curricula. They are also becoming incorporated into the everyday function of the clinical teams in which students learn. However, there are no published descriptions of such model curricula or their evaluation. In fact the most recent review of the subject by Green (1999) identifies critical appraisal as the most consistently named objective in graduate clinical epidemiology curricula; only a minority targeted other skills of importance to EBM such as those of question formulation and literature searching.

If programmes are to move beyond teaching critical appraisal skills in typical journal clubs to teaching all the steps of EBM in the students' or residents' established clinical venues, the following will be required:

♦ access to on-site electronic information;

♦ a faculty which monitors their students' and residents' behaviour; and

♦ institutions which assist the faculty in learning how to role model and teach EBM in real time.

Educational strategies in any venue must begin with actual current clinical questions (Green 1999). A potentially interesting (though not yet evaluated) CME approach to evidence-based practice is PEARLS™ run by the College of Family Physicians of Canada (www.cfpc.ca/pearlsE.htm). It consists of an exercise to take learners through a 5-step reflective learning process comprising: formulation of a specific practice reflection question; literature search; critical appraisal of key articles; a practice decision based on the evidence; evaluation of impact of decision two months later. Members receive a supporting manual and an option to access expert facilitators for personal advice.

Putting it together: a workshop model

Over the course of the past year we have developed a workshop model for teaching the skills of 'informed shared decision making' (ISDM). It comprises a short introduction to basic concepts and the rationale, followed by a live demonstration of ISDM through a 10-minute encounter between one of the workshop facilitators and a simulated patient, followed by feedback from the simulated patient and a group discussion. The demonstration not only serves to illustrate ISDM in practice but gives participants a preview of the format for the remainder of the workshop in which they will have a chance to practice with different simulated scenarios and get feedback in small groups. It also sets the tone for the workshop: that it is acceptable to make mistakes or experiment (there is no single 'right' way), and that the simulated patients are an integral part of the teaching team and the ultimate authority when it comes to giving feedback.

We have developed five simulated scenarios, selected to highlight different aspects of ISDM or different patient characteristics (e.g. dependent/independent). The scenarios depict typical decisions in primary care and are 'low stakes'. For example:

> Beth is a menopausal woman in desperate need of symptomatic relief for hot flushes. She is also an 'information junkie' and arrives with large quantities of information from the Internet on hormone replacement therapy, but which she finds very confusing. She has heard about an increased risk of breast cancer. She is also interested in the possibilities of alternative or complementary therapies.

The simulated patients are trained to give feedback specific to the ISDM competences: in particular whether they feel informed, they have been given choices, the decision has been shared, communication has been explicit, the encounter is complete (with action plan), and whether they feel their autonomy has been increased. Our preliminary results have shown the workshop model to be acceptable and useful for family practitioners and family practice residents.

Barriers towards achieving change

Communication skills curriculum

There is inadequate communication skills teaching about decision making. Most formal communication skills teaching occurs in the first year or two of medical school, and the emphasis is on the first half of the interview: taking a history in order to make a diagnosis (Elwyn *et al.* 1999b; Novack *et al.* 1993). Maguire *et al.* (1986) studied 40 young doctors, half of whom had had feedback training in interviewing skills as students five years previously. All were equally poor in giving information and advice and very few obtained and took any account of patients' views and expectations. The doctors agreed that their poor performance was due to lack of clear guidance about how to give information and advice to patients, either while or since they were medical students.

The lack of explicit teaching about aspects of the interview of most relevance to EPBC is one part of the problem; the other is that the communication skills which are taught, with their emphasis on history taking, may be counter to the goals of EBPC. As is indicated by socio-linguistic studies, such as those by Waitzkin (1984) and Mishler (1984), standards of thoroughness in clinical history taking encourage a style of high control and frequent interruptions initiated by professionals. They tend to de-emphasize

Table 15.3 Evidence-based patient choice: goals and barriers in education and training

	What to teach	Problems
Undergraduate (UG)	Prerequisites, e.g.: – Promote attitudes towards involving patients – Basics of Evidence-based Medicine (EBM) – Basic communication skills – Ethics – informed consent or informed choice – Evidence for EBPC and patient involvement	Effect of professionalization on attitudes Hospital-based clinical training Emphasis on first half of interview (history taking, making diagnosis) Little explicit teaching of communication skills in clinical years Inadequate role models
Postgraduate (PG)	Putting EBPC into practice Model conceptual framework Advanced communication skills	Inadequate role models Lack of explicit supervision or examination for EBPC Attitudes of patients to professional 'uncertainty'
Continuing Medical Education (CME)	Putting EBPC into practice Keeping up-to-date with the evidence and new sources of information How to teach others (UG; PG) EBM (still new for some)	Defensive response to implied criticism of communication skills How to get them in the door? Working environment that does not support EBPC (no time, gatekeeper receptionist) Lack of supporting patient information or decision aids Providing low cost effective CME No incentives to change

patients' concerns that do not contribute to diagnosis and treatment. Research shows that the interrogative mode is a subtly dominating format: professionals rarely explain the rationale behind their questions to patients who often become confused or mystified. Learning the standards of medical history taking involves a set of cognitive processes in the professional that are different from those the patient brings to the encounter. The drive for thoroughness and technical comprehension that is internalized during medical education may interfere with professionals' sensitivity to patients' needs.

The survey by Novack *et al.* (1993) of the current state of medical interviewing and interpersonal skills teaching in US medical schools showed that in introductory courses (during the first two years) the main topics taught are the medical interview (83%), physical examination (46%), the professional–patient relationship (37%), and the medical record (25%). There was little co-ordination of skills teaching throughout the curriculum and various barriers were identified to teaching a progressive sequence of skills (e.g. basic skills in first year, psychosocial hypothesis generation and testing in second and third year, psychosocial therapeutic skills and patient education in third and fourth years). These barriers included lack of curriculum time (61%), lack of trained faculty support (50%), and lack of faculty interest (39%).

In the survey by Hargie *et al.* (1998) 16 of 19 UK medical schools reported having experienced problems when implementing communication skills training. These covered resource problems (facilities, money for simulated patients, and tutors), staff matters (availability, training, opposition), lack of curriculum time, and negative student attitudes.

Role models, supervision, and feedback

These two latter surveys also pointed to a lack of good role models for professional–patient communication in general, and this is borne out by other surveys. For example, in a study by Beaudoin *et al.* (1998) in three Canadian medical schools, only 46% of students agreed that their teachers displayed patient-centred characteristics and 53% agreed that their teachers were good role models in teaching the professional–patient relationship, although junior doctors were slightly less critical.

During clinical training (undergraduate or postgraduate) on the wards, communication skills are rarely observed and students receive little feedback. Burack *et al.* (1999) found that senior doctors did not explicitly discuss attitudes, refer to moral or professional norms, 'lay down the law', or call attention to their modelling, and rarely gave behaviour-specific feedback. Reasons for not responding to problematic behaviours in students or junior doctors included lack of opportunity to observe interactions, sympathy for learner stress, and the unpleasantness, perceived ineffectiveness, and lack of professional reward for giving negative feedback.

We held a focus group with medical students shortly before graduation and asked them what they had learned about each of a set of exit competences for communication skills. In response to the competence 'Demonstrate techniques of shared decision making in formulating a management plan', the students responded that as far as treatment is concerned 'you learn what your attending senior doctor wants or likes'. When asked about discussion of treatment with patients, there was a big silence. When asked specifically about shared decision making, they laughed and said that sometimes their seniors 'shared with us what they were going to do for the patient.' We do not think our experience is unique. The opportunities to see EBPC modelled by senior doctors are limited. Moreover, if these seniors have not been trained in EBPC then it is unlikely that they can identify specific behaviours in the students to give constructive feedback.

Culture of medical education and training

There is some evidence that the ability of students to communicate well with patients deteriorates as they proceed through medical school. Major sociological studies such as those by Becker *et al.* (1961) and Mizrahi (1986) in the USA, and Sinclair (1997) in the UK, suggest that medical schools and teaching hospitals have de-humanizing effects on medical students and postgraduates, with deleterious consequences for their relationships with patients. Sparr *et al.* (1988) prospectively studied perceptions of the professional–patient relationship among junior doctors in two US medical schools. At the beginning of the year the doctors were quite positive about the doctor–patient relationship and preferentially endorsed collegial models. As the year progressed they endorsed significantly fewer positive and more negative models.

The reasons for the adverse effects of medical schools on professional–patient relations are still not fully understood, though likely factors include the process of professionalization, emotional and educational stress, the pressure of work and competing educational priorities during clinical training, and verbal and other abuse. Oratz (1982), in an article written while a medical student, examines the socialization of students during the transition from pre-clinical to clinical training in an attempt to understand how medical education shapes students' attitudes and affects future professional–patient relationships. For example, she identifies two coping mechanisms, intellectualization and emotional detachment, and occupational rituals, which students adopt to respond to the anxieties of ward-based clinical training. These serve to increase the emotional distance between students and patients and engender disillusioned and cynical attitudes.

However, it must be pointed out that the nature of medical education and the culture of medical schools has certainly changed and improved since many of these studies were done; that there are studies which show no decline in students' attitudes towards patients; and that there is some evidence that the deleterious effects of medical education are transitory and that more positive attitudes prevail once in independent practice. However, it is also clear that the hospital in-patient environment in which much of clinical education takes place, does little to support a 'patient-centred' approach to communication (Thistlethwaite and Jordan 1999), let alone notions of patient autonomy and choice.

Patient autonomy and professional authority

Kaufman (1982) identifies several reasons why minimal communication with patients persists as an informal norm of professional practice. Firstly, physicians are trained to assume authority and responsibility for the medical care of the patient, and the concept of responsibility is deeply ingrained in students through their clinical training experiences. Effective communication requires that the student confront his or her own feelings about the patient and the illness, and the uncertainties and ambiguities that are an unavoidable feature of the treatment process. Secondly, medical knowledge is seen as part of the professional property of the physician. Sharing information with patients may be construed as undercutting the status and authority of the physician in the treatment relationship. These issues are explored more fully in Chapter 6 (Bellaby). Restricting patients' access to knowledge about their treatment may be a necessary expedient for student physicians who are unsure of their status as doctors.

These barriers are well illustrated by one of the few studies to directly address health professionals' views of informed patient choice. Oliver *et al.* (1996) piloted the introduction of evidence-based leaflets on routine ultrasonography in early pregnancy. The ultrasonographers doubted the credibility of the evidence and were concerned that the leaflets would raise women's anxiety, reduce uptake of scans, and reinforce media messages about the poor safety record of ultrasonography. This case study highlights the resistance of some health professionals to evidence-based health care. It also identifies the underlying conflicts with the principle of professional autonomy allied with concern that informed choice may create anxiety.

Changing physician behaviour

Recent reviews have shown the limitations of most CME in changing physician behaviour and improving the quality of care and patient outcomes: there are 'no magic bullets' (Oxman *et al.* 1995). Davis *et al.* (1992) did, however, identify a direct relationship between the intensity of the educational intervention and the number of studies with positive outcomes. Studies that use practice enabling or reinforcing elements were more effective in changing outcomes. Change was facilitated when the intervention addressed a perceived clinical need, performance gap, or barrier to performance change

(Davis *et al.* 1995). In a survey of CME needs of family doctors and specialists, Mann and Chaytor (1992) found that decisions to acquire new skills or knowledge rose internally from curiosity, externally from problems encountered in practice, or from a combination of these factors. But how do you convince professionals they need to learn about EBPC?

Organization of health care

Kaufman (1982) also identifies some barriers to the involvement of patients in decision making which result from the organization of clinical practice. In the busy office or clinic students learn to 'process' patients quickly and efficiently. All health professionals must strike a balance between the desirability of answering patients' questions and the necessity of keeping up with a busy appointment schedule. There is a perception among physicians that involving patients more in the consultation (e.g. asking about their concerns and expectations, inviting questions) would take more time. However, perhaps this should still be viewed as a research question. There is certainly some evidence that effective communication by trained physicians takes no longer (Roter *et al.* 1995) and may result in reductions in health care utilization (Clark *et al.* 1998). However, in most of those studies mean consultation times of both trained and untrained physicians were relatively long (15 minutes plus). It seems likely that the oral presentation of information to support EBPC may not be realistic within the limitations of the typical 6–10 minute family practice encounter, and that the patient needs to view the professional as only one of a variety of information sources.

Family doctor trainees in the study by Edwards *et al.* (1999) noted the lack of data and difficulty in keeping up with information on risk as major barriers. Doctors in the studies by McColl *et al.* (1998) and Salisbury *et al.* (1998) also identified lack of personal time as the major barrier to practising EBM. Organizational factors may also restrict participation in CME. Mann and Chaytor (1992) found that the most important barrier to CME for family practitioners was practice responsibility (71%), followed by loss of income and timing (68%). Specialists rated all barriers less highly than did family practitioners; their perceived greatest barrier was timing of programmes (60%).

Strategies to promote the practice of EBPC

Beyond the educational solution

Education alone will not solve the problem. Even if we were able to effectively train all professionals, there would still be practical problems in implementing EBPC which go beyond educational solutions. We can predispose professionals to the practice of EBPC and help them to make more effective and efficient use of resources such as time and information. But education will not solve the barriers to EBPC inherent in the organization of health care.

Doctors in the study by McColl *et al.* (1998) thought the most appropriate way to move towards evidence-based family practice was by using evidence-based guidelines and proposals developed by colleagues skilled in accessing and interpreting evidence. They did not feel that all doctors should be taught about literature searching and critical appraisal. As described above, one service development which concords with these views is the ATTRACT service for family practice professionals in Wales [http://www. tripdatabase.com]. Others can work on the evidence. This may allow the professionals to focus more on the skills required for EBPC in practice.

Parallel to the challenge of providing health professionals with efficient access to evidence-based information is a need to provide patients with good quality information to support EBPC. Unfortunately most current information materials are inadequate for the task (Coulter *et al.* 1999) and we have found that print materials available in physicians' offices and given to patients during the consultation rated fair to low on the DISCERN tool designed to evaluate the quality of written patient health information on treatment choices (Charnock 1998). Patients and physicians need access to a wide range of good quality health information to directly support decision making within the consultation. This will allow physicians to use time efficiently and give patients the opportunity to digest the information at leisure and discuss it with family and friends.

Legislation, accreditation, licensing

In recent years the courts of law of Canada, the USA, Australia, and the UK have placed increasingly greater weight on the patient's perspective. They are requiring high standards of disclosure in matters of informed consent, amounting to a principle of informed choice. These trends are now being reflected in the policies and guidelines of medical organizations, for example the recent policy statement from the Canadian Medical Association in conjunction with other national associations (Canadian Health Care Association, *et al.* 1999). Objectives relating to informed choice have been included recently in the Medical Council of Canada licensing examinations taken at the end of medical school. Some postgraduate training schemes, especially those for family doctors, include assessments of communication skills through videotape review. The UK Royal College of General Practitioners assesses professional competence using direct observation of actual performance in the usual place of work via video tape recording (Tate *et al.* 1999). There is potential to broaden and deepen the criteria related to treatment decision making in these video assessments.

Handfield-Jones and Kocha (1999) provide a useful overview of what medical organizations in Canada are currently doing to support and emphasize the importance of good quality communication skills. Criteria for accreditation at undergraduate and postgraduate levels include communication skills in general. Recognizing that many established professionals have had only limited exposure to communication skills training (including CME) and may be resistant to or threatened by such training, they propose a number of schemes. These include:

♦ the establishment of certification of communication skills;

♦ linking reimbursement of professionals to patient satisfaction and/or evaluation of communication skills (this is already happening in some US Health Maintenance Organizations); and

♦ reduced insurance premiums for physicians who participate in strategies to improve communication skills.

They note that although rewards are preferable to coercion, there is increasing pressure from licensing and certification bodies, with strong support from patients, to impose some level of communication skill competence. It must be noted though, that the communication skills referred to by these medical organizations are as yet very basic and broadly defined. With the exception of specific mention of 'ensuring a patient-centred approach', there is nothing that addresses the need for patient involvement in evidence-based decision making and the skills involved.

Consumers as change agents

Feedback has been shown to be a powerful method of bringing about changes in professional practice. In a study by Fidler *et al.* (1999), a higher number of physicians initiated changes in response to feedback from patients in the areas of 'communication and patient support' than in any of the other major areas of practice studied (office staff and systems, collegial communication, clinical skills and resource use, professional development, and personal stress management). The highest proportion of physicians initiated changes relating to increased explanations about medication side-effects (17%), how to avoid illness (15%), and made printed health materials available (15%). Patients were more powerful change agents than other physicians or co-workers.

In medical education patients have traditionally been assigned a passive role but there are some recent examples of more active patient involvement in undergraduate curricula. So for example, students are encouraged to interact with 'consumers' or 'citizens' who exercise some degree of control over the educational process as teachers or evaluators (Wykurz 1999; Hendry *et al.* 1999; Hajioff and Birchall 1999). In our studies we have found feed-back by simulated patients is more acceptable and authoritative than that from peers: only a patient can say if his autonomy has been increased or if she feels informed about treatment choices.

Patients may well have an important influence in stimulating health care professionals towards more 'patient-centred' care models, and in particular towards engaging patients more in decisions about their treatment and care. It may be, though, that many patients have fairly low expectations of the care provided at present. The stimulus for professionals to change the way they provide care will not be so great in this situation. There may be a specific role here for consumer-representative groups, both local and national. They may be able to influence the types of training that take place and the way health care is delivered, to promote EBPC models of care. Consumer groups should recognize the influence they can have, and their responsibilities as change agents to achieve the type of health care they desire.

Conclusion

Whether one takes the view that professionals should engage in all the steps of evidence-based health care or not, it is clear that professionals have responsibilities to acquire and maintain good communication skills. Specific competences have been identified for 'shared decision making' and informed patient choice models of care. It is clear that there is a wide gulf between these ideals and current practice, though various educational strategies have been developed to bridge this gap. The uptake of such education, and the acquisition of skills appears very modest in general, and in particular among senior professionals. Various barriers to the implementation of EBPC orien-tated training and models of care can be identified and should be addressed. Some of the solutions may not be educational but more structural, including legislative requirements. The roles of patients, both individually and in repre-sentative groups, in encouraging professionals to practice evidence-based patient choice models of care cannot be underestimated.

References

Alguire PC (1998). A review of journal clubs in postgraduate medical educa-tion. *Journal of General Internal Medicine* **38**: 347–53.

Becker HS, Geer B, Hughes EC and Strauss AL (1961). *Boys in white: student culture in medical school*. Chicago and London, University of Chicago Press.

Beaudoin C, Maheux B, Cote L, Des Marchais JE, Pierre J and Berkson L (1998). Clinical teachers as humanistic caregivers and educators: perceptions of senior clerks and second-year residents. *Canadian Medical Association Journal* **159**: 765–9.

Boon H and Stewart M (1998). Patient–physician communication assessment instruments: 1986 to 1996 in review. *Patient Education and Counseling* **35**: 161–76.

Bottorff JL, Ratner PA, Johnson JL, Lovato CY and Joab SA (1998). Communicating cancer risk information: the challenges of uncertainty. *Patient Education and Counseling* **33**: 67–81.

Braddock CH III, Edwards KA, Hasenberg NM, Laidley TL and Levinson W (1999). Informed decision making in outpatient practice. *Journal of the American Medical Association* **282**(24): 2313–20.

Burack JH, Irby DM, Carline JD, Root RK and Larson EB (1999). Teaching compassion and respect. Attending physicians' responses to problematic behaviors. *Journal of General Internal Medicine* **14**: 49–55.

Canadian Health Care Association, Canadian Medical Association, Canadian Nurses Association, Catholic Health Association of Canada (1999). Joint statement on preventing and resolving ethical conflicts involving health care providers and persons receiving care. *Canadian Medical Association Journal* **160**(12): 1757–60.

Charnock D (1998). *The DISCERN handbook. Quality criteria for consumer health information on treatment choices.* Oxford, Radcliffe Medical Press.

Clark NM, Gong M, Schork A, Evans D, Roloff D, Hurwitz M, *et al.* (1998). Impact of education of physicians on patient outcomes. *Pediatrics* **101**: 831–6.

Coulter A, Entwistle V and Gilbert D (1999). Sharing decisions with patients: is the information good enough? *British Medical Journal* **318**: 318–22.

Davis DA, Thomson MA, Oxman AD, Haynes RB (1992). Evidence for the effectiveness of CME. A review of 50 randomized controlled trials. Journal of the American Medical Association, 268: 111–117.

Davis DA, Thomson MA, Oxman AD and Haynes RB (1995). Changing physician performance. A systematic review of the effect of continuing medical education strategies. *Journal of the American Medical Association* **274**: 700–5.

Davis P, Russell AS and Skeith KJ (1997). The use of standardized patients in the performance of a needs assessment and development of a CME intervention in rheumatology for primary care physicians. *Journal of Rheumatology* **24**: 1995–9.

Edwards A, Elwyn G and Gwyn R (1999). General practice registrar responses to the use of different risk communication tools in simulated consultations: a focus group study. *British Medical Journal* **319**: 749–52.

Elwyn G, Edwards A, Gwyn R and Grol R (1999a). Towards a feasible model for shared decision making: focus group study with general practice registrars. *British Medical Journal* **319**: 753–6.

Elwyn G, Edwards A and Kinnersley P (1999b). Shared decision making in primary care: the neglected second half of the consultation. *British Journal of General Practice* **49**(443): 447–82.

Fidler H, Lockyer JM, Toews J and Violato C (1999). Changing physicians' practices: the effect of individual feedback. *Academic Medicine* **74**: 702–14.

Fox E, Arnold RM and Brody B (1995). Medical ethics education: past, present, and future. *Academic Medicine* **70**(9): 761–9.

Green L, Kreuter M, Deeds S and Partridge K (1980). *Health education planning: a diagnostic approach*. Palo Alto, California, Mayfield Press.

Green ML (1999). Graduate medical education training in clinical epidemiology, critical appraisal, and evidence-based medicine: a critical review of curricula. *Academic Medicine* **74**(6): 686–94.

Hajioff D and Birchall M (1999). Medical students in ENT outpatient clinics: appointment time, patient satisfaction and student satisfaction. *Medical Education* **33**: 669–73.

Handfield-Jones R and Kocha W (1999). The role of medical organizations in supporting doctor–patient communication. *Cancer Prevention and Control* **3**(1): 46–50.

Hargie O, Dickson D, Boohan M and Hughes K (1998). A survey of communication skills training in UK Schools of Medicine: present practices and prospective proposals. *Medical Education* **32**: 25–34.

Hendry GD, Schreiber L, Bryce D (1999). Patients teach students: partners in arthritis education. *Medical Education* **33**: 674–7.

Hope T (1996). *Evidence-based patient choice*. London, King's Fund.

Hope T, Fulford KWM and Yates A (1996). *The Oxford practice skills course*. Oxford, Oxford University Press.

Hulsman RL, Ros WJG, Winnubst JAM and Bensing JM (1999). Teaching clinically experienced physicians communication skills. A review of evaluation studies. *Medical Education* **33**: 655–68.

Johnson SM, Kurtz ME, Tomlinson T and Fleck L (1992). Teaching the process of obtaining informed consent to medical students. *Academic Medicine* **67**: 598–600.

Kaufmann CL (1982). Medical education and physician–patient communication. In: *Making health care decisions. The ethical and legal implications of informed consent in the patient–practitioner relationship. Vol. 3: Appendices (Studies on the foundations of informed consent)*. Washington DC, President's Commission for the Study of Ethical Problems in Medicine and Biomedical and Behavioral Research, USA.

Kurtz SM, Laidlaw T, Makoul G and Schnabl G (1999). Medical education initiatives in communication skills. *Cancer Prevention and Control* **3**: 37–45.

Kurtz SM and Silverman JD (1996). The Calgary-Cambridge observation guides: an aid to defining the curriculum and organizing the teaching in communication training programmes. *Medical Education* **30**: 83–9.

Kurtz S, Silverman J and Draper J (1998). *Teaching and learning communication skills in medicine*. Oxford, Radcliffe Medical Press.

Laxdal OE (1982). Needs assessment in continuing medical education. *Journal of Medical Education* **57**: 827–34.

Lirenman DS (1996). A survey of perceived learning needs of primary care physicians in British Columbia. Report to the Division of Continuing Medical Education Advisory Committee. January.

McAlister FA, Graham I, Karr GW and Laupacis A (1999). Evidence-based medicine and the practising clinician. *Journal of General Internal Medicine* **14**(4): 262–4.

McColl A, Smith H, White P and Field J (1998). General practitioners' perceptions of the route to evidence-based medicine: a questionnaire survey. *British Medical Journal* **316**: 361–5.

McManus IC, Vincent CA, Thom S and Kidd J (1993). How to do it: teaching communication skills to clinical students. *British Medical Journal* **306**: 1322–7.

Maguire P, Fairbairn S and Fletcher C (1986). Consultation skills of young doctors: II. Most young doctors are bad at giving information. *British Medical Journal* **292**: 1576–8.

Makoul G, Arntson P, Schofield T (1995). Health promotion in primary care: physician–patient communication and decision making about prescription medications. *Social Science and Medicine* **41**(9): 1241–54.

Mann KV and Chaytor KM (1992). Help! Is anyone listening? An assessment of learning needs of practising physicians. *Academic Medicine* **67**(10, Supplement): S4–S6.

Morris LA (1990). Communicating therapeutic risks. New York, Springer-Verlag.

Mishler EG (1984). *The discourse of medicine: dialectics of medical interviews*. Norwood NJ, Ablex Pub Corp.

Mizrahi T (1986). *Getting rid of patients. Contradictions in the socialization of physicians*. New Jersey, Rutgers University Press.

Norman GR and Shannon SI (1998). Effectiveness of instruction in critical appraisal (evidence-based medicine) skills: a critical appraisal. *Canadian Medical Association Journal* **158**(2): 177–81.

Novack DH, Volk G, Drossman DA and Lipkin M, Jr (1993). Medical interviewing and interpersonal skills teaching in US medical schools. *Journal of the American Medical Association* **269**: 2101–5.

Oliver S, Rajan L, Turner H, Oakley A, Entwistle V, Watt I, *et al.* (1996). Informed choice for users of health services: views on ultrasonography leaflets for women in early pregnancy, midwives and ultrasonographers. *British Medical Journal* **313**: 1251–5.

Oratz R (1982). Achieving aesthetic distance: education for an effective doctor–patient relationship. In: *Making health care decisions. The ethical and legal implications of informed consent in the patient–practitioner relationship. Vol. 3: Appendices (Studies on the foundations of informed consent)*. Washington DC, President's Commission for the Study of Ethical Problems in Medicine and Biomedical and Behavioral Research, pp. 143–73.

Oxman AD, Thomson MA, Davis DA and Haynes RB (1995). No magic bullets: a systematic review of 102 trials of interventions to improve professional practice. *Canadian Medical Association Journal* **153**(10): 1423–31.

Roter DL, Hall JA, Kern DE, Barker LR, Cole KA and Roca RP (1995). Improving physicians' interviewing skills and reducing patients' emotional distress. A randomized clinical trial. *Archives of Internal Medicine* **155**: 1877–84.

Sackett DL and Parkes J (1998). Teaching critical appraisal: no quick fixes. *Canadian Medical Association Journal* **158**(2): 203–4.

Sackett DL, Richardson WS, Rosenberg W and Haynes RB (1997). *Evidence-based medicine. How to practice and teach EBM*. London, Churchill Livingstone.

Salisbury C, Bosanquet N, Wilkinson E, Bosanquet A and Hasler J (1998). The implementation of evidence-based medicine in general practice prescribing. *British Journal of General Practice* **48**: 1849–51.

Silverman J, Kurtz S and Draper J (1998). *Skills for communication with patients*. Oxford, Radcliffe Medical Press.

Sinclair S (1997). *Making doctors. An institutional apprenticeship*. Oxford, Berg.

Sparr LF, Gordon GH, Hickam DH and Girard DE (1988). The doctor–patient relationship during medical internship: the evolution of dissatisfaction. *Soc Sci Med* **26**(11): 1095–101.

Stewart M, Brown JB, Weston WW, McWhinney IR, McWilliam CL and Freeman TR (1995). *Patient-centered medicine. Transforming the clinical method*. Thousand Oaks, California, Sage Publications.

Tate P, Foulkes J, Neighbour R, Campion P and Field S (1999). Assessing physicians' interpersonal skills via video-taped encounters: a new approach for the Royal College of General Practitioners membership examination. *Journal of Health Communication* **4**(2): 143–53.

Thistlethwaite JE and Jordan JJ (1999). Patient-centred consultations: a comparison of student experience and understanding in two clinical environments. *Medical Education* **33**: 678–85.

Towle A and Godolphin W (1999). Framework for teaching and learning informed shared decision making. *British Medical Journal* **319**: 766–71.

Tuckett D, Boulton M, Olson C and Williams A (1985). *Meetings between experts – an approach to sharing ideas in medical consultations*. London, Tavistock Publications.

Waitzkin H (1984). Doctor–patient communication. Clinical implications of social scientific research. *Journal of the American Medical Association* **252**(17): 2441–6.

Waitzkin H (1985). Information giving in medical care. *Journal of Health and Social Behaviour* **26**: 81–101.

Wykurz G (1999). Patients in medical education: from passive participants to active partners. *Medical Education* **33**: 634–6.

Young JM and Ward JE (1999). General practitioners' use of evidence databases. *Medical Journal of Australia* **170**(2): 56–8.

16 Moving to the mainstream

Margaret Holmes-Rovner, Hilary Llewellyn-Thomas,
and Glyn Elwyn

Introduction

Evidence-based patient choice (EBPC) may well be the future framework for health care, but it is definitely not yet in place in the clinical settings we observe. Evidence-based medicine (EBM) has had unparalleled influence over medicine, but its recent extension to encompass the realm of patient choice has not yet gained widespread acceptance. It may be an even more arduous journey than that faced by the pioneers of EBM. In this chapter, we explore the expected difficulties that lie ahead and speculate about the possible solutions, such as:

♦ electronic management of evidence and the provision of more and better decision aids to underpin the movement towards EBPC; and

♦ active teaching of EBPC skills across the entire range of public and clinical health information systems.

This chapter has three sections:

Section 1

'Existing and Emerging Problems' lays out three areas that appear to thwart moving EBPC into the mainstream. The first area, 'Is choice a slippery slope?', suggests that introducing unfettered choice may generate unbridled and inappropriate consumer demand for health care. The treatments demanded may overstretch agreed-upon resources and may frequently be counter intuitive in view of existing evidence about benefits and harms. The second area, 'Health system contexts', argues that choice must be bounded by health care constraints and publicly set priorities. The third area, 'Resistance in the field', acknowledges that clinical practice has proved to be very resistant to change and that the concept of 'patient choice' may not have sufficient inherent force to overcome that resistance.

Section 2

The second section serves as a bridge to some proposed solutions, and is ironically entitled, 'How health professionals and patients came to embrace uncertainty and love difficult choices'. Here, we mean to emphasize the magnitude of the obstacles to moving EBPC into the mainstream. Individuals find it difficult to embrace uncertainty. Facing choices requires shouldering the anxieties and fears that may accompany the active consideration of information. Furthermore, an explicit decision making process raises the issue of resource thresholds. 'Consumers' frequently don't like being told they cannot have things, and a frequent consequence of consumerism is the creation of greater demands. The challenge is to convince the public that their interests could be better served if they demand only those technologies that, overall, do more good than harm at a reasonable cost. This section attempts to identify steps around these obstacles to the successful implementation of EBPC.

Section 3

In the 'Solutions' section, we argue that better decision aids (O'Connor 1999 *et al*. 1999*a* and 1999*b*) and a concerted effort to educate the public are the best ways of promulgating EBPC. Schools, patient interest groups, journalists, and others all need to be engaged in the effort to communicate the uncertainties and limits of medical technologies in a more open and balanced way. They need to be convinced that more is not always better and that the essence of good choice involves supporting the use of only demonstrably effective technologies. The section has two parts. In the first part, 'Better tools', we describe the necessary minimum elements that should be incorporated into effective evidence-based patient decision aids, and argue that these elements should constitute the informational core for patient choice. In the second part, 'Moving the tools into the mainstream', we make a strategic argument for how to provide the tools across the groups who can expand evidence-based patient choice. Access to good quality evidence-based information could empower patients and foster evidence-based decision making within the current resource constraints, but this will require the active engagement of an expanding community of practitioners of evidence-based, consumer-sensitive health care.

1 Existing and emerging problems

Is 'choice' a slippery slope?

Can the terms 'evidence-based' and 'patient choice' really be brought together? Is it possible simultaneously to commit to using only effective technologies while inviting individual choice? Is it possible to engage patients, consumer groups, clinicians, policy makers (and, in the background, commercial interests) together in sorting out the medical evidence and making optimal choices? The initial assumptions by the pioneers of shared decision making regarding the 'enlightened' patient may have been overly optimistic (Wennberg *et al.* 1993; Holmes-Rovner *et al.* 1999). Patients appear not to choose consistently the least invasive, and therefore least expensive, technology. Often, full and accurate information about harms as well as benefits is not placed before the patient, or is not portrayed in ways that make it easy for individuals to assess the relevance and threat. Even when they have full, comprehensible information, patients, like their health care professionals, frequently prefer expensive new technologies that are only marginally better than older ones.

Furthermore, commercial and professional interests influence the availability of different treatment options, the information that is provided about them, and the dynamics of professional–patient interactions. Their interests have traditionally been in fostering the increased use of efficacious technologies, regardless of cost. In 1999, the first year of direct advertising by pharmaceutical companies to patients in the US, sales of drugs doubled and pharmaceutical medications now represent the largest proportion of the US health care budget. Another prime example is the way that hormone replacement therapy (HRT) is 'marketed' in some sections of the popular media, whilst another body of opinion from alternative health care argues against hormonal 'manipulation'.

A doctrine of patient choice could turn quickly to unbridled consumerism, putting pressure on governments and insurers to provide services that are beyond their means. These issues are at the centre of intense political debate, particularly in health care systems in which participants are well informed about new technologies but experience tight limits on their health care budgets. In the UK, for instance, the National Institute for Clinical Excellence (NICE) was subjected to intense public criticism due to a proposal not to recommend payment for beta-interferon for treatment of multiple sclerosis. For these clinical decisions, the question becomes not, 'Is this the optimal choice under conditions of limited resources?' but 'Who is to blame for denying patients access to health care?' Are these tensions the inevitable repercussions of suggesting that 'evidence-based patient choice' frameworks should inform health care decisions?

We suggest that if EBPC is to contribute to, rather than sabotage, health care systems, we must acknowledge openly that evidence of effectiveness comes before choice, and that there are explicit cost thresholds which determine the availability of some treatments. Some political systems allow a much more open and transparent debate to be held on these issues whilst others still struggle to frame the economic arguments coherently. If we accept the principle that ultimately 'evidence' has ascendancy over 'choice', then in many circumstances promoting patient choice is reasonable. But where treatments are necessary and different therapies have similar results in terms of morbidity and mortality, then promoting patient choice is especially appropriate (Coulter 1997; Elwyn *et al.* 1999, 2001). This position of 'equipoise' is similar to that which faces patients who are asked to enter clinical trials.

In this complex area where individual benefits are pitted against public costs, coherent EBPC policies could be of most value as a way of informing the 'rationing' debate (Coulter and Ham 2000). All treatment and screening decisions should involve assessments of harm and benefits at both the individual and societal levels. They should be considered against accepted thresholds for public expenditure of funds. The proponents of EBPC believe that debate should be framed in terms of the relative weights of harms and benefits, which involves evaluating trade-offs between length and quality of life, attitudes towards risk, preferences for invasiveness, impact on cultural beliefs, and other attributes of the interface between people and technologies.

Health system contexts for choice

The effective dissemination of EBPC, particularly if it occurs via the World Wide Web (WWW), will require explicit recognition of the inherent contextual issues in different health care systems. Such systems comprise supranational agreements, say within the European Union (EU), national systems, like the UK NHS, subscriber systems, like an American Health Maintenance Organization (HMO), or a village where local policy makers control resource allocation.

If health care systems do not openly acknowledge and defend their resource allocation decisions, then the principles of patient choice do not have a sustainable framework within which to work, and are subject to a wide variety of forces. Attempts to introduce EBPC are occurring in regions of the world in which the culture of health care may in some aspects be quite similar, yet in others widely divergent. Societies vary in terms of the definition of good health, the importance attributed to health status, the acceptability of various ways of trying to achieve good health, and the extent to which health care is regarded as a citizen's right. There is also variance in cultural assumptions about clinician and patient roles and responsibilities, in patients' regard for clinicians and attitudes about patient autonomy, and in the degree to which traditional perceptions are becoming further entrenched or subject to challenge. Furthermore, health care systems are organized at differing levels, sometimes at national but often at smaller divisions (state or regions). These systems are imbued with values from their host culture but also face particular local issues of policy definition, accessibility, and accountability. Health care institutions or agencies, in turn, have their own histories, informational and referral networks, and resource constraints. Played out against this complex background is the fact that attitudes towards uncertainty in medical care vary as well as judgements about the feasibility of providing explicit medical evidence summaries to patients. Finally, the ways EBPC is enacted in actual clinical encounters can be profoundly affected by variability in language, in ethnicity, in literacy, and in 'numeracy'.

Each health care system will have to develop solutions that respect and engage the local context because, ultimately, all policy deliberations are determined and delivered by local interactions among participants. For example, New Zealand's approach to rationing under the National Health Committee is based on the philosophy that the provision of publicly-funded core services must be consistent with the wider values of 'communities' rather than those of individuals, yet the systems have to find a way of ensuring that these policies are implemented consistently at the individual level (National Health Committee 1993).

Therefore, developers of decision aids for a particular health system need to explicitly acknowledge its policy. In the UK, for example, the PSA (prostatic specific antigen) test is not advocated as a screening procedure for prostate cancer but other health care systems have taken differing stances. However, PSA tests, when performed, still require patients to be informed about the pros and cons of having the investigation, and a relevant UK-based decision aid should reiterate the underlying policy context as well as providing an evidence-based synopsis of the harms and benefits, the long-term consequences of screening, and the role of personal preferences. This argument implies that those who wish to promote the principles of EBPC must consider simultaneously the underlying clinical evidence, the health system policy, its rationale, and the resulting patient choice problem. If any of these context issues are ignored, then EBPC advocates are thrown back into a tug-of-war over who is being denied what, rather than fostering a deliberative process.

The Internet could support the positive potential of EBPC. The WWW could present health technology and outcome data for the creation of new decision aids, as well as store well developed ready-to-use decision tools. However, it will be necessary to adapt such tools to fit into the relevant policy frameworks of local health care systems. Such a Web-based capability could also inform local efforts by describing others' successful and unsuccessful priority setting initiatives based on medical evidence and consumer involvement.

Resistance in the field

Introducing the idea of explicit shared decision making in academic discourse, promulgating patient choice policies at political levels, and developing decision aids to support the concept have not led to a widespread acceptance and implementation within clinical settings. While the ideas of shared decision making and consumer education may be widely supported (Laine and Davidoff 1996; Coulter 1999), decision aids (and the implementation of shared decision making consulting styles) have been adopted primarily in academic settings (O'Connor *et al.* 1999b).

In a recent experiment to evaluate the potential of shared decision making programmes to improve the quality of care outside academic and HMO settings, a health insurer (Blue Cross and Blue Shield of Michigan) introduced shared decision making in its fee-for-service hospital systems (Holmes-Rovner *et al.* 2001). The insurer's objectives were to:

◆   provide a high-quality, cost-effective benefit to the insurer's members;

◆   improve quality of care, including patient and provider satisfaction; and

◆   help manage health care utilization and costs.

The study was of two multimedia Shared Decision making Programs® (SDP) (Foundation for Informed Medical Decision Making, 2000), one for the surgical treatment choices for early stage breast cancer, and the other for moderate ischaemic heart disease treatment choices, and took place in three hospitals in Michigan, USA. The SDP programmes were judged to be clear, accurate, contained the correct amount of information, and were of acceptable duration. Professionals were seemingly neutral about patients' desire to participate in treatment decision making and reported that they were happy to refer patients to the SDPs. However, the survey and participant observation data revealed a much lower patient usage of the SDPs than predicted. When this low rate of referral was investigated, the reported barriers mainly involved time pressures and the potential disruption to care processes. The physicians were seemingly reluctant to add tasks that disrupted their typical patient pathways.

We can also speculate that professionals may have other objections to SDPs and decision aids that are not as overtly acceptable as the assertion that 'time is short' and 'we are busy clinicians'. Decision aids contain detailed information about clinical outcomes (usually derived from population data) and take the conceptual stance that patients should be offered the opportunity to become engaged in the task of decision making. On the other hand, individual clinicians may challenge 'population' derived data ('my figures are different'), may feel threatened by the degree of variability that surrounds the probabilistic reporting of uncertainty, and may feel that decision aids interfere with the satisfactory enactment of the clinician role.

Clinicians may not admit to such feelings, sensing that paternalism of this type is not typically welcomed. These covert attitudes may represent much more fundamental barriers to EBPC than the glib comment that time is too short, however true that assertion is in many contexts. Although there have been trials in decision support in which large numbers have been successfully recruited (Man-Son-Hing *et al.* 1999), advocating the involvement of patients in decisions and the use of decision aids could be regarded as a minority interest primarily pursued in settings researching the effects of increasing patient autonomy.

2   How health professionals and patients came to embrace uncertainty and love difficult choices

Could this become the storyline for EBPC in the next decade? Although there are no comprehensive surveys available, we are on safe ground when we declare that the promotion of patient involvement in decisions is not yet widely accepted. The principles of EBPC may challenge many unvoiced assumptions in health care. Health professionals today frequently go into medicine because they enjoy the challenge of taking uncertainty out of health problems through their diagnostic and treatment skills. Patients come to health professionals to have vexing problems solved. Moving from a culture of 'dependency' on professional expertise to a more 'questioning' and deliberative interaction presupposes that the skills to undertake this shift are going to be embraced by patients and professionals alike. Society at large may be ready to shift towards a more interactive partnership, but we cannot assume that this change will be sudden or painless.

The unprecedented access to information is going to be one of, if not *the,* most powerful influence on this process. Other levers will be the gradual accumulation of evidence-based decision aids (making it easier to share options with patients). However, merely introducing evidence-based approaches to health care decision making could create paradoxical situations. Increasing the explicitness of treatment effectiveness rates does not usually reduce uncertainty about health care outcomes. The very fact that many people must be treated in order to generate one positive outcome (the number needed to treat) is a disconcerting concept for many patients when it is fully realized. If, at the same time, professionals also introduce the concept of equally feasible treatment options for any given situation, then the concept of EBPC could intensify disquiet.

Furthermore, as professionals and health care managers encounter increased pressures for explicit accountability, greater tensions are likely to surface. Episodes of professional error and poor judgement have been documented and widely discussed in both the UK and the US. Health care interventions are more effective and yet paradoxically more criticized than ever before (see also Chapter 6 by Bellaby). At the same time, there is considerable confusion about necessary medical uncertainty, unnecessary interventions, and unacceptable incompetence. It is difficult for the public to distinguish between real 'error' and the poor outcomes that will occur precisely because medical care has in-built rates of ineffectiveness and unpredictability. Without this clarification, distrust of professionals will increase if, as incidents are highlighted, the public attributes 'uncertainty' to untrustworthy physicians rather than to imperfect information and the random effects of probability.

Distinctions need to be drawn, therefore, between 'error' (admittedly unacceptably high at between 3% and 7% of hospital admissions in the US and UK) and the inevitable variation in outcomes that occurs as a consequence of medical uncertainty. Consumers and policy makers need to know how to make these distinctions. Unfortunately, the knowledge base and analytic skills to do so are currently taught, when they are taught at all, only in health professional training. They are not widely dispersed to the media, policy makers, and consumer advocates who increasingly need them.

Patients report that clinicians rarely engage in a detailed discussion about options, side-effects, and the benefits of treatment. At the same time, health care professionals tend to report new technologies optimistically (Entwistle *et al.* 2000). 'New' is often perceived as better, with risks and side-effects often underemphasized or not mentioned at all. Patients are therefore not able to anticipate problems and treatment failures. This could result in compliance problems, and even premature rejection of the technology (Entwistle *et al.* 1998).

Furthermore, this lack of information results in a diminution of consumer autonomy. Most patients have no real experience of what would constitute a positive experience of being truly involved in their health care management. It is, of course, important to respect the rights of patients who wish not to be involved in treatment decisions. Our ethical position in this chapter is that of 'optional autonomy' not 'mandatory autonomy'; that is, the patient's preference for involvement should determine the clinical interaction, not a fixed ethical stance (Schneider 1998).

In this regard, it is noteworthy that some empirical reports regarding patient role preference in decision making have been based on 'hypothetical' surveys (Benbassat *et al.* 1998; Guadagnoli and Ward 1998). These reports may not represent the distributions of actual preferences that could emerge when the decision situation is presented skilfully to patients facing actual choices, and the relevance of accepting some responsibility in the decision making process is clearly outlined. Nevertheless, it is vital to point out that patients will find it difficult to indicate whether they want to be involved in treatment decision making if they have not first been presented with information about the decision space – the range of uncertainties and the probabilities (Elwyn *et al.*, 2001).

Taken together, the arguments outlined above highlight how the advocates of EBPC need to augment their work involving decision aids with strategies in intensive public education. This would involve explicit plans for promoting public discussion of the principles of EBPC and for providing patients with the deliberative skills required to engage in effective decision making.

3 Solutions

Better tools: promoting transparency through a minimal set of patient choice elements

As O'Connor and Edwards report in Chapter 14, when patients use 'decision aids' their knowledge and satisfaction with the decision process is increased (O'Connor *et al.* 1999c). But we must be careful not to suggest that all decision aids are the same. Decision aids need to be critically appraised, like all other 'technologies' in health care. There is evidence that various kinds of decision aids are being used by pharmaceutical companies to inform patients about their products and procedures. The design of these aids is susceptible to conflicts of interest, and biases may be introduced into their presentation (Edwards *et al.* 2001).

It is therefore very important to establish clear standards for the development of decision aids, and as the empirical experience with these tools accumulates, the required quality criteria are becoming clearer (O'Connor *et al.* 1999b). Decision aids must be constructed to display the patient choice problem, and present all reasonable options (within the policy constraints described earlier), including doing nothing or watchful waiting. Evidence-based statements about the benefits and harms associated with each option should be derived from credible sources; the quality and consistency of the underlying empirical studies should be described. They should be explicit about uncertainties and controversies, and point out value trade-offs. They should do this in a balanced way, using concise, jargon-free language. Decision aids must be clear about publication date and be revised when new evidence emerges. They must be explicit about authorship and sponsorship.

To facilitate their broad use, these characteristics should be developed into an agreed set of required standards for decision aids. More generally, perhaps these standards should be applied to all sources of patient information. One way to promote the adoption of such standards is to develop an accepted instrument to appraise materials. Efforts to develop explicit minimum quality criteria for patient information have been made by numerous groups and one of the best is the DISCERN instrument (Charnock *et al.* 1999) (and see Chapter 3 Entwistle and O'Donnell), which generates a 'quality' score to help consumers judge the quality of materials. However, we propose moving beyond scales like these. We would advocate a standard for appraising materials that has been designed to facilitate patient choice. Although this approach may run the risk of being perceived as the latest brand of political correctness, it may help to identify materials that have been developed using weak methods or that have promotional biases. Two provisional sets of standards are described, one for treatment and one for screening decisions. Both will be further developed over time as they are applied to actual decision aids.

Transparency is now required within health care settings. Accordingly, patients and health professionals should expect clear summaries of the information (and the sources and samples from which it is derived) used to

Table 16.1 Criteria for evaluating patient information materials: treatment decisions

Element	Data Requirement
Clinical condition reported	All data specific to clinically important subgroups
Patient decision situation	Describe all options among: surgical therapies, medical therapies, watchful waiting, complementary therapies
Treatment description(s) (for each subgroup)	For each treatment describe therapeutic mode, duration, nature of patient involvement
Outcomes and probabilities	Lifetime outcome rates for each outcomes including ◆ absolute number improved ◆ improvement rate (relative risk change) Time period specific outcome rates for (i.e. 5 years) ◆ absolute number improved ◆ improvement rate Side-effect rates
Value issues	◆ Trade-offs between length of life and quality of life ◆ Trade-offs among the inconveniences, costs, chances of side/toxic-effects, etc., in order to gain a benefit like symptom relief ◆ Descriptions of patients' experiences ◆ Cultural values of ethnic minorities that differ from majority values
Authorship	◆ Author of a decision aid ◆ Authors of the underlying studies
Sponsorship	◆ Financial supporter(s) of any decision aid ◆ Has the sponsor(s) acknowledged and addressed conflicts of interest?
Health system policy	◆ Health system policy re: service provision ◆ Explanation for provision or non-provision of one or more services

Table 16.2 Criteria for evaluating patient information materials: screening decisions

Element	Data Requirement
Clinical condition to be prevented	◆ Expected incidence of the disease in 1, 5, 10, and 20 years among untreated patients ◆ Identification of the clinically important subgroups at risk ◆ Probabilities of key patient-orientated outcomes (harms and benefits) caused by the disease in an untreated population
Prevention options	◆ Screening/early detection ◆ Watchful waiting ◆ Medical preventive strategies ◆ Lifestyle preventive strategies
Follow-up treatment effectiveness	◆ Probabilities of key patient-orientated harms and benefits, in terms of difference from the rates in the unscreened population ◆ Absolute risk reduction ◆ Relative risk reduction
Screening test(s) characteristics	◆ Sensitivity, specificity ◆ Side-effects and rates ◆ Follow-up tests and procedures(s)
Value trade-offs	◆ Trade-offs between potential anxiety of screening and treatment now to prevent a disease in the future ◆ Impact of the screening process on family and professional life (including legal and health coverage implications) ◆ Cultural values of ethnic minorities that differ from majority values
Authorship	◆ Author of a decision aid ◆ Authors of the underlying studies
Sponsorship	◆ Financial supporter(s) of any decision aid ◆ Has the sponsor(s) acknowledged and addressed conflicts of interest?
Health system policy	◆ Health system policy re: service provision ◆ Explanation for provision or non-provision of one or more services

answer questions about a specific intervention like, 'Do the benefits outweigh the harms?' These are clearly enormous challenges, particularly if one of the critical aims is to ensure that the materials are also easy to use in discussions between patients and professionals.

Moving the new tools into the mainstream: the opportunities

It may be naïve to suggest that one way to promote EBPC and a wider use of decision aids is to teach critical appraisal skills to the public. But we suspect that there may be greater merit to this approach than is at first apparent. It does at least have the advantage that this approach has not been tried with any degree of consistency in the past. Public debate on health care issues can be broadly caricatured as selling and lobbying, rather than public engagement and deliberation over the extent and quality of evidence. For the clinical encounter to change, we perceive that the process of public dialogue has to change. If the first and only encounter with shared decision making skills occurs when people are anxious about a major illness, it is far too late to expect a patient to learn to deliberate carefully over information that is potentially disconcerting and complex. Skills such as these need to be introduced at an early stage of a patient's 'career', with less 'threatening' problems so that the concepts of uncertain outcomes and the benefits of taking an active role are realized in young adulthood when critical faculties can be fully engaged and learnt. A multi-faceted strategy would help the public to understand a priori that health care budgets are limited and technologies imperfect. It would help ensure that the concepts of EBPC and shared decision making become *embedded* into the discourse of health care encounters.

There are many opportunities to implement this strategy. Fig. 16.1 illustrates how the minimum standards for decision aids could be implemented via the Internet. Consumers increasingly seek online information and, as the penetration of this medium increases, it provides for vastly improved equity of access to information. Its public availability also would ensure that quality could be monitored if the information elements suggested in Tables 16.1 and 16.2 were consistently provided. To help this happen, organizations such as the Cochrane Collaboration that support systematic secondary research could formulate an explicit policy to support EBPC. For instance, as a matter of course, each review could report its results so that a balanced patient-orientated synopsis appears on the Internet, and could provide links to formal decision aids that have been developed and evaluated as these become available.

Examples of the expanding set of electronic networks that provide resources appear in Fig. 16.1. We think that members of the groups illustrated here, when they access overviews of evidence, also should be able to gain access to patient-focused summaries created according to the criteria outlined in Tables 16.1 and 16.2. The idea of linking repositories of evidence, professionals, patients, and the tools that support SDM and EBPC holds considerable promise. It allows us to make all the components required for an effective 'patient involvement' process available to all the relevant parties,

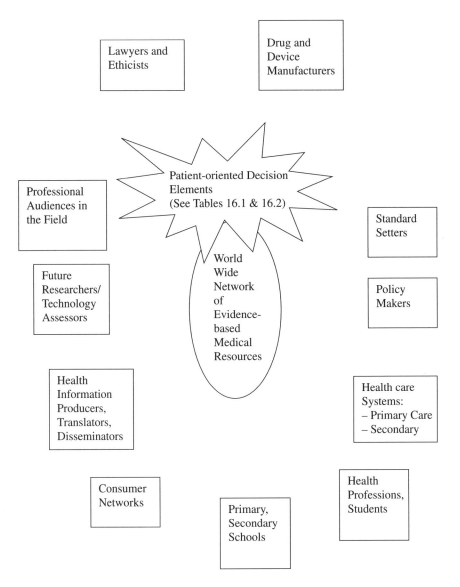

Fig. 16.1 Opportunities to promote evidence-based patient choice.

thus levelling the playing field to a much greater degree than has been previously possible. This kind of organized initiative will help to provide the path from synthesized medical information described by Gray in Chapter 2 towards the kind of evidence-based patient decision making described by Eysenbach and Jadad in Chapter 17.

Reorientating the presentation of medical information to support patient decisions is a great challenge. For that reason, this responsibility must be dispersed and shared, hopefully in an organized and systematic fashion. An important step forward is to understand the opportunities to redesign the ways in which currently available clinical evidence can be placed before patients. Provided that these tools are well linked into the new electronic networks, then the effort could successfully bring the cross-currents of consumerism, accountability, and evidence-based medicine into a constructive force for change.

Health professionals in the field

Experienced health professionals are among the most important and yet the most sceptical of potential advocates of evidence-based patient choice. They are the direct users of medical technologies and have their own preferences for therapeutic modalities. At the same time, when 'evidence' is either new or contested, many individual clinicians may not have access to, or be aware of, the latest best evidence. On a personal level, many clinicians may not wish to introduce experimental techniques, including decision aids, when it does not suit their practice or is in accord with their attitudes. Given this attitudinal predisposition, it is likely that many clinicians will acknowledge the existence of decision aids with a polite nod and continue their practice without them.

The best model for successful implementation of EBPC may be the deliberate use of professional networks and short problem-based workshops that have so successfully fostered the dissemination of evidence-based medicine among established health professionals (O'Connor *et al.* 1999b). This strategy depends to a large extent on the 'readiness' of professionals to develop their skills in 'sharing' decisions about screening, testing, and offering treatment choices (see Elwyn and Charles, Chapter 8). This kind of caveat may be relevant even when professionals are asked to supply decision aids for patients to use outside the consultation, since there will always need to be subsequent contact to confirm option choice.

Health professionals in training

Many health professional curricula already incorporate communication skills training. These courses could be adapted to include shared decision making skills, or separate courses can be developed. O'Connor maintains that there are core and disease-specific clinician skills in 'decision support' which can be systematically taught, and has devised a clinical course at the University of Ottawa (Ottawa Health Decision Centre). This course is outlined here as one example of clinical training in shared decision making.

Box 16.1 **Preparing professionals to provide decision support**

The professionals learn about:

1. *The concept of decisional conflict and its defining characteristics.* These include inadequate or misunderstood information, lack of clarity about personal values, inadequate support or undue pressure from others, and inadequate or missing resources for decision implementation (O'Connor AM, 1995).

2. *The processes of systematically assessing patients' needs for decision support.* For example, how to determine whether a patient needs: a) more help understanding information; b) help to clarify and communicate his or her values to the clinician or others; c) more social support or relief from undue pressure from others when grappling with the decision problem; and/or d) the resolution of problems with inadequate or missing resources for decision implementation.

3. *The concepts and skills involved in tailoring interventions to patients' needs.* The systematic appraisal outlined above indicates whether the situation calls for the provision of information about a recommended action, or the engagement with an actual choice. Then, for patients facing an actual choice, the professional helps him/her to engage in deliberation about the decision at hand. The professional gains particular skills to help with this deliberation; these skills may or may not involve using a particular kind of formal decision aid.

4. *The background work that supports successful incorporation of a decision aid into a particular practice environment.* Those professionals who are interested in the development and use of a new decision aid for their practice setting then learn about a) the differentiation between Eddy's three kinds of practice policies ('Standards', 'Guidelines', and 'Options' (Eddy DM, 1992)); b) how formal decision aids play a greater role in situations involving Guidelines and Options; and c) the importance of carrying out a careful prior 'needs assessment' of the attitudes and opinions of clinicians and patients before launching the design, testing, and implementation of a new decision aid.

International collaboration on the WWW could create the educational infrastructures to support courses modelled along these lines in basic medical or nursing curricula, in conjoint or international degree programmes, and in distance education programmes. Such courses could also be made available in condensed form in professional societies' continuing education programmes. As the field grows, academic centres could establish fellowships for the development of deeper expertise in the principles of SDM and EBPC.

Journalism and the popular press

In 1999 Irwig and colleagues at the University of Sydney published a book that seeks to foster EBPC by providing patients with an explicit knowledge structure and tactics to help them interact with their clinicians. There are other signs that these issues surrounding clinical uncertainty are being made accessible to patients. Wolford (2000) introduced the concepts of test fallibility in a book with the provocative title, *'False Positives Can Kill You'*. When terms such as 'false positives' and 'false negatives' start appearing on popular book covers and patients take legal action about the consequences of being falsely reassured by unspecific tests, then we can be fairly certain that the paternalistic culture ascribed to medicine is rapidly changing.

Woloshin and Schwartz (1999) are developing techniques to familiarize patients with the various ways in which risk can be described. Their objective is to create a 'primer' that could be incorporated into the initial phases of a patient's encounter with a formal decision aid. Devices like these are designed to help consumers understand the concept of uncertainty in medical care and to become aware of the kinds of judgement heuristics to which they and their clinicians are susceptible (Redelmeier *et al.* 1993). These efforts need to be more broadly accepted. We propose that a wide body of scientists – particularly in the fields of health care, decision psychology, and clinical epidemiology – could work with journalists to raise their critical awareness and willingness to present complex issues that impinge on health care decisions.

Broadcast media

Another, largely unexploited, opportunity for placing these concepts before the public is to create a good working relationship with those who work at the editorial level in broadcasting and to suggest television series or special presentations on EBPC. These programmes could be built around high-interest issues such as a debate about the quality of the evidence in alternative medicine and the uncertainties involved in screening programmes.

Revising the school curricula

Additional effort could be invested in EBPC by working with the next generation of patients and health professionals, *before* they actually encounter difficult decisions in real life. The forces of consumerism, abundance and complexity of choice are likely to increase over time. Education policy makers, decision scientists, and teachers in mathematics and social sciences should work together to create an integrated curriculum. This would seek to provide today's students with critical appraisal skills that can be used as they encounter the choices ahead of them, particularly in health care situations. The material can be based on high-interest situations like the controversies in genetic research, AIDS prevention and management, and the conduct of clinical trials. Interactive electronic technologies involving computer programmes, CD-ROMs, and the Internet also could be used to engage interest. This could, if successfully implemented, transform the whole landscape of EBPC for future generations.

Conclusion

In this chapter, we considered how best to move EBPC into the mainstream of health care, and identified the many obstacles. We then argued that a common set of minimum quality standards for decision aids should be incorporated into patient education materials designed to support EBPC. There are multiple opportunities for using this set of criteria to develop EBPC materials for both health service and educational organizations. We also propose that the underlying mechanism that should be used to develop and promote EBPC is the WWW. It has unprecedented ability to link policy frameworks, consumers, patient groups, and health professionals with validated decision aids based on validated evidence derived from empirical studies. We recognize that we are enthusiasts, and that the socio-political milieu surrounding these opportunities is complex and dynamic. We therefore believe that any strategy to promote EBPC needs to recognize and work with this complexity to systematically place appraisal skills and decision aids in the hands of patients and health care professionals simultaneously.

References

Benbassat J, Pilpel D and Tidhar M (1998). Patients' preferences for participation in clinical decision making: a review of published surveys. *Behavioural Medicine* **24**: 81–8.

Charnock D, Shepperd S, Needham G and Gann R (1999). DISCERN: an instrument for judging the quality of written consumer health information on treatment choices. *Journal of Epidemiology and Community Health* **53**: 105–11.

Coulter A (1997). Partnerships with patients: the pros and cons of shared clinical decision making. *Journal of Health Services Research and Policy* **2**: 112–21.

Coulter A (1999). Paternalism or partnership? *British Medical Journal* **319**: 719–94.

Coulter A and Ham C (2000). *The global challenge of health care rationing.* Buckingham, Open University Press.

Eddy DM (1992*). A manual for assessing health practices and designing practice policies: the explicit approach.* Philadelphia, American College of Physicians.

Edwards A, Elwyn G, Covey J, Mathews E and Pill R (2001). Presenting risk information – the effects of 'framing' and other manipulations on patient outcomes. *Journal of Health Communication.* **6**: 1–22.

Elwyn G, Edwards A and Kinnersley P (1999). Shared decision making: the neglected second half of the consultation. *BJGP* **49**: 477–82.

Elwyn G, Edwards A, Kinnersley P and Grol R (2001). Shared decision making and the concept of equipoise: defining the competences of involving patients in health care choices. *BJGP*, in press.

Entwistle VA, Sheldon TA, Sowden IS and Watt IS (1998). Evidence-informed patient choice: issues of involving patients in decisions about health care technologies. *International Journal of Technology in Health Care* **14**: 212–25.

Entwistle VA, Watt IS and Johnson F (2000). The case of Norplant as an example of media coverage over the life of a new health technology. *Lancet* **355**: 1633–6.

Foundation for Informed Medical Decision Making (2000). www: healthdialog.com.

Guadagnoli E and Ward P (1998). Patient participation in decision making. *Social Science and Medicine* **47**(3): 329–39.

Holmes-Rovner M, Kroll J, Rovner D, Breer L, Schmitt N, Rothert ML, *et al.* (1999). Patient decision support intervention: increased consistency with decision analytic models. *Medical Care* **37**: 270–84.

Holmes-Rovner M, Valade D, Orlowski C, Draus C, Nabozny-Valerio B and Keiser S (2001). Shared decision making programmes in fee-for-service environments: implementation barriers and opportunities. *Health Expectations*, in press.

Irwig J, Irwig L and Sweet M (1999). *Smart health choices: how to make informed health decisions.* St Leonards, Allen and Unwin.

Laine C and Davidoff F (1996). Patient-centred medicine: a professional evolution. *Journal of the American Medical Association* **275**: 152–6.

Man-Son-Hing M, Laupacis A, O'Connor A, Biggs J, Drake E, Yetisir E, *et al.* (1999). A randomized trial of a decision aid for patients with atrial fibrillation. *Journal of the American Medical Association* **282**: 737–43.

National Health Committee (1993). *The best of health 2.* Wellington, New Zealand, National Advisory Committee on Core Health and Disability Support Services.

O'Connor AM (1995). Validation of a decisional conflict scale. *Medical Decision Making* **15**: 25–30.

O'Connor AM, Drake ER, Fiset V, Graham I, Laupacis A and Tugwell P (1999*a*). The Ottawa patient decision aids. *Effective Clinical Practice* **2**: 163–70.

O'Connor AM, Fiset V, Degrasse C, Graham I, Evans W, Stacey D, *et al.* (1999*b*). Decision aids for patients considering health care options: evidence of efficacy and policy implications. *Journal of the National Cancer Institute* **25** Monograph: 67–80.

O'Connor AM, Rostom A, Fiset V, Tetroe J, Entwistle V, Llewelyn-Thomas H, *et al.* (1999c). Decision aids for patients facing health treatment or screening decisions: systematic review. *British Medical Journal* **319**: 731–4.

Ottawa Health Decision Centre Decision Support Courses http://www.lri.ca/programs/ceu/ohdec, University of Ottawa.

Redelmeier DA, Rozin P and Kahneman D (1993). Understanding patients' decisions. Cognitive and emotional perspectives. *Journal of the American Medical Association* **270**: 72–6.

Schneider CE (1998). *The practice of autonomy: patients, doctors, and medical decisions*. New York, Oxford University Press.

Wennberg JE, Barry MJ, *et al.* (1993). Outcomes research, PORTs, and health care reform. *Ann N Y Acad Sci* **703**: 52–62.

Wolford G (2000). *False positives can kill you*. California, University of California Press.

Woloshin S and Schwartz LM (1999). How can we help people make sense of medical data? *Effective Clinical Practice* **2**: 176–83.

17 Consumer health informatics in the Internet age

Gunther Eysenbach and Alejandro R Jadad

Introduction

For the past 100,000 years, people have been able to produce, distribute, and process information in a synchronized manner. About 500 years ago, the situation started to change rapidly. With the advent of the mobile type press, our ability to produce and distribute information started to accelerate, outpacing our capacity to process information. During the past 10 years, we have witnessed how the Internet and the World Wide Web have led to a hyper-production and hyper-distribution of information, which have clearly overwhelmed our capacity to process it.

In this chapter we will explore current access to and barriers to further information for consumers. We will discuss how computers and other developments in information technology are ushering in the *era of consumer health informatics,* and the potential that lies ahead. It is clear that this will be a period in which the public will have unprecedented ability to access information and to participate actively in evidence-based health care.

We propose that consumer health informatics be regarded as a whole new academic discipline, one that should be devoted to the exploration of the new possibilities that informatics is creating for consumers in relation to health and health care issues. In its broadest sense, consumer health informatics should involve the following (Eysenbach 2000*a*):

- analysing, formalizing, and modelling consumer preferences and information needs;
- developing methods to integrate these into information management in health promotion, clinical, educational, and research activities;
- investigating the effectiveness and efficiency of computerized information, (tele)communication, and network systems for consumers in relation to their participation in health- and health care-related activities;

♦ studying the effects of these systems on public health, the patient–professional relationship, and society.

We will discuss the responses that are required of the health care professions and individual practitioners. There are also potentially helpful checks and balances on the nature of information now available to consumers. We will outline some of these and explore how all these developments may come together. None of these developments in information occur in isolation. They must be seen within the context of other changes, particularly the shifting emphasis away from the traditional paternalistic model of health care. These other changes are addressed more fully in other chapters of this book so will not be discussed in detail here. We will describe the development in information availability, but want the reader to place these issues in the broader context of moves towards greater informed choice for consumers in their health care decisions.

Current access to information by consumers: the gap between the ideal and the real

Ideally (as long as they wish), all consumers should be able to access valid and relevant information about their health status. They should be able to judge the advantages and disadvantages of all possible courses of action, according to their values, beliefs, preferences, and their personal circumstances (for example, their perceived state of health, their socio-economic status).

In reality, we are far from this ideal state, as many barriers prevent consumers from accessing the information they need, when they need it, where they need it, and in the amount and format in which they need it. The following is a brief description of some of the most prominent barriers. We do not pretend to include an exhaustive list, but a selection of those that, in our opinion, are preventing consumers from participating meaningfully in evidence-based decision making. We have separated the barriers depending on whether they relate to providers, to the consumers *per se*, to the information available, to the health care system, and to information technology. As a theme in the titles of the following sections we will draw an analogy from the supply of water.

Barriers related to providers: keeping the consumer thirsty

Despite a strong international trend to shift towards a shared decision making model, many consumers in both developed and developing countries still find themselves interacting with providers who favour the 'classical', authoritarian, paternalistic, asymmetrical model of consumer–provider interaction. In these situations, consumer access to information is prevented by health care providers who adopt the role of main purveyors of knowledge. The professional acts not only as the sole holder of the consumer's data but also as the filter for other types of information needed by the consumer to participate in decisions about their health and health care. In other cases, consumers face providers who prefer an 'informed choice' decision making model, in which they give consumers as much information as they think they need to make a decision, but the professionals do not participate directly in the decision. A shared decision making approach goes beyond this, placing consumers and providers as active participants in the decision making process, with two-way exchange of information and working as partners. These models are discussed more fully in Chapter 8 (Elwyn and Charles).

Even if providers wish to shift from the authoritarian or informed models to a shared one, however, many remain unable to do it because of inadequate communication skills, lack of time, or lack of financial incentives. A combination of the above factors may explain why many providers do not even think that consumers could benefit from the Internet. A survey from the US shows striking figures: only 39% of all professionals see the Internet as a valuable health information source for consumers. This sharply contrasts with the value consumers give to web-education: 70% of consumers retrieving health information on the Internet agree that 'the Internet empowers me to make better choices in my life' (*source*: cyberdialogue/ findsvp survey, reproduced in Reents and Miller (1998)).

Various factors probably contribute to the low esteem in which professionals hold the Internet as an educational tool. These include the (partly justified) concerns about the quality of Internet information and discomfort about having to deal with a consumer who is perhaps better informed than oneself. The Wilson study (1999) illustrates the extent of this: an amazing 65% of the family doctors said that the information presented by consumers was new to them (see Table 17.1).

Barriers related to consumers: a rocky road, few shoes and no maps to find the wells

Lack of easy-to-access sources of high-quality relevant information

Until very recently, databases such as Medline were available only to experts (sometimes not even to them). Although consumers were always 'passively' exposed to health information in the mass media, the possibilities to actively perform targeted literature searches were limited. Not only did consumers have limited insights into and access to the whole body of medical knowledge, but usually they also had virtually no access to their own medical records.

Table 17.1
Survey among family doctors and practice nurses about consultations with consumers
holding Internet health care information (Wilson, 1999)

	Family doctor No. of Staff	(%)	Practice Nurse No. of Staff	(%)
The consumer participates more actively in his/her treatment	65	(78.3%)	26	(83.9%)
The consumer has higher expectations	75	(85.2%)	26	(78.8%)
The information is accurate	59	(73.8%)	24	(75%)
The length of consultation is increased	68	(77.3%)	24	(72.7%)
This type of consumer is a welcome challenge	46	(55.4%)	24	(72.7%)
The consultation is more interactive than usual	43	(50.6%)	22	(68.8%)
The consumer correctly interpreted information	38	(44.7%)	19	(59.4%)
The consumer is more demanding	50	(58.8%)	14	(42.4%)

To date, it has been the 'traditional' responsibility of the professional to integrate all types of information in the personal interaction with the consumer. Thus they would give consumers details about their conditions and distil and present the relevant external information on the available options. Increasingly, however, the traditional professional – filter and sole provider of information – is being bypassed by consumers, who now have direct access to both the external evidence and their personal health record (Fig. 17.1). This process is likely to accelerate and evolve quickly, thanks to powerful forces which are shaping health and health care, of which the Internet is perhaps the most prominent (Braddock *et al.* 1999). These changes are already facing resistance from the provider community. Many professionals are concerned that consumers may misinterpret information and will not arrive at the information that is relevant to them (intersection of Fig. 17.1) but get lost in a stew of irrelevant and low-quality information. Vignettes of how the influence of information affects the models of care are illustrated in Fig. 17.2.

The problem of low health literacy

Low health literacy frequently impairs consumers' understanding of health messages and limits their ability to care for their health problems (AMA Ad Hoc Committee on Health Literacy for the Council on Scientific Affairs 1999). This is a problem especially prevalent among the elderly (Gazmararian *et al.* 1999). Consumers with inadequate health literacy have a complex array of communications difficulties, which may lead to poor health outcomes. Individuals judged to be 'functionally illiterate' (estimated to include 30 to

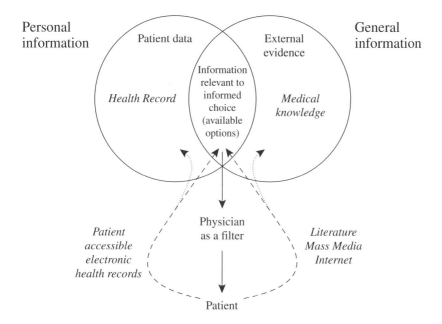

Fig. 17.1 Consumer data and external evidence are the two categories of information that need to be integrated by the professional and consumer to arrive at a health care decision. Increasingly, consumers can bypass the professional as a filter (and moderator) and have direct access to parts of this information. This may be problematic, if the consumer accesses not only information that is relevant for their informed decision process, but also low-quality and irrelevant information. At the same time this is also an opportunity for evidence-based health care, as consumers are now able to question the evidence-base of professionals.

50% of the adult population in the US and Canada) have been shown to report worse health status and have increased risk of hospitalization (Baker *et al.* 1997). To compound this, much consumer education material has been produced which is at a higher reading level than the estimated average reading level of the American public (Vivian and Robertson 1980) and most patient information on the WWW is written at even higher reading levels (Graber *et al.* 1999). Unsurprisingly such material may fail to communicate the basic information intended.

Twenty-five years ago Tudor Hart (1971) described the inverse care law, stating that 'the availability of good medical care tends to vary inversely with the need for it in the population served'. In analogy, we may postulate an '*inverse information law*' (Eysenbach 2000*a*) stating that access to appropriate information varies inversely with the need for it. In other words, it is likely that access to high-quality relevant information is particularly difficult for those who would need it most. At present, people with low health literacy do not benefit from advances in consumer health informatics and cybermedicine, as they lack access to or understanding of these technologies. A

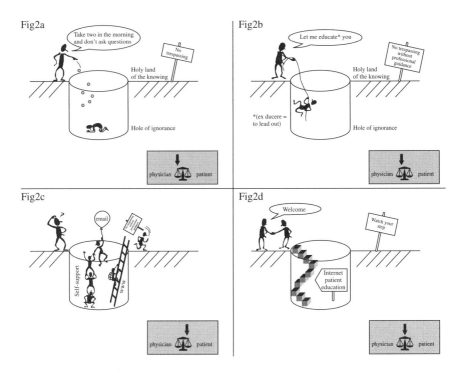

Fig. 17.2 Different models of the consumer–professional relationship: a) paternalistic, b) educational, c) Internet-age, and d) consumer-as-partner.

sequence can be envisaged in which low health literacy leads to poor health, poor health leads to low income, and low income limits access to modern information technology. Thus, one fundamental problem of telemedicine and using the Internet for health education is that those who are at highest risk of preventable or treatable health problems have the greatest need for information and are the least likely to have access to such technologies (Eng *et al.* 1998).

Public policies are needed to actively fight this pervasive inequality. It is also important to realize that there needs to be greater awareness about the problem of health literacy. The American Medical Association's Ad Hoc Committee on Health Literacy for the Council on Scientific Affairs concluded that 'professional and public awareness of the health literacy issue must be increased, beginning with education of medical students and professionals and improved consumer–professional communication skills' (AMA Ad Hoc Committee on Health Literacy for the Council on Scientific Affairs 1999). In addition to efforts to increase awareness, we also need to develop better methods of screening consumers to identify those with poor health literacy, more effective health education techniques, and more research on outcomes and costs associated with poor health literacy, and the causal pathway of how poor health literacy influences health.

Limited access to the Internet

Even if there were resources that provided high-quality information easily on the Internet, regardless of their literacy levels, a major barrier that would still need to be overcome is the broader barrier of access, described in detail below ('Barriers related to technology'). Thus, the inverse information law is true both on the macrolevel – the poorest countries have the worst access to information and communication (UNDP 1999) – and on the individual level (microlevel), with disadvantaged individuals within a society having the poorest health, inferior health literacy, and the worst access to information.

Barriers related to the information: hydrants with muddy water

Unlimited access to poorly organized information

In the past, health professionals had to cope with information overload, while consumers had to cope with information deficit. Today, consumers have many opportunities to access information in abundance, through mass media, self-support groups, and particularly the Internet (Fig. 17.2c). The directed, intentional process of active 'health education' (Fig. 17.2b) is now being counteracted by an anarchical process of uncontrolled information retrieval by the consumer.

For the first time in the history of medicine, consumers have equal access to the knowledge bases of medicine – and those 'connected' are making heavy use of this. An example of this is the fact that the number of Medline searches performed by directly accessing the database at the National Library of Medicine increased from 7 million in 1996 to 120 million in 1997, when free public access was opened. The new searches are attributed primarily to 'non-professionals' (Sieving 1999). It has been argued that 'a driving force behind demand for online health information is the shortage of information easily obtained from traditional channels' (Reents and Miller 1998). With the duration of an average consultation still only seven minutes in the UK (and twelve minutes in the US) it comes as little surprise that professionals routinely fail to address the information needs of consumers (Braddock *et al.* 1999). While most professionals do not understand or have access to these modern information technologies, or simply lack sufficient time to familiarize themselves with the Internet, consumers have all the time in the world to search the Internet for relevant information.

This new 'reversed' information asymmetry creates new conflicts – the fact that consumers are taking the initiative to look out for the latest research results 'stands on its head the tradition in which a doctor gives orders and the consumer obeys', as an article in the *New York Times* put it. 'And that makes some doctors nervous' (Hafner 1998). Some of the concern is well founded. It is likely, for instance, that health professionals may find themselves in the middle of unnecessary conflicts if consumers find information on the Internet that is unknown to the professional, contradicts their recommendations, or that suggests the use of an effective intervention that is unavailable.

In a postal questionnaire survey among 160 family doctors and 96 practice nurses in Scotland (Wilson 1999), 58% of doctors and 34% of nurses stated that they have been approached by consumers with Internet health care information. Only 39% of the doctors and 31% of the nurses felt 'positive' about these consumers, the remainder were 'indifferent', 'uncomfortable', or 'not sure'. About half of the respondents were concerned about the reliability of Internet information and a similar percentage were concerned that consumers did not interpret information correctly (Wilson 1999). On the positive side, the majority of health professionals feel that when consumers bring information they participate more actively in their treatment, that the consultation is more interactive, and that overall 'this type of consumer is a welcome challenge' (see Table 17.1).

The almost unlimited access to information offered by the Internet also creates other potential problems. Seeking desired information on the Internet is often time-consuming. Consumers often experience confusion and anxiety caused by the virtually unlimited amount of information available, which is poorly organized and has quite variable quality and relevance.

Few mechanisms to control the quality of the information

Currently there is no agreed mechanism for ensuring the accuracy, currency, or completeness of the information presented to consumers (Hersey *et al.* 1997). A quality control process, both when preparing information and when accessing it, has been demanded from different sides. A recent review of 54 consumer information materials concluded that 'current information materials for consumers omit relevant data, fail to give a balanced view of the effectiveness of different treatments, and ignore uncertainties; moreover, many information materials adopt a patronizing tone – few actively promote a participative approach to decision making' (Coulter *et al.* 1999).

On the Internet, there have been numerous studies evaluating the quality of information given on different venues such as websites (Impicciatore *et al.* 1997), newsgroups (Culver *et al.* 1997) and email-consultations (Eysenbach and Diepgen 1998a, b). While the Internet offers a huge amount of health information, many of the authors are not trained in medicine or even health education. In many situations, the intention of information provision is not to educate, but to sell something.

The lack of reliability is a particular concern. In addition to this, the Internet poses special problems for consumers, which have been summarized as 'lack of context' (Eysenbach and Diepgen 1998c), meaning that the Internet poses additional problems for consumers and health professionals to assess and apply the material, compared to critical appraisal of traditional information. This is due to the following characteristics of the Internet (Eysenbach and Diepgen 1999a):

- There are no clear markers such as traditional publishing which allow consumers to recognize:
  1. the target group of a document (consumers/professionals)
  2. the intention (advertisement or objective information);
- The anonymity (of authors) makes it difficult to appraise information based on the credentials of the authors;
- Internationality: information valid in foreign health care systems may not be applicable locally (Coiera 1996).

These characteristics of the Internet may explain why consumers have difficulties finding information that relates to them and why the majority of physicians say that the consumer has difficulties interpreting information correctly (Wilson 1999).

While it has been pointed out that we still know very little about the impact of the Internet on public health (Coiera 1998), there are many ways that Internet information could do harm (Science Panel on Interactive Communication and Health 1999):

- Misinformation can lead consumers with life-threatening conditions to lose trust in their provider, and take actions that undermine the effectiveness of their treatment (such as by taking substances that interact in a negative way with prescribed medications).
- Consumers may use their limited time with their health care provider unproductively, or in ways that ultimately increase costs of care, and even abandon a provider delivering high-quality care to pursue ineffective therapies.
- Vulnerable people may also be victimized by biased or incomplete information from those with a financial interest in the information they provide.

Such risks are present in most media, but on the WWW this problem reaches a new dimension.

Barriers related to technology: few pipes, few glasses, and complex taps

If consumers are to take full advantage of the Internet, access to it should be easy, affordable, and available in all settings. This is still far from reality.

Despite an unprecedented rate of penetration in developed countries, the majority of people in the world remain without access to computers and the Internet. The Internet is still available to less than 50% of people in North America, the region with the highest proportion of users in the world. In developing countries, the main barriers are the high cost of computers and poor telecommunications infrastructure. In both developed and developing countries, many consumers still perceive computer-based systems as difficult to use.

The end result is that rather than levelling the playing field, the rapid development of the Internet is contributing to widening inequalities across the world (UNDP 2000). Even in developed countries, there is some evidence of a similar widening gap across groups with different socio-economic and demographic profiles (UNDP 1999). There is a clear digital divide between the information rich (such as Whites, Asians/Pacific Islanders, those with higher incomes, those more educated, and dual-parent households) and the information poor (such as those who are younger, those with lower incomes and education levels, certain minorities, and those in rural areas or central cities) (Irving *et al.* 1999). The levels of access appear to be increasing rapidly in other parts of the world, particularly in Western Europe and in the developed countries of Australasia. Although the data are very poor, it seems that the developing world is lagging behind, creating an increasingly wide access gap.

While the information society offers tremendous potential for reducing the knowledge gap between professionals and patients, it also brings a risk of a widening of the gap between those who have access to new technology and those who have been excluded. Therefore the field must not be left to market forces alone and active policy is required to push information technology to those who are underserved (Eysenbach 2000*a*).

Striving for the ideal: bridging the gaps through information technology

Developing advanced approaches to knowledge representation

So far, most (if not all) of the Internet-based applications to promote transfer of knowledge to consumers are a mere transition from paper-based to electronic-based means to process and distribute information in text form. The true 'revolution' (in the sense of going full circle), however, is likely to come from ongoing and future increases in bandwidth that will enable all people to communicate through the Internet more effectively. The next generation Internet (see www.ngi.gov) will operate at speeds up to a thousand times faster than today. Sight, sound, and even touch will be integrated through powerful computers, displays, and networks. With these developments we will be able to go beyond text to more 'natural' or primal ways of representing and exchanging knowledge. Soon we will be able to put together and deliver relevant and valid information, of different types, using more engaging ways to package the messages and multisensory modes of communication. The effectiveness and efficiency of these new modalities to organize information will be optimized through inexpensive Internet appliances (such as fridges and microwave ovens with Internet access), personal portable or wearable computers, and wireless access to the Internet (Jadad *et al.* 2000).

Another trend will lead to a 'quality leap': the perspective of 'machine understandable information'. Key to this development is the widespread use of metadata. Recent developments and Internet standards, such as the eXtensible Markup Language (XML), Dublin Core metadata (Malet *et al.* 1999), MedPICS (Eysenbach and Diepgen 1998*c*, 1999*a*), and RDF (Resource Description Framework), will make relations between information pieces 'understandable' for computers, allowing software for example to perform intelligent searches, filter information automatically, or to tailor information to the individual. The Web would evolve into a global medical knowledge base that is easily navigable and searchable across languages and continents (Eysenbach *et al.* 1999).

Promoting team work

It is time for health professionals 'to embrace the concept of informed consumers and use their web-surfing skills' (Pemberton and Goldblatt 1998) (see also Box 17.1) rather than seeing them as threatening intruders trespassing into a forbidden zone. For the providers, this requires the acquisition of skills in the use of the Internet, familiarization with sources of high-quality information (Shepperd *et al.* 1999), and confidence with the use of aids and tools to engage in shared decision making.

On a public health level, 'stairways' for the consumer should be built, guiding consumers to high-quality information, as illustrated in Fig. 17.2d. Examples include 'Healthfinder', a government-sponsored health portal in the US (www.healthfinder.gov) or the National electronic Library for Health (NeLH) in the UK. The latter's mission is 'to improve health and health care, consumer choice, and clinical practice', and it includes NHS Direct Online, a service to provide consumers with information such as 'How can I stay healthy, feel better, and reduce the risk of disease?', 'Do I need to see a doctor for this problem?', and 'How can I learn more about my condition, contribute to my care, and make the best use of health services?' (Gray and de Lusignan 1999). Clearly, the demand for such information is vast, as can be seen in the large number of patient requests doctors on the Internet receive via email (Widman and Tong 1997; Eysenbach and Diepgen 1998*a*, 1999*b*).

Box 17.1 **Suggestions for providers to interact with Internet-literate consumers (Pemberton and Goldblatt, 1998)**

Do

♦ Try to react in positive manner to information from the Internet
♦ Warn about the variability in the quality and reliability of material from the Internet
♦ Warn about time constraints that may limit your ability to address all the information found on the Internet
♦ Develop a strategy for dealing with Internet information before the encounter (e.g. get consumers to email summary of issues before consultations)
♦ Accept consumer contributions as valuable
♦ Accept that they may find relevant and valid information previously unknown to you.

Don't

♦ Be dismissive or paternalistic
♦ Be derogatory of comments made by others on the Internet
♦ Refuse to accept information found on the Internet
♦ Feel threatened

Giving consumers control over their own information

One of the most radical steps towards consumer empowerment will involve making the electronic health records (at least parts of them) available to consumers on the Internet. Once this occurs, consumers will be able to do 'online-doctoring', just as they do 'online-banking' and 'online-shopping' today (Eysenbach 2000a).

To put the records into the hands of consumers is not a new idea. More than 25 years ago it was already advocated that 'patients' should be able to take their records home (Coleman 1984). Baldry *et al.* (1986) conducted an early experiment with giving consumers in the waiting room their medical records to read. The international trend is to allow consumers to inspect their records and to allow them to make copies thereof (McQuoid-Mason 1996). The European Union Data Directive (applicable October 1998) required all member countries to enact legislation enabling subject access to medical records, if not already enacted.

Consumer health informatics developments offer further opportunities for this process, with the potential to grant consumers access to information which is relevant to them and to integrate their personal data with explanatory information. For example, a system called SeniorMed allows elderly consumers access to their electronic medication lists via the WWW. Such systems may be integrated with drug information (Rind *et al.* 1999). MedicaLogic, a company based in the US, is also testing a concept called 'Internet Health Record', a service that lets consumers privately access information from their real medical records over the Internet. The information is embedded in a system that lets them research health conditions, refill prescriptions, and communicate with their professional's office. Consumer records could be linked with glossaries, and be linked to information on the Internet (for example, if the problem list contains 'smoking', links could refer to 'how-to-quit-smoking' health promotion sites or to Medline). Consumers could also change or comment on certain entries (http://www.medicalogic. com/services/about_98point6.html).

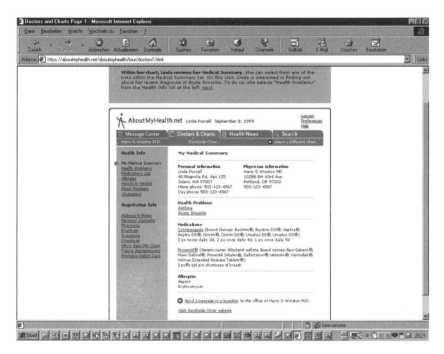

Fig. 17.3 Internet accessible consumer health record.

Ensuring better quality control

In the field of Internet publishing, many instruments to evaluate health information exist, but none of them have been validated. In addition, it is unclear whether they should exist in the first place, whether they measure what they claim to measure, or whether they lead to more good than harm (Jadad and Gagliardi 1998).

The Swiss Health on the Net foundation has compiled some consensus ethical principles for publishers of health information, the so-called HON Code of Conduct (http://www.hon.ch/HONcode/). Information providers who agree to implement these ethical principles display the HON logo on their websites. However, there are no mechanisms for controlling or enforcing the adoption of such principles. As a result, it is not clear how many of the several thousand sites displaying the logo have actually implemented the principles. The HON Code is often misinterpreted (also in the peer-reviewed literature!) as an award-system, rating system, or as 'quality criterion' which allows consumers to appraise the quality of a website. It is however not possible for a third party (that is, the user of a website) to verify for example that a principle such as 'privacy and confidentiality' or 'honesty in disclosing sources of funding' is observed.

A systematic review on different quality criteria used to assess information on the Internet has been published recently (Kim *et al.* 1999). Consumers may for example use indirect quality criteria such as popularity, expressed as number of visitors or 'webcitations' (Eysenbach and Diepgen 1998c; Hernández-Borges *et al.* 1999). There are now several tools available on the Internet for use by consumers which help users to assess the quality themselves (http://hitiweb.mitretek.org/iq/default.asp, http://www.discern.org.uk, http://www.quick.org.uk).

DISCERN is a standardized index to judge the quality of health information. This instrument is targeted at producers, health professionals, and consumers to appraise written information on treatment choices. Crucial in the development was the determination of inter-rater agreement among different user groups. Questions with insufficient inter-rater agreement, such as those concerning design or reading level ('the information is easy to understand'), were eliminated from the final instrument. However, the validity of DISCERN in terms of the relationship between a DISCERN score and impact of the information on consumer outcomes have not yet been determined. It should also be noted that the inter-rater reliability for DISCERN was rather low when it was used by consumers. Thus it is not yet clear whether DISCERN is a truly useful instrument for consumers to distinguish good from bad information.

In the near future, an international system of accreditation or 'quality seals' (evaluative meta-information assigned by trusted raters) may help consumers to identify high-quality information on the Internet. A European Union (EU) funded project, 'G7 ENABLE', has described 'Barriers To A Global Information Society For Health'. It made the following observations to the EU Commission: 'A great deal of health-related information on the Web is poor, misleading and much positively harmful. This substantially diminishes the benefits that the Internet could potentially deliver'.

What is required is an internationally-recognized scheme whereby the public can identify, and search for, high-quality Internet health information. These should carry the authority of clinical bodies, which are recognized as having the clinical standing to be trusted. Such a filtering and rating system is currently being implemented in a new EU project called MedCERTAIN (MedPICS Certification and Rating of Trustworthy Health Information on the Net, http://www.medcertain.org), funded under the EU Action Plan for safer use of the Internet (Eysenbach *et al.*, forthcoming). The aim of this project is to establish trust and improve the quality of health information on the Internet by the 'four E's' (Eysenbach 2000*b*):

♦ *Educating* the public (teaching critical appraisal skills to consumers);

♦ *Encouraging* self-governance, for example encouraging health information providers to obey ethical codes for health (Eysenbach 2000*b*) and promoting self-labelling (disclosure of important information such as authorship and sponsors, also with metadata);

♦ *Evaluation* and certification of information (offer a framework for third party rating, so that interested medical societies and bodies can assign 'quality seals' to trustworthy information);

♦ *Enforcement* (Network of Hotlines for consumers).

The international MedCERTAIN trustmark will be established in close collaboration with all interested agencies and relevant national organizations which pursue similar aims. These would include, for example, bodies such as OMNI (Organizing Medical Networked Information, http://www. omni.ac.uk/) or the UK Centre for Health Information Quality. A basic principle is inter-operability of existing rating services and the creation of metadata exchange standards.

The future

The vast potential of the Internet to promote health information and to foster consumer–professional communication is far from being realized. The Internet has both the clientele (consumers who really want to learn something about their health) and the technical prerequisites (the reach of a mass-medium, combined with the possibility for interactivity to tailor information specific to the individual) to be an ideal medium to promote consumer education and decision support. An interesting future perspective is the linkage of the personal online-accessible health record with general health information from evidence-based resources. The convergence of technology and knowledge will be greatly enhanced by the use of multimedia and artificial intelligence. Further contributions will come from the advent of low cost portable and wearable computers. These will allow access to knowledge at the right time and in the right place through ubiquitous computer networks and wireless connections to the Internet. Among other challenges (Jadad 1999), development and proper evaluation of these tools and making them accessible to those who need them most will be the main themes of consumer health informatics in the information age.

References

AMA Ad Hoc Committee on Health Literacy for the Council on Scientific Affairs (1999). Health literacy: report of the Council on Scientific Affairs. Ad Hoc Committee on Health Literacy for the Council on Scientific Affairs, American Medical Association. *Journal of the American Medical Association* **281**(6): 552–7.

Baker DW, Parker RM, Williams MV, Clark WS and Nurss J (1997). The relationship of patient reading ability to self-reported health and use of health services. *Am J Public Health* **87**(6): 1027–30.

Baldry M, Cheal C, Fisher B, Gillett M and Huet V (1986). Giving patients their own records in general practice: experience of patients and staff. *British Medical Journal (Clin Res Ed)* **292**(6520): 596–8.

Braddock CH, Edwards KA, Hasenberg NM, Laidley TL and Levinson W (1999). Informed decision making in outpatient practice: time to get back to basics. *Journal of the American Medical Association* **282**(24): 2313–20.

Coiera E (1996). The Internet's challenge to health care provision. *British Medical Journal* **312**(7022): 3–4.

Coiera E (1998). Information epidemics, economics, and immunity on the Internet. We still know so little about the effect of information on public health. *British Medical Journal* **317**(7171): 1469–70.

Coleman V (1984). Why patients should keep their own records. *J Med Ethics* **10**(1): 27–8.

Coulter A, Entwistle V and Gilbert D (1999). Sharing decisions with patients: is the information good enough? *British Medical Journal* **318**(7179): 318–22. (http://wwwbmjcom/cgi/content/full/318/7179/318)

Culver JD, Gerr F and Frumkin H (1997). Medical information on the Internet: a study of an electronic bulletin board. *J Gen Intern Med* **12**(8): 466–70.

Eng TR, Maxfield A, Patrick K, Deering MJ, Ratzan SC and Gustafson DH (1998). Access to health information and support: a public highway or a private road? *Journal of the American Medical Association* **280**(15): 1371–5.

Eysenbach G and Diepgen TL (1998a). Responses to unsolicited patient email requests for medical advice on the World Wide Web. *Journal of the American Medical Association* **280**(15): 1333–5.

Eysenbach G and Diepgen TL (1998*b*). Evaluation of cyberdocs. *Lancet* **352**(9139): 1526.

Eysenbach G and Diepgen TL (1998*c*). Towards quality management of medical information on the Internet: evaluation, labelling, and filtering of information. *British Medical Journal* **317**(7171): 1496–500. (http://www.bmj.com/cgi/content/full/317/7171/1496)

Eysenbach G and Diepgen TL (1999*a*). Labeling and filtering of medical information on the Internet. *Methods Inf Med* **38**(2): 80–8.

Eysenbach G and Diepgen TL (1999*b*). Patients looking for information on the Internet and seeking teleadvice: motivation, expectations, and misconceptions as expressed in e mails sent to physicians. *Arch Dermatol* **135**(2): 151–6.

Eysenbach G, Sa ER and Diepgen TL (1999). Shopping around the Internet today and tomorrow: towards the millennium of cybermedicine. *British Medical Journal* **319**(7220): 1294. (http://www.bmj.com/cgi/content/full/319/7220/1294)

Eysenbach G (2000*a*). Consumer health informatics. *British Medical Journal* **320**(7251): 1713–6. (http://bmj.com/cgi/content/full/320/7251/1713)

Eysenbach G (2000*b*). Towards ethical guidelines for e-health: JMIR Theme Issue on eHealth Ethics. *J Med Internet Res* **2**(1): e7. (http://www.symposion.com/jmir/2000/1/e7/)

Eysenbach G, Yihune G, Lampe K, Cross P, and Brickley D (2001) MedCERTAIN: quality management, certification and rating of health information on the Net. *Proc AMIA Symp*, forthcoming.

Gazmararian JA, Baker DW, Williams MV, Parker RM, Scott TL, Green DC, *et al.* (1999). Health literacy among Medicare enrollees in a managed care organization. *Journal of the American Medical Association* **281**(6): 545–51.

Graber MA, Roller CM and Kaeble B (1999). Readability levels of patient education material on the World Wide Web. *J Fam Pract* **48**(1): 58–61.

Gray JA, de Lusignan S (1999). National electronic library for health (NeLH). *British Medical Journal* **319**(7223): 1476–9. (http://www.bmj.com/cgi/content/full/319/7223/1476)

Hafner K (1998) Jul 9. Can the Internet cure the common cold? *The New York Times; Sect Technology*. (http://www.corporateserver.com/qiodemo/nyt.htm)

Hart JT (1971). The inverse care law. *Lancet* **1**(7696): 405–12.

Hernández-Borges AA, Macías-Cervi P, Gaspar-Guardado MA, Torres-Álvarez de Arcaya ML, Ruiz-Rabaza A and Jiménez-Sosa A (1999). Can examination of WWW usage statistics and other indirect quality indicators help to distinguish the relative quality of medical websites? *J Med Internet Res* **1**(1):e1. (http://www.symposion.com/jmir/1999/1/e1/index.htm)

Hersey JC, Matheson J and Lohr KN (1997) Sep. Consumer Health Informatics and Patient Decision making. Rockville, MD: Agency for Health Care Policy and Research; Report nr AHCPR Publication No. 98-N001. (http://www.ahcpr.gov/research/rtisumm.htm)

Impicciatore P, Pandolfini C, Casella N and Bonati M (1997). Reliability of health information for the public on the World Wide Web: systematic survey of advice on managing fever in children at home. *British Medical Journal* **314**(7098): 1875–9.

Irving L, Klegar-Levy K, Everette DW, Reynolds T and Lader W (1999) Jul. Falling through the Net: defining the digital divide. A report on the telecommunications and information technology gap in America. Washington, DC, National Telecommunications and Information Administration, US Dept of Commerce. (http://www.ntia.doc.gov/ntiahome/fttn99/contents.html, http://www.ntia.doc.gov/ntiahome/fttn99/FTTN.pdf)

Jadad AR (1999). Promoting partnerships: challenges for the Internet age. *British Medical Journal* **319**(7212): 761–4. (http://www.bmj.com/cgi/content/full/319/7212/761)

Jadad AR and Gagliardi A (1998). Rating health information on the Internet: navigating to knowledge or to Babel? *Journal of the American Medical Association* **279**(8): 611–4.

Jadad AR, Haynes RB, Hunt DL and Browman GP (2000). The Internet and evidence-based decision making: a needed synergy for efficient knowledge management in health care. *Canadian Medical Association Journal* **162**(3): 362–5. (http://www.cma.ca/cmaj/vol-162/issue-3/0362.htm)

Kim P, Eng TR, Deering MJ and Maxfield A (1999). Published criteria for evaluating health related websites: review. *British Medical Journal* **318**(7184): 647–9.

McQuoid-Mason D (1996). Medical records and access thereto. *Med Law* **15**(3): 499–517.

Malet G, Munoz F, Appleyard R and Hersh W (1999). A model for enhancing Internet medical document retrieval with 'medical core metadata'. *J Am Med Inform Assoc* **6**(2): 163–72.

Pemberton PJ and Goldblatt J (1998). The Internet and the changing roles of doctors, patients and families. *Med J Aust* **169**(11–12): 594–5.

Reents S and Miller TE. (1998). The health care industry in transition – the online mandate to change. http://www.cyberdialogue.com/free_data/white_papers/intel_health_day.html. Cyber Dialogue.

Rind DM, Kim JH and Sturges EA (1999). SeniorMed: Connecting patients to their medication records. *Proc AMIA Symp* (1–2): 1147.

Science Panel on Interactive Communication and Health. (1999) Apr. Wired for health and well-being; the emergence of interactive health communication. Washington, DC, US Department of Health and Human Services, US Government Printing Office

Shepperd S, Charnock D and Gann B (1999). Helping patients access high-quality health information. *British Medical Journal* **319**(7212): 764–6. (http://www.bmj.com/cgi/content/full/319/7212/764)

Sieving PC (1999). Factors driving the increase in medical information on the Web – One American perspective. *J Med Internet Res* **1**(1): e3. (http://www.symposion.com/jmir/1999/1/e3)

UNDP (1999). *Human development report 1999.* Oxford, Oxford University Press. (http://www.undp.org/hdro/report.html)

UNDP (2000). *Human development report 2000.* Oxford, Oxford University Press. (http://www.undp.org/hdr2000/english/HDR2000.html)

Vivian AS and Robertson EJ (1980). Readability of patient education materials. *Clin Ther* **3**(2): 129–36.

Widman LE and Tong DA (1997). Requests for medical advice from patients and families to health care providers who publish on the World Wide Web. *Arch Intern Med* **157**(2): 209–12.

Wilson SM (1999). Impact of the Internet on primary care staff in Glasgow. *J Med Internet Res* **1**(2): e7. (http://www.symposion.com/jmir/1999/2/e7/)

18 The future

Angela Coulter

In September 1999 the British Medical Journal published a special theme issue entitled 'Embracing patient partnership'. Following its publication visitors to the BMJ's website were asked to respond to a brief questionnaire asking their views on consulting styles (BMJ 16/10/99). The survey ran over a two-week period from 17 September to 4 October. The results are shown in Table 18.1.

Visitors to the BMJ website are certainly not representative of the general population. Predominantly medically trained professionals, they constitute a particularly well informed and influential group. It is not particularly surprising, therefore, that respondents to this survey indicated a preference for a participative role in decisions about their own care, but the disjunction between the way in which they said they wanted to be treated when they were patients and their views of how most other patients are treated currently was striking. Even more noteworthy was their sense that paternalistic consultation styles are on the way out, to be replaced by shared decision making or informed choice as the dominant modes.

If these survey respondents are correct, the next ten years will see a profound change in relationships between health professionals and their patients. The factors driving the change include rising educational standards, improvements in public access to health information, and a decline in deference to professional authority. Government action has fuelled the change. Consumerism has been promoted as a central plank of health policy in the belief that consumer pressure and competition would both drive up quality standards and increase value for money in the health services. In the UK this has been accompanied by various policy initiatives designed to channel the demand for health care to the most appropriate and cost-effective providers. But costs have continued to rise and there has been an upward trend in the number of complaints and law suits by dissatisfied patients, suggesting either that services have deteriorated or that people are now more likely to seek redress when things go wrong. This chapter looks at the implications of the change in public expectations of health services and the opportunities and challenges this poses for professionals and for health policy makers.

Table 18.1 Responses to BMJ questionnaire on consultation styles[1]

	Doctor decides	Doctor and patient decide together	Patient decides
As a patient, which consulting style do you prefer?	56 (6.6%)	737 (87.0%)	54 (6.4%)
Which consulting style predominates today?	503 (59.6%)	298 (35.3%)	43 (5.1%)
Which consulting style do you think will predominate in 10 years' time?	75 (8.9%)	546 (64.7%)	223 (26.4%)

1. http://www.bmj.com/ 24th October 1999

Public access to health information

The Internet is already beginning to exert an influence on clinical practice and this effect seems set to increase rapidly as computer literacy becomes widespread and more and more people gain access to the World Wide Web. By the end of 1999, 15% of the UK population used the Internet, while in the USA the proportion was 25% in the country as a whole, rising to more than 50% in some urban areas (CyberAtlas 1999). Of these just over half used the Internet to access health information. At the current rate of growth it seems likely that by 2010 the majority of patients will be Internet users and a high proportion will have sought information from health-related websites. Doctors are even more likely to use the Internet. A 1999 survey of US physicians found that 85% were Internet users, an increase of 875% from 1997 (CyberAtlas 1999). In addition 33% of those surveyed said they had used email to communicate with patients.

As mentioned in the previous chapter, the rapid spread of multiple television channels and the convergence of digital television, email, and other computer-based technologies will greatly enhance the potential for interactive communications. Members of the public will be able to make their own diagnoses, inform themselves about treatment options and risks, seek and receive medical advice, and educate themselves about self-management of their condition, all without stirring from their armchairs. By the time they reach the doctor's clinic they will be much more knowledgeable than today's patients and quite likely to have formed their own views about what should be done. They will expect a different type of relationship with the health care professionals they consult and they will be more likely to want to be actively involved in decisions about their care.

Access to information is an essential underpinning for evidence-based patient choice. The Internet will greatly enhance public access to health information, but there is a downside to this information explosion. The majority of the health information available on the Internet is provided or sponsored by commercial companies whose main interest is to sell their products. The online health care industry is dominated by pharmaceutical companies who have seized on the potential offered by the Internet for direct-to-consumer advertising. The Americans currently lead the world in e-commerce. The market for online consumer health sales in the USA is projected to grow to $2.1 billion by 2003 (Jupiter Store 1999). The Internet is much more difficult to regulate than print media because it transcends national boundaries. Direct-to-consumer advertising of prescription drugs is currently outlawed in the UK, but this type of regulation will seem increasingly irrelevant as people turn to commercially sponsored websites for health information. Pressure is already mounting from both industry and consumer groups to remove the advertising restrictions (Cardy *et al.* 1999). The arguments for increased liberalization are finely balanced, but it is clear that commercial companies would not be campaigning for a change in the law if they did not think that direct-to-consumer advertising would enable them to influence clinical decisions. The potential to increase demand for medical interventions and health care services is seen as a great business opportunity. Whether it will benefit the health of the public depends on the quality of information that will be made available.

There is good reason to believe that information available from these sources may not conform to the highest evidence-based standards. Even non-commercial providers of health information for patients often provide an overly-optimistic view of the benefits of medical care (Coulter *et al.* 1998). Companies which are trying to sell products are unlikely to want to advertise their negative aspects by providing, for example, information about risks and side-effects. Inaccurate, biased, or out-of-date information could cause harm to users who are unable to verify its reliability. Several studies have found that accessing reliable information from websites is a hit-and-miss affair and users can easily be misled, sometimes with serious consequences (Weisbord *et al.* 1997; Impicciatore *et al.* 1997).

A number of solutions to this problem have been proposed including accreditation of websites by third parties and dissemination of quality checklists for use by website users. These approaches have a number of drawbacks, some of which may eventually be overcome by the introduction of electronic filters which could evaluate information on the Internet and provide warnings of biases and inaccuracies (Eysenbach and Diepgen 1988). But policy makers and clinicians ought to take this issue seriously as it has the potential to distort the demand for health care to serve the commercial interests of information providers. Access to good quality evidence-based information has the potential to empower patients and to channel use of health care resources more appropriately, but this will not happen by default. Initiatives to improve the quality of the information and to help people discriminate between reliable and unreliable information must be put in place if the benefits are to be realized. Governments should invest in public education programmes to encourage people to critically appraise health information. For their part health care professionals will need to be aware of the range and quality of information sources that may be used by their patients so they can advise them appropriately.

Information about health service quality

People's choice of health care provider is also likely to be influenced by the information revolution. Publication of various statistical indicators of quality is becoming commonplace for public services, including health care. Performance league tables are published in daily newspapers attracting the attention of politicians and the public. In the future performance indicators for individual hospitals, specialist departments, and primary care groups will be easily accessible via websites. Intended as a spur to quality improvement, it seems likely that these lists will exert an influence on where patients seek help and who they choose to consult. The trends are already obvious in education where parents in the UK are beginning to base their choice of school on a comparison of pupils' exam results. Once health outcomes information is more readily available, patients will be able to make comparisons between hospitals and general practices, and possibly between individual clinicians. They will start to act more like discriminating customers of health services, expecting a say in referral decisions and choice of specialist. Provider units will be prompted to market their services to attract custom and poor performers will have to raise their standards or go out of business.

That, at least, is the theory which led many governments to introduce market-based competition in health care systems. In practice competitive markets in health care have not resulted in improved standards for all. Patients have not tended to act like informed consumers, perhaps because they have not been provided with the information they need to judge the quality of care, nor the means to act on it. Purchasers have been slow to use financial levers to influence quality standards or to increase efficiency, and providers have not responded to market signals in the predicted manner (Enthoven 1999).

Whatever one thinks about market competition as a means of allocating health care resources, attempts to measure value for money and account for performance are generally welcome in a democratic society. But this approach to public accountability does have pitfalls. Just as schools league tables place greatest emphasis on exam results while ignoring other aspects of education quality, so health care league tables tend to measure the things that are most easily measured instead of the less tangible factors which may be important to patients.

The experience of the UK *Patient's Charter* standards is a case in point. These have attracted criticisms from NHS staff and from patients. They focused on access issues, largely because they were easily measurable, but staff felt under pressure to give priority to patients with minor problems over those with more serious clinical needs, just to avoid looking bad in the waiting list statistics. They also felt the Charter encouraged unrealistic expectations among patients and led to an increase in the rate of complaints. Patients too were critical of the standards. Many said they would prefer to be given information about their entitlement to good quality clinical care, how they could recognize it and where they could find it, instead of the almost exclusive emphasis on access and waiting times (Farrell *et al.* 1998). Although the Charter promised patients the right to full information and the opportunity to participate in decisions about their care, the reality for most patients fell far short of the aspiration. But since there was no measurable standard for this aspect of the Charter, it was not seen as a priority.

Members of the public have a legitimate interest in the quality of the services provided for their use. Information about service availability and performance ought to be a key component of the evidence on which to base informed choices. But this type of evidence can give a misleading picture. The *Patient's Charter* standard which aimed to reduce waiting times in accident and emergency clinics led some hospitals to employ so-called 'hello' nurses who greeted patients within the five minutes laid down by the Charter standard. The statistics looked good but patients still had to wait long hours before they were attended to by a doctor. Simple performance indicators can give a false sense of the relative performance of different providers. Outcome measures need to incorporate case mix adjustment if fair comparisons are to be drawn and attention needs to be paid to possible perverse incentives brought about by the tendency on the part of providers to 'game' the system. When published mortality rates were used as a quality comparator in the USA, there were reports that some hospitals were discriminating against high-risk patients in order to secure their position at the top of the league table. Mortality rates turn out to be an unsatisfactory measure of the quality of care (Hofer and Hayward 1996) and process measures, such as surveys of patients' experience of care, provide more reliable measures (Cleary 1999). Those using the league tables to choose between health care providers should understand their limitations if they want to make truly informed choices.

New tensions in professional–patient relationships

So the future patient will approach the health care professional armed with a great deal more information, but we should not take it for granted that they will be well informed or that their expectations will be realistic. For a moment, though, let us suppose this problem will be overcome as a result of government action to ensure that high-quality information is available. In this future utopia patients will have access to reliable and comprehensive information about their illness, its causes, and the treatment options. What effect will this have on relations between professionals and their patients?

We should expect a very different professional–patient relationship from that which prevails today. The patient of the future will be less deferential, more aware of the risks inherent in medical treatments, and more choosy. They will have higher expectations and a greater desire to participate actively in decisions that affect them. It would be wrong to imagine that the information asymmetry between professional and patient will be completely eliminated however. Several hours spent searching through websites by someone with no medical training is unlikely to match years of professional training. It is more likely to generate questions than answers. Professionals will have to hone their educational skills if they are to satisfy patients' desire to understand what is happening to them and they will have to ensure that they are sufficiently well informed to answer patients' questions or to guide them to reliable information sources.

If both professionals and patients have access to the same information sources and both agree on the factors to be taken into account in deciding how to manage the problem, the quality and appropriateness of patient care could be considerably enhanced. If, on the other hand, they disagree on the approach or base their decisions on conflicting sources of information, the potential for mistrust and conflict will be increased. There are a variety of reasons why the relationship might become difficult:

- The health care professional may feel threatened by a well informed or 'demanding' patient;
- Either or both parties may be misinformed because they are unable to discriminate between reliable and unreliable information or because they have misunderstood the information they have obtained;
- Patient and professional may make different interpretations of the same evidence;
- Either or both parties may be unwilling to share decision making;
- Patients may be unsuccessful at communicating their preferences or professionals may not want to listen;

- Patients may be unwilling to accept external constraints imposed by the health system, e.g. time constraints, budgetary constraints, limitations on access, or on the availability of treatments;

- Either or both parties may be unwilling to accept responsibility for the cost consequences of their decisions and the potential knock-on effects on other patients.

Ultimately a patient cannot force a professional to provide treatment which the professional considers undesirable, but unresolved disagreement could do serious damage to the therapeutic relationship. Faced with a busy workload and conscious of the risk of litigation the professional may be tempted to concede to the patient's demands rather than risk a breakdown in the relationship. Alternatively the patient may give up the struggle to influence the treatment decision. Either way the outcome is likely to be unsatisfactory for at least one party and the therapeutic effect of the treatment may be diminished in the process.

It is tempting to think that this type of conflict might be resolved by resorting to the evidence. Evidence-based clinical guidelines, especially if they have the backing of nationally recognized organizations, could be helpful but they are not a panacea. Even the best scientific evidence gathered by the most rigorous methods has its limitations. It will often be insufficiently complete to provide guidance on what to do in every clinical situation and insufficiently reliable to eliminate the need for judgement. Expert opinion can vary when it comes to devising guidelines and the most careful consensus development procedures cannot rule out the possibility that different groups of experts will arrive at different conclusions after scrutinizing the same data. Patients may therefore receive conflicting advice from different clinicians simply because clinicians' preferences vary. Many guidelines will be incomprehensible to patients because they were developed by, and for the use of, clinicians. Patients rarely have an input into guideline development and their perspectives may be completely absent from the evidence sources on which the guidelines are based (Coulter 1995). So use of a traditional clinical guideline may not be helpful in resolving differences between professionals and patients.

Specially designed patient decision aids are a more useful alternative. Leaflets, videos, decision boards, and computer-based decision support systems, which both inform patients and provide them with a systematic means of determining their preferences for alternative outcome states, have been shown to have value. As reviewed also in Chapter 14 (O'Connor and Edwards), trials have shown that they improve patients' knowledge about treatment options, reduce their decisional conflict, and stimulate them to take a more active role in decision making without increasing their anxiety (O'Connor et al. 1999). Doctors who have made them available to their patients report improvements in the decision making process (Murray *et al.* 2000). If these were to become widely available in doctors' surgeries, and ultimately in patients' homes via interactive television or the Internet, they could play an important role in facilitating evidence-based patient choice. They are only an aid to decision making though, not a substitute for good interpersonal communication. They can speed up the process of information transfer, but if conflict is to be minimized the length of consultation time will have to increase.

In 1998 a mixed group of American clinicians, patients, and communications experts was convened to devise a strategy for minimizing the risk of conflict in the professional–patient relationship and for dealing with it when it arose (Levinson *et al.* 1999). They stressed the need for openness on the part of professionals and transparency about the basis for clinical decisions. They listed four key skills which professionals should use to resolve communications difficulties:

- Understanding patients' worries and concerns;
- Expressing empathy;
- Encouraging patients to take an active role in discussing options in care;
- Negotiating differences of opinion when necessary.

These essential components of good communication may strike readers as too obvious to be worth restating, but research shows that many consultations still fail to meet these standards (Williams *et al.* 1998). With average consultation times in UK general practice running at only eight minutes (Howie *et al.* 1999) and outpatient consultations being even shorter (Waghorn and McKee 1999), it is hard to see how shared decision making could be accommodated without a fundamental change in the organization of care. The informed patients of the future will almost certainly require more consultation time, not less, if their expectations are to be met.

Individual versus population needs

The decreasing willingness to accept medical advice at face value may have been fuelled by governments' attempts to foster consumerism and competition as a means of improving efficiency and containing costs. Meanwhile consultation rates, referral rates, admission rates, and health care costs have been steadily rising. The increasing gap between public expectations and the supply of services has led governments to consider new ways in which demand for health care can be managed to ensure that limited resources are used efficiently and equitably. Health care professionals play a key role in shaping the demand for health care. The patient consults with a health problem and the professional's advice translates this request for help into a request for a particular treatment or intervention. So a demand management strategy needs to take account of two key decision points: the decision to consult and the choice of treatment.

The UK government has attempted to tackle the former by introducing telephone helplines such as NHS Direct where patients can get advice about the severity of their problem and be guided towards the most appropriate source of help. They are also keen to promote self-help among those with chronic diseases, to increase public understanding of risk to limit the effects of health scares, and to encourage responsible use of services (Secretary of State for Health 1999). But to date they have been reluctant to spell out for members of the public the financial consequences of their demands. Politicians prefer to propagate the idea that all demands could be met if only efficiency could be increased. Rationing remains a dirty word largely because it conjures up war-time images of shortages, queues, and tokens. This is an old-fashioned view. Rationing is the process of choosing which beneficial services should be offered to whom, and which should not (New 1996). It is, and always has been, a feature of health care delivery in every country, but successive British governments have been reluctant to admit to its existence. If the NHS had access to unlimited resources, rationing would not be an issue, but a service which has to operate within budget limits cannot avoid the need to make hard choices. Government spokesmen prefer to talk about priority setting – a less alarming word which serves to obscure the fact that access to some potentially beneficial treatments or services has to be restricted.

Mechanisms for restricting access include *denial* of treatment, *selection* by restricting treatments to particular groups, *deflection* to a different service, *deterrence* by raising barriers to access, *delay* through queues or waiting lists, *dilution* by restricting the quantity or quality of care, or *termination* by early discharge from treatment (Klein *et al.* 1996). All these mechanisms are used in the NHS, but rationing by delay (waiting lists) has attracted most attention from politicians and the public. This has been seen as evidence of inefficiency rather than as a rationing mechanism. For the most part rationing has been implicit rather than explicit, and priorities have been determined behind closed doors instead of being publicly debated.

This situation is beginning to change as it becomes clear that the potential for medical technologies to achieve beneficial effects for larger numbers of people with a wider range of conditions and ailments is increasing faster than the public's willingness to pay for them. Governments have therefore recognized that health care professionals, patients, and the public must be brought onside in the attempts to contain costs and agree priorities. Recent years have seen a worldwide trend in health policy towards initiatives designed to align clinical and financial responsibility by devolving budgets down to the clinical level. Examples in Britain have included clinical budgeting, general practice fundholding, clinical governance, and shared responsibility for prescribing and purchasing costs by primary care groups. These attempts to get professionals to take account of the financial consequences of their decisions have been accompanied by greater freedom to set priorities locally. Many health authorities and primary care groups have been making considerable efforts to consult their local populations and involve them in the decision making process (Coulter 1999). This is a welcome development, but if local groups make different decisions about what they are prepared to pay for, the result will be variations in what is available to patients in different parts of the country. Inequalities in access to particular treatments, dubbed 'post-code prescribing' by the media, seem to offend against the key NHS values of equity and fairness.

Media interest in post-code prescribing has centred on individual patients denied access to specific high-cost treatments such as interferon beta for multiple sclerosis, taxanes for ovarian and breast cancer, donepezil for Alzheimer's disease, and in-vitro fertilization to treat infertility. Denial of these treatments to patients on the basis of non-clinical criteria such as where they happen to live has been seen (correctly) as an example of rationing in action. Health authorities under pressure to meet budget targets have made different decisions about which expensive treatments they will pay for. Press stories about patients in neighbouring authorities apparently having different entitlements to treatment have proved shocking to a public accustomed to thinking about the NHS as a fair and equitable service. When budgets are fully devolved to primary care groups and trusts it will be harder for clinicians to avoid responsibility for these decisions, placing even greater pressure on their relationships with patients.

The government's response has been to establish the National Institute for Clinical Excellence (NICE) to provide guidance to the NHS on clinical effectiveness, cost-effectiveness, and clinical audit methods. Its aim is to 'produce clear guidance for clinicians about which treatments work best for which patients' (NHS Executive 1998). It is envisaged that NICE will eventually produce a range of clinical guidance 'products', some of which will focus on the treatment of specific conditions, while others will provide guidance on new treatments or products including pharmaceuticals, devices, diagnostic tests, and surgical procedures. The hope is that inequalities in the availability of particular treatments will be eliminated when health care professionals and patients have access to national guidelines and standards based on rigorous reviews of the scientific evidence.

The important development is the recognition that this evidence-based guidance must be made available to patients as well as professionals. If clinical guidelines are to have an impact on rationing practices, they must be perceived as legitimate by patients and the public (Norheim 1999). That means that patient representatives should be involved in developing them, they should take account of evidence which is patient-centred (reflecting the patient's point of view on the relative importance of different health outcomes), the basis for the recommendations (including any value judgements) should be transparent, and they should allow scope for individual preferences in choosing between alternatives.

How much scope should be allowed for individual choice remains a matter for debate. In spite of the British public's concern about equity, opinion can be easily swayed when special cases seem to demand special resources. The case of Jaymee Bowen (Child B) was a recent high-profile example (Ham 1999). Her father's refusal to accept the recommendations of doctors and the health authority that further treatment was not in her best interests, attracted great public sympathy. The media likes to champion the individual versus the bureaucrats, even if the bureaucracy – in this case the health authority – has tried its best to represent the interests of the local population. It was easier to identify with the tragic case of one attractive ten-year-old, than to empathize with the unknown people who might be denied treatment if Jaymee's care had been allowed to consume a considerable proportion of the health authority's resources. This type of tension is unlikely to diminish in the future, indeed it may increase considerably, but it will not become any easier to handle if policy makers (and clinician purchasers) try to push the issues under the carpet. Just as decision making at the one-to-one level of the clinical consultation must take account of the principles of shared decision making, so must those responsible for allocating health care resources seek legitimacy by involving the public and ensuring that the basis for their decisions is transparent and open to challenge if necessary.

Threats and opportunities

I have argued that public expectations are changing and that clinical practice and the organization of health care delivery must change too if the consensual basis for publicly-funded health care systems is to survive. Paternalistic approaches to communication will no longer be tolerated by patients, and health care professionals will find that they need to devote far more time to explaining and negotiating. Some professionals will feel threatened by these changes which seem to challenge their authority. They may fear that their role will be reduced to that of facilitator rather than decision maker, devaluing their clinical expertise and their status. They must be persuaded that the clock cannot be turned back. The changes we see in patients' expectations are mirrored by changes in other fields. Consumerism is becoming a more powerful force – it will not go away. The promotion of evidence-based patient choice could be a significant factor in helping health systems and health care providers to adapt to the new world. What steps should be taken to ensure that this is achieved?

Firstly, it is important to recognize that a move in the direction of more patient choice does not imply abrogating responsibility to the patient or slavish adoption of one mode of decision making. Some patients may not want the responsibility, or burden, of decision making and it would be inappropriate to offer choices to patients in every situation. For example, emergency situations often require quick decisions when there is no time to involve the patient. Sometimes it may be appropriate to leave the choice of treatment entirely to the patient, with the clinician's role relegated to information provider only. Examples might include a woman's choice of contraceptive method – assuming she has full information about the efficacy of the different methods, and the risks, and there are no relevant contra-indications, the woman who wants to should be allowed to decide for herself. In most cases though, the goal will be to reach a shared decision in which the patient's values and preferences are given due weight and, where appropriate, patients are offered the opportunity to participate in treatment choices if they wish to do so.

This implies that the principles and practice of shared decision making must be fully understood by all health care professionals. Communications skills will have to be accorded much greater priority in training programmes and clinical care will have to be reorganized to allow more time for professional–patient discussion. Professionals will need to ensure that patients understand the basis for their recommendations and must be willing to accept that patients' priorities and values may differ from theirs. Patients will also need help to enable them to become more discriminating users of health care. It will be important to ensure that information available to patients via electronic media or by other means is of high quality and reliability. This should be accompanied by public education programmes which focus on how to understand and deal with health risks, how to manage health problems, and where to find appropriate information and help.

Secondly, if evidence-based patient choice is to be truly relevant to patients it will be important to adopt a broad approach to what is accepted as evidence. Patients want evidence about the clinical efficacy of medical treatments, but they also want self-help information and information about the performance and quality of different health care providers. These different types of evidence must incorporate patients' perspectives so patients' representatives should be actively involved in generating it. Experience shows that when patients are involved in the research process as colleagues and co-investigators rather than as subjects or objects of the research, the quality and relevance of the studies improves (Goodare and Lockwood 1999). Patients' evaluations of health care can also be crucial in assessing performance and improving quality (Cleary 1999).

The third key point is the need to situate individual clinical decisions in the wider context of resource availability and public priorities. This balancing act of individual needs versus population requirements should not be done in secrecy by those responsible for purchasing health services. Patients and citizens need to understand the choices confronting policy makers and need to be involved in determining priorities. Evidence-based patient choice cannot be divorced from its societal context and when individual expectations clash with population priorities there must be a mechanism for resolving the conflict. The challenge is to harness its potential to improve the effectiveness of medical care, while ensuring that it does not undermine the principles of solidarity and fairness which underpin public health care systems.

References

BMJ (1999). Poll results. *British Medical Journal* **319**: 1026.

Cardy P, Cayton H, Edwards B and Gay H (1999). *Keeping patients in the dark: should prescription medicines be advertised direct to consumers?* London, IEA Health and Welfare Unit.

Cleary P (1999). The increasing importance of patient surveys. *British Medical Journal* **319**: 720–1.

Coulter A (1995). Assembling the evidence: patient-focused outcomes research. *Health Libraries Review* **2**: 263–8.

Coulter A (1999). Seeking the views of citizens. *Health Expectations* **2**: 219–21.

Coulter A, Entwistle V and Gilbert D (1998). *Informing patients*. London, King's Fund.

CyberAtlas (1999). http://cyberatlas.internet.com (accessed 21/11/99).

Enthoven A (1999). *Rock Carling lecture*. Nuffield Trust, London.

Eysenbach G and Diepgen T L (1998). Towards quality management of medical information on the Internet: evaluation, labelling, and filtering of information. *British Medical Journal* **317**: 1496–500.

Farrell C, Levenson R and Snape D (1998). *The Patient's Charter: past and future*. London, King's Fund.

Goodare H and Lockwood S (1999). Involving patients in clinical research. *British Medical Journal* **319**: 724–5.

Ham C (1999). The role of doctors, patients and managers in priority setting decisions: lessons from the 'Child B' case. *Health Expectations* **2**: 61–8.

Hofer TP and Hayward RA (1996). Identifying poor quality hospitals. *Medical Care* **34**: 737–53.

Howie JGR, Heaney DJ, Maxwell M, Walker J, Freeman GK and Rai H (1999). Quality at general practice consultations: cross-sectional survey. *British Medical Journal* **319**: 738–43.

Impicciatore P, Pandolfini C, Casella N and Bonati M (1997). Reliability of health information for the public on the World Wide Web: systematic survey of advice on managing fever in children at home. *British Medical Journal* **314**: 1875–81.

Jupiter Store (1999). http://www.jup.com (accessed 21/11/99).

Klein R, Day P and Redmayne S (1996). *Managing scarcity.* Milton Keynes, Open University Press.

Levinson W, Gorawara-Bhat R, Dueck R, Egener B, Kao A, Kerr C, *et al.* (1999). Resolving disagreements in the patient–physician relationship. *Journal of the American Medical Association* **282**: 1477–83.

Murray E, Davis H, SeeTai S, Coulter A, Gray A and Haines A (2000). A randomized controlled trial of an interactive multimedia decision aid on benign prostatic hypertrophy in primary care. *British Medical Journal.* In press

New B (1996). *The rationing agenda in the NHS*. London, King's Fund.

NHS Executive (1998). *A first class service: quality in the new NHS.* London, Department of Health.

Norheim OF (1999). Health care rationing – are additional criteria needed for assessing evidence-based clinical practice guidelines? *British Medical Journal* **319**: 1426–9.

O'Connor AM, Roston A, Fiset V, Tetroe J, Entwistle V, Llewellyn-Thomas H, *et al.* (1999). Decision aids for patients facing health treatment or screening decisions: systematic review. *British Medical Journal* **319**: 731–4.

Secretary of State for Health (1999). Saving lives: our healthier nation. London, HMSO.

Waghorn A and McKee M (1999). Surgical outpatients: are we allowing enough time? *International Journal for Quality in Health Care* **11**: 215–19.

Weisbord SD, Soule JB and Kimmel PL (1997). Poison online – acute renal failure caused by oil of wormwood purchased through the Internet. *New England Journal of Medicine* **337**: 825.

Williams S, Weinman J and Dale J (1998). Doctor–patient communication and patient satisfaction: a review. *Family Practice* **15**: 480–92.

Index